Familial Breast and Ovarian Cancer
Genetics, Screening and Management

This book surveys the profound and far-reaching ramifications that have arisen from the very significant advances in our understanding of the genetic basis of familial breast and ovarian cancer. Written by international experts from Europe and North America, it provides the busy clinician with a contemporary and wide-ranging guide to the latest developments in the diagnosis, genetics, screening, prevention and management of familial breast cancer. In this rapidly advancing field, this book provides an unrivalled source of information, including sections on ethical and insurance issues and the different cultural aspects of breast cancer. The use of recently devised cancer genetics clinics and different referral criteria and patterns to these clinics are also detailed. This accessible book will be of immense value to all clinical geneticists, oncologists and healthcare professionals involved in screening and counselling programmes.

Familial Breast
and Ovarian Cancer
Genetics, Screening and Management

Edited by

Patrick J. Morrison
Belfast City Hospital Trust, Belfast, UK

Shirley V. Hodgson
Guy's Hospital, London, UK

and

Neva E. Haites
University of Aberdeen, Aberdeen, UK

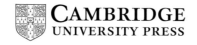
CAMBRIDGE
UNIVERSITY PRESS

PUBLISHED BY THE PRESS SYNDICATE OF THE UNIVERSITY OF CAMBRIDGE
The Pitt Building, Trumpington Street, Cambridge, United Kingdom

CAMBRIDGE UNIVERSITY PRESS
The Edinburgh Building, Cambridge CB2 2RU, UK
40 West 20th Street, New York, NY 10011-4211, USA
477 Williamstown Road, Port Melbourne, VIC 3207, Australia
Ruiz de Alarcón 13, 28014 Madrid, Spain
Dock House, The Waterfront, Cape Town 8001, South Africa

http://www.cambridge.org

First published 2002

Printed in the United Kingdom at the University Press, Cambridge

Typeface Minion 10.5/14pt   *System* Poltype® [V N]

A catalogue record for this book is available from the British Library

Library of Congress Cataloguing in Publication data

Familial breast and ovarian cancer: genetics, screening, and management / [edited by]
Patrick J. Morrison, Shirley V. Hodgson, Neva E. Haites.
    p.   ;   cm.
Includes bibliographical references and index.
ISBN 0 521 80373 X
1. Breast – Cancer.   2. Breast – Cancer – Genetic aspects.   3. Ovaries – Cancer.
4. Ovaries – Cancer – Genetic aspects.   I. Morrison, Patrick J. (Patrick John), 1963–   II. Hodgson, S. V.
III. Haites, Neva E. (Neva Elizabeth), 1947–
[DNLM: 1. Breast Neoplasms – genetics.   2. Ovarian Neoplasms – genetics. WP 870 F198 2002]
RC280.B8 F355 2002
616.99'449–dc21   2002025937

ISBN 0 521 80373 X hardback

To all of the families with hereditary cancer who have worked with us to begin to understand the problem, and for their patience while we search for the answers.

Contents

Contributors

Bernard Asselain
Department of Biostatistics,
Institut Curie,
Paris,
France

A. D. Baildam
Department of Surgery,
Withington Hospital,
Manchester, UK

Heiko Becher
University of Heidelberg,
Department of Tropical Hygiene
and Public Health,
Im Neuenheimer Feld 324,
69120 Heidelberg,
Germany

Alison Bish
Psychosocial Oncology Group,
Cancer Research UK,
London, UK

Dirk Brinkmann
Gynaecological Oncology Unit,
St Bartholomew's and The Royal London
School of Medicine and Dentistry,
Charterhouse Square,
London, UK

Lucy Brooks
Department of Medical Genetics,
St Mary's Hospital,
Manchester, UK

Jenny Chang-Claude
Division of Epidemiology,
German Cancer Research Centre,
Im Neuenheimer Feld 280,
69120 Heidelberg,
Germany

Pierre O. Chappuis
Room L10–120, Montreal General Hospital,
1650 Cedar Ave,
Montreal,
Quebec,
Canada

Diana M. Eccles
Department of Human Genetics,
Princess Anne Hospital,
Southampton, UK

Charis Eng
Clinical Cancer Genetics Program,
Ohio State University,
Human Cancer Genetics,
420 West 12th Avenue,
Suite 690 TMRF Columbus,
Ohio, USA

D. G. R. Evans
Department of Medical Genetics,
St Mary's Hospital,
Hathersage Road,
Manchester, UK

Adrienne M. Flanagan
Department of Histopathology,
Royal Free and University College Medical
School,
Rockefeller Building,
University Street,
London, UK

William D. Foulkes
Division of Medical Genetics,
Montreal General Hospital,
1650 Cedar Ave,
Montreal,
Quebec,
Canada

Jonathon Gray
Institute of Medical Genetics,
University Hospital of Wales,
Heath Park,
Cardiff, UK

Helen Gregory
Department of Medical Genetics,
Grampian University Hospitals Trust,
Foresterhill,
Aberdeen, UK

Neva E. Haites
Department of Medical Genetics,
University of Aberdeen,
Foresterhill,
Aberdeen, UK

Shirley V. Hodgson
Division of Medical and Molecular Genetics,
Guy's Hospital,
London Bridge,
London, UK

Ian Jacobs
Department of Obstetrics and Gynaecology
St Bartholomew's and The Royal London
School of Medicine and Dentistry,
London, UK

Patrick G. Johnston
Department of Oncology,
Belfast City Hospital Trust,
Belfast, UK

Richard Kennedy
Department of Oncology,
Belfast City Hospital Trust,
Belfast, UK

Sunil R. Lakhani
The Breakthrough Toby Robins Breast
Cancer Research Centre,
Institute of Cancer Research,
Mary-Jean Mitchell Green Building,
Chester Beatty Laboratories,
Fulham Road,
London, UK

F. I. Lalloo
Department of Medical Genetics,
St Mary's Hospital,
Hathersage Road,
Manchester, UK

Usha Menon
Gynaecological Oncology Unit,
St Bartholomew's and The Royal London
School of Medicine and Dentistry,
Charterhouse Square,
London, UK

Pål Møller
Unit of Medical Genetics,
The Norwegian Radium Hospital,
N-0310 Oslo,
Norway

Patrick J. Morrison
Department of Medical Genetics,
Belfast City Hospital Trust,
Belfast, UK

M. A. Nooy
Leiden University Medical Centre,
Rijnsburgerweg 10,
Poortgebouw Zuid,
2333 AA Leiden,
The Netherlands

Barnaby Rufford
Gynaecological Oncology Unit,
St Bartholomew's and The Royal London
School of Medicine and Dentistry,
Charterhouse Square,
London, UK

Andrew Shenton
Department of Medical Genetics,
St Mary's Hospital,
Manchester, UK

C. Michael Steel
School of Biological and Medical Sciences,
Bute Medical Building,
St Andrews,
Fife, Scotland

Dominique Stoppa-Lyonnet
Unité de Génétique Oncologique Institut
Curie,
Section Médicale,
26 Rue d'Ulm,
75231 Paris,
France

Steven Sutton
Health Behaviour Unit,
Epidemiology and Public Health,
Brook House,
2–16 Torrington Place,
London, UK

H. F. A. Vasen
Netherlands Foundation for the Detection
of Hereditary Tumours,
Rijnsburgerweg 10,
Poortgebouw Zuid,
2333 AA Leiden,
The Netherlands

Foreword

I am very pleased to have been asked to write the Foreword to this important and timely book. As Chair of the Human Genetics Commission I am only too aware of the impact of familial breast cancer, or indeed many other familial cancers, on our work.

The issues raised by an increased understanding of the genetics of breast cancer have formed part of our thinking on how to deal with issues of privacy and confidentiality, such as the provision of genetic information to family members. Moving beyond the clinical, we have also considered some of the issues concerning patenting of gene sequences, taking as one example the continuing debate about the BRCA1 and BRCA2 gene patents. In addition, we have considered familial breast cancer as one of several conditions on the radar of insurance companies before underwriting life or health insurance.

I am therefore pleased to see that a fellow member of the Human Genetics Commission, Professor Patrick Morrison, and his colleagues have so carefully and clearly set out many of these important issues in this book. I hope that it will be widely read by clinicians and those responsible for policy in all of these areas and that they will take note of the important messages herein.

May 2002   **Baroness Helena Kennedy QC**

Preface

Cancer genetics is a new field where medical knowledge is developing rapidly, and there is a continuing need to assess the implications of new research into the genetic aspects of breast and ovarian cancer for clinical management.

Clearly, many individuals have a family history of cancer, but only a small proportion have inherited genes conferring a high risk of developing specific cancers. The development of services to identify individuals at high risk for genetic assessment/testing and management, and to offer those at moderately increased risk appropriate surveillance and follow-up for cancer, is a major organizational challenge which must be shared between clinicians at all levels – from primary care to the specialist geneticist.

Because this field is developing so rapidly, there are scanty up-to-date, concise and accessible sources of information to which interested professionals (whether clinical geneticists, surgeons, oncologists, psychologists or other professionals) can turn. This book has been written to address this.

It is divided into three parts. Part 1 deals with summaries of the molecular biology and natural history of hereditary breast and ovarian cancer. Part 2 examines current screening recommendations, how services have been set up, the characteristics of patients referred, and how services differ in different cultures. Part 3 deals with management of breast and ovarian cancer in mutation carriers and those at high risk, and also includes chapters on ethical, social and insurance issues, psychosocial aspects, and preventative surgery.

We hope this volume will be regularly updated and will be of value to all those involved in cancer genetic screening, counselling and management programmes.

2002   **Patrick J. Morrison**

Acknowledgements

We are particularly grateful to our secretaries, Joanne Hazlett, Elizabeth Manners and Liza Young, for reformatting and typing parts of the manuscript, and to our families for tolerating us beyond the bounds of reasonable duty, during the writing of this book.

Part 1

Molecular biology and natural history

Introduction

Patrick J. Morrison[1], Shirley V. Hodgson[2] and Neva E. Haites[3]

[1]Belfast City Hospital Trust, Belfast, UK
[2]Guy's Hospital, London, UK
[3]University of Aberdeen, UK

It has long been recognized that some very rare forms of cancer, such as retinoblastoma and neurofibromatosis, are caused by inherited genes. It is only within the last few years, however, that rapid progress has been made in understanding the role that inherited genes also play in determining a proportion of the more common cancers, including breast, colorectal and ovarian cancer. Although there is still uncertainty about the precise contribution of inherited predisposition genes to the incidence of these cancers, the available evidence suggests that breast, colorectal and ovarian cancer have a number of common genetic features.

- A small proportion of these cancers (about 5%) are caused by inherited genes which, though comparatively rare, confer very high lifetime risks of developing cancer. In some cases these lifetime risks may be as high as 80%.
- Cancers caused by these high penetrance genes are more likely to occur at an early age than sporadic cancers, and 15–20% of the cancers diagnosed in people under the age of 50 years may be accounted for by these genetic mutations.
- Carriers of known genetic mutations, which confer high lifetime risks of developing breast or ovarian cancer, are also at significantly increased risk of developing certain other forms of cancer.
- A further 10–20% of breast, ovarian and colorectal cancers are likely to be caused by inherited polymorphisms in predisposition genes, which are commoner but less penetrant but which confer some increased risk (more than three times the general population risk). These 'medium risk' genes have not yet been clearly identified.
- Familial clustering of the more common cancers may also be influenced by environmental and lifestyle factors as well as by chance.

Services for cancer genetics

Cancer genetics is a new field and the organization of services in this area may be initiated by clinical genetics services or through oncology and other departments, where individuals with a special interest in cancer genetics arrange to see individuals with a family history of cancer, estimate their cancer risks and arrange surveillance and genetic testing as appropriate.

In many parts of Europe, cancer genetics clinics have been established for many years, and most specialized genetic counselling for cancer susceptibility is organized from genetics centres. However, the organization and quality of such services vary, depending on the economic status and healthcare systems of the country. There is increasing awareness that education and referral guidelines for primary care physicians are important. This would allow a collaborative relationship to be developed with primary healthcare services, helping them act as gatekeepers for the prioritization of referrals for genetics services.

Growing public awareness of the familial risks of cancer has led to a rapid increase in demand for advice about these risks and in the number of referrals to genetics clinics in all parts of Europe. Many of these clinics lack the resources to meet this demand and as a result of this and a desire to provide the 'best' service possible to high-risk patients, clinics need to ensure that the service they provide is evidence based. Where evidence is lacking, an audit of 'best practice' guidelines is essential to provide the information. In order to obtain sufficient information, a very large cohort of at-risk individuals, well documented for family history, needs to be followed up for many years. Such an audit is only possible with large multicentre trials, and the emerging European and North American collaborations are an ideal forum for this.

The basic aims of genetic services for people concerned about familial risks of breast or ovarian cancer are: (1) to provide advice and counselling about familial risks, and (2) to identify those who are at an increased risk. Where possible, molecular tests for mutations in genes such as *BRCA1* and *BRCA2* may be possible, and predictive testing will allow the identification of very-high-risk individuals. Once identified, these individuals will need to be enrolled in effective protocols for the management of their risk and for the treatment of cancers detected. Large-scale evaluation of such management is facilitated by European collaborative studies.

This collection of chapters sets out guidelines for assessing whether individuals are at an increased risk of developing cancer on the basis of their family history. The initial point of contact for many individuals concerned about familial cancer risks is the family doctor. Hence guidelines could be provided to family doctors and their staff to assist them in the assessment of risks. Individuals considered to be at sufficiently high risk could be referred to genetics clinics, where a more detailed assessment would be carried out.

Individuals who are assessed as being at an increased risk of developing cancer, but often where no *BRCA1* or *BRCA2* mutation can be identified, should be offered regular screening. Suggested screening protocols for the management of these individuals, covering the age range, frequency and type of screening, are outlined in chapters benefiting from the collective experience of groups from many European countries and from the USA and Canada.

Cancer genetics is an area where medical knowledge is developing rapidly, and there will be a continuing need to assess the implications of new research into the genetic aspects of breast and ovarian cancer for the screening programmes currently recommended. The implications of research into the genetic aspects of other forms of cancer may also need to be assessed. The benefit of the experience of different countries and cultures in implementing the health strategies suggested by the results of such research is important.

Eleven centres in Europe worked together from 1997 on an EU-funded demonstration project entitled: 'Familial Breast Cancer: Audit of a New Development in Medical Practice in European Centres'.

The chapters included in this book were generated, in part, from the work of this project and provide guidelines, evidence and consensus views for a variety of aspects of patient care within a cancer genetics clinic. The other chapters originate from colleagues worldwide who are providing evidence in other areas of cancer genetics on which patient care can be based.

As a final outcome of the EU demonstration project, the 'International Collaborative Group on Familial Breast and Ovarian Cancer' was established. This worldwide group will continue the work of the project and will, in addition, collaborate and integrate with other groups and individuals who share a common interest in producing evidence to develop our understanding of the inherited cancers and hence improve the care of patients and their families.

2

Overview of the clinical genetics of breast cancer

Neva Haites and Helen Gregory

University of Aberdeen, UK

Introduction

Breast cancer is the most common cancer in women, accounting for 20% of all new cases of cancer. The lifetime risk to a woman in the UK is 1 in 12 females, with an incidence of less than 10 per 100 000 women aged under 30 years, rising to 300 per 100 000 in women aged over 85 years. Breast cancer can occur in sporadic and hereditary forms, and both forms are associated with modification to the genetic material. In the case of hereditary forms, a constitutive mutation in a specific gene predisposes individuals to cancer. In sporadic forms, mutations in somatic cells accumulate and result in transformation of a normal cell to one with malignant potential.

Statistical analysis of epidemiological data is compatible with a dominant gene (or genes) predisposing to breast cancer in certain families, with 5–10% of breast cancer being due to highly penetrant, dominant genes (Easton and Peto, 1990; Claus et al., 1991). Approximately 10% of isolated cases presenting under 35 years may be due to such a gene but only 1% of cases presenting over 80 years (Langston et al., 1996; Ford et al., 1998).

Table 2.1 lists genetic syndromes that may predispose to breast cancer, some of which will be discussed in this chapter and in some greater detail in subsequent chapters.

Family history as an indicator of predisposition to breast cancer

A history of breast cancer among relatives has been found, in epidemiological studies, to be an indication of breast cancer risk. Familial breast cancer is characterized by: a younger age at diagnosis than sporadic forms, increasing numbers of affected family members, an increased risk of bilateral breast cancer, and a strong association with ovarian cancer.

Table 2.1. Genetic syndromes associated with breast cancer susceptibility

Syndrome	Gene/chromosome
1. Site-specific hereditary breast cancer	*BRCA1, BRCA2, +*
2. Breast/ovarian cancer	*BRCA1, BRCA2*
3. Li–Fraumeni syndrome	*TP53*
4. Ataxia-telangiectasia syndrome	*ATM*
5. Cowden disease	*PTEN*
6. Klinefelter's syndrome	47, XXY
7. Muir–Torre syndrome	*MSH2, MLH1*
8. Peutz–Jeghers syndrome	*STK11/LKB1*

If a woman has a first-degree relative (mother, sister or daughter) who has developed breast cancer before the age of 50 years, her own risk of developing the disease is increased two-fold or greater, and the younger the relative the greater is the risk. If a woman has two first-degree relatives with the disease, her risk may be increased four- to six-fold, and again, the younger the relative the greater is the risk (Claus et al., 1996; McPherson et al., 2000). It must also be remembered that males can pass on genes predisposing to breast cancer and hence it is also relevant to consider the history of breast cancer in female relatives of the father of a consultand.

Studies of familial breast cancer

It has been recognized for many years that there is an association in certain families between breast and ovarian cancer. The risk for epithelial ovarian cancer was found to be significantly elevated in patients with first-degree relatives affected with breast cancer (twice the population risk) (Muderspach, 1994; Claus et al., 1996). Similarly, the risk for breast cancer was found to be elevated in patients who had first-degree relatives with ovarian cancer.

Following international studies of large families with an excess of both early-onset breast cancer and of ovarian cancers, Mary Clair King's group demonstrated linkage between inherited susceptibility to early-onset breast cancer and a polymorphic marker on chromosome 17q21.3 (Hall et al., 1990). Predisposition to breast and ovarian cancer was also found with this locus in many families around the world, but it was also clear that other families existed with an excess of early-onset breast cancer that did not segregate with this locus (Narod et al., 1995). Subsequently, by studying, among others, families with male and female breast cancer, a second locus was found on chromosome 13q12–13 (Wooster et al., 1994).

It is now clear that there are other families with a predominance of breast cancer who are not linked to either of these loci, and hence it is likely that other genes exist that predispose individuals to breast cancer (Bishop, 1994).

Molecular features

Following the linkage studies, two genes were identified that are implicated in the pathogenesis of breast and ovarian cancer: *BRCA1* localized to chromosome 17q21 (Hall et al., 1990; Miki et al., 1994) and *BRCA2* localized to chromosome 13q12–13 (Wooster et al., 1994). These two genes would appear to account for almost all families with breast and ovarian cancer predisposition and also for approximately 50% of families with predisposition to breast cancer alone (Ford et al., 1994).

Genes implicated in breast cancer predisposition

BRCA1

The *BRCA1* gene on chromosome 17q21 was identified by positional cloning methods and found to have 5592 coding nucleotides that are distributed over 100 000 bases of genomic DNA and has 22 coding exons. These encode a protein of 1863 amino acids. Loss of the wild-type allele was found in over 90% of tumours from women with a germline mutation in *BRCA1*, and hence it is regarded as a tumour suppressor gene. In addition, transfection of wild-type *BRCA1* into breast/ovarian cell lines decreased cell proliferation, whereas mutant *BRCA1* did not (Koonin et al., 1996).

Sequence analysis of *BRCA1* indicates that it has a C3HC4 zinc-binding RING-finger domain at the amino terminus of the protein, a classic simian virus 40-type nuclear localization sequence in exon 11, and two regions resembling the transactivating domain of a number of transactivation factors called 'BRCT' (*BRCA1* carboxyl-terminal) domains. Other proteins with similar domains function in cell cycle control and DNA damage repair pathways (Bork et al., 1997; Callebaut and Mornon, 1997).

Mutations

More than 500 sequence variations have been identified in *BRCA1*, and of these, more than 80% of all *BRCA1* mutations are frameshift or nonsense mutations that alter the codon reading frame and result in a 'stop' codon producing a premature protein termination (Futreal et al., 1994; Gayther et al., 1995; FitzGerald et al., 1996; Szabo and King, 1997; Liede et al., 1999). Genetic susceptibility to breast cancer is thought to occur when one *BRCA1* allele is inactivated in the germline

Table 2.2. Prevalence of *BRCA1* and *BRCA2* genes

	Gene mutation	General population (%)	Breast cancer (%)	Age group (years)
Ashkenazi	*BRCA1:* 185del AG	0.8	20	<42
	BRCA1: 5382insC	0.4		
	BRCA2: 6174delT	1.2	8	<42
Icelandic	*BRCA2:* 999del5	0.6	24	<40
British	*BRCA1:* all mutations	0.11	3.1	<49
	BRCA2: all mutations	0.12	3.0	<49

From Peto et al. (1999); Johannesdottir et al. (1996); Struewing et al. (1997).

and subsequently the other allele is lost in somatic breast tissue. The most common mutations, so far discovered, are 185delAG and 5382insC (Table 2.2). In addition, germline deletions have been found, and may be associated with the high frequency of 'Alu' repeats in the introns. In the Dutch/Belgium population, three large deletions have been identified and account for 30% of all germline mutations in Dutch families. Four novel deletions have recently been found in the regulatory regions of the *BRCA1* gene in French and American families (Peelen et al., 1997; Petrij-Bosch et al., 1997; Puget et al., 1999a, 1999b).

Penetrance and prevalence

Collaborative studies by the Breast Cancer Linkage Consortium (BCLC) have examined multiple families with germline mutations in *BRCA1* and *BRCA2* to establish the penetrance of mutations in these genes and the risks of other cancers (Ford et al., 1994; Ford et al., 1998; Puget et al., 1999a) (Figure 2.1). These studies suggest that carriers of mutations in *BRCA1* have an associated cumulative breast cancer risk of 80–85% by age 80 years. Once affected with a first breast cancer, such gene carriers have a subsequent risk of contralateral breast cancer estimated to be up to 48% by age 50 years and 64% by age 70 years. Similarly, the risk of ovarian cancer in carrier women is 60% by age 80 years as compared with a population risk of around 1%. Colon cancer risk is increased to 6% by the age of 70 years and prostate cancer may occur three times more often than expected in male *BRCA1* mutation carriers, with an absolute risk of 6% by age 74 years (Ford et al., 1998).

There is a correlation between the position of the mutation within the gene and the ratio of breast to ovarian cancer incidence in a family. It has been noted that mutations in the 3′ third of the gene are associated with a lower proportion of ovarian cancer (Futreal et al., 1994), although it is not known whether this is due

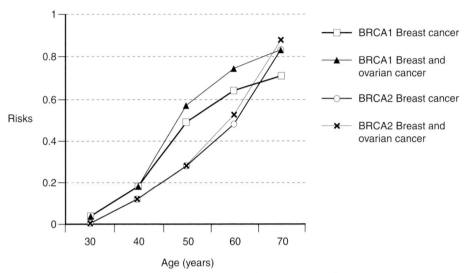

Figure 2.1   Breast cancer and breast and ovarian cancer risks in *BRCA1* and *BRCA2* mutation carriers (Breast Cancer Linkage Consortium, 1999).

to a difference in penetration of the mutation for breast cancer, ovarian cancer or both (Gayther et al., 1995; Rahman and Stratton, 1998).

Germline mutations in *BRCA1* account for 15–45% of hereditary breast cancer and around 80% of breast/ovarian cancer families (Table 2.3). In addition, as is seen in Table 2.4, there is evidence for an increased risk of colorectal and prostate cancer (Ford et al., 1998). Studies suggest that *BRCA1* accounts for about 1% of breast cancer in the general population (Peto et al., 1999) but about 3% of those breast cancers occurring in women aged less than 49 years and 0.49% of women aged more than 50 years (Table 2.5).

BRCA2

A second breast cancer susceptibility gene (*BRCA2*) was localized to chromosome 13q12–13 (Wooster et al., 1994). In these families, cases of male breast cancer were found to be a part of the *BRCA2* tumour spectrum, and in addition, the risk of ovarian cancer is lower than in families with *BRCA1*.

BRCA2 was cloned and found to be a large gene (Easton et al., 1995; Wooster et al., 1995). It has 11 385 coding nucleotides that are distributed over 70 000 bases of genomic DNA and has 27 exons coding for a protein of 3418 amino acids. It bears no clear homology to previously described genes and its protein has no previously defined functional domains. Eight copies of a 30–80 amino acid repeat (BRC repeat) are coded in the portion of the protein encoded by exon 11. These domains are highly conserved and are postulated to be involved in the binding of *RAD51* to *BRCA2* protein (Callebaut and Mornon, 1997).

Table 2.3. Heterogeneity analysis

	Family type	No. of families	BRCA1	BRCA2	Other
Families with female breast cancer only (no ovarian cancer or male breast cancer)	All	117	0.28	0.37	0.35
	6+ breast cancers	34	0.19	0.66	0.15
	4–5 breast cancers	83	0.32	0.09	0.59
Families with breast/ovarian cancer	All	94	0.80	0.15	0.05
	2+ ovarian cancers	52	0.88	0.12	0.00
	1 ovarian cancer	42	0.69	0.19	0.12
Families with at least one male breast cancer	All	26	0.19	0.77	0.04
All families	All	237	0.52	0.35	0.13
	6+ breast cancers	83	0.46	0.50	0.04
	4–5 breast cancers	154	0.55	0.12	0.33

From Ford et al. (1998).

Table 2.4. Risks of cancers other than breast/ovarian cancers in BRCA1 and BRCA2 mutation carriers

	Cancer type	Relative risk
BRCA1	Colon	3.30
	Prostate	4.11
BRCA2	Stomach	2.59
	Pancreas	3.51
	Gallbladder	4.97
	Melanoma	2.58
	Prostate	4.65

From Ford et al. (1998); Breast Cancer Linkage Consortium (1999).

Mutations

Like *BRCA1*, more than 250 distinct mutations in *BRCA2* have been identified, scattered throughout this gene. To date, insufficient evidence is available for the risk associated with most missense mutations to be calculated with certainty and

Table 2.5. Prevalence of *BRCA1* and *BRCA2* mutations in cases of early-onset breast cancers in England and Wales

	Age (years)		
	0–49	50–69	0–69
BRCA1 prevalence (%)	3.12	0.49	1.19
BRCA2 prevalence (%)	3.23	0.94	1.55

Peto et al. (1999).

hence all mutations definitely associated with predisposition to cancer result in truncation of the *BRCA2* protein (Wooster et al., 1995; Takahashi et al., 1996; Tavtigian et al., 1996). Mutations in both *BRCA1* and *BRCA2* are recorded in the Breast Cancer Information Core (BIC) website: http://www.nhgri.nih.gov/ Intramural_research/Lab_transfer/Bic/Member/index/html

Penetrance and prevalence

BRCA2 carriers have an increased lifetime risk of developing breast cancer of 80–85% by 80 years of age and a lifetime risk of developing ovarian cancer of 27% by 80 years of age (Figure 2.1). Multiple other cancers occur in excess in carriers of *BRCA2* and are described in Table 2.4.

About one-half of hereditary site-specific breast cancer families are linked to mutations in the *BRCA2* gene, especially those with cases of male breast cancer (Wooster et al., 1994; Wooster et al., 1995; Ford et al., 1998) (Table 2.3). However, ovarian cancer was thought to occur less commonly, although the number of ovarian cancers resulting from mutations in the *BRCA2* gene may be higher than was previously estimated (Takahashi et al., 1996). In two population-based studies of women with breast cancer, the result of mutation analysis suggested that *BRCA2* mutations are associated with 3.0% of patients less than 50 years of age and 0.12% of older women (Peto et al., 1999) (Table 2.5).

Founder effects involving *BRCA1* and *BRCA2*

Specific *BRCA1/2* mutations are highly prevalent in population subgroups, such as those identified among Jewish women of central European (Ashkenazi) origin. Approximately 10% of mutations in *BRCA1* (Struewing et al., 1997; Bar-Sade et al., 1998; Fodor et al., 1998) found in cases of breast cancer are accounted for by 185delAG and 5382insC mutations. With the *BRCA2* mutation, 6174delT, these three mutations together may account for a quarter of all cases of early-onset breast cancer and two-thirds of early-onset breast cancer in the setting of a family history of breast/ovarian cancer among Ashkenazi Jewish women (Johannesdottir et al., 1996) (Table 2.2).

Observations suggest that the penetrance of 185delAG (that is, the likelihood that a person with the mutation will actually develop cancer) is significantly greater than the penetrance of 6174delT. This supports the possibility that some breast cancer gene mutations are associated with a higher risk than others, a finding that further complicates genetic counselling in this setting (Struewing et al., 1997). In Icelandic and Finnish populations, the *BRCA2* mutation 999del5 is a founder mutation with evidence from a shared haplotype of a common founder (Johannesdottir et al., 1996). Similar founder mutations have been found in other populations and mutations such as large deletions may also be specific to founder populations (Szabo and King, 1997; Liede et al., 1999).

Function of *BRCA1* and *BRCA2* proteins

Studies of the normal function of *BRCA1* suggest that it encodes a protein involved in the cellular response to DNA damage, a role in transcription and cell cycle control. *BRCA1* has been found to be part of a subnuclear focus known to contain *RAD51*, a human homologue of the yeast DNA damage checkpoint gene, thought to be involved in homologous recombination and double-strand break repair. It is also thought to have a role in regulating apoptotic cell death. From studies on human cell lines containing only mutant *BRCA1* there is a suggestion that they have increased sensitivity to ionizing radiation, and are defective for transcription-coupled repair but not for double-strand repair. Evidence indicates a link between *BRCA1* phosphorylation by Chk2 and ATM. This suggests that *BRCA1* may link DNA repair functions of *BRCA2* to pathways that signal DNA damage or incomplete DNA replication (Oddoux et al., 1996; Bertwistle et al., 1997; Hsu and White, 1998; Abbott et al., 1999; Chen et al., 1999).

Heterogeneity

As can be seen in Table 2.3, Ford et al. carried out heterogeneity analyses using *BRCA1/2* linkage data. With the Cancer and Steroid Hormone (CASH) model being assumed for all genes, they estimated the proportions of families linked to each gene depending on the family structure and prevalence of cancer. This suggested that 52% of breast cancer in families was due to *BRCA1* and 35% to *BRCA2*.

They also estimated the proportions under the assumption that *BRCA1* confers the risks estimated in previous Breast Cancer Linkage Consortium studies. In general, both methods gave very similar results with the exception that families with male breast cancer were not included in the latter calculations, as the penetrance in males is not known for all genes. The largest difference between the two methods is that, with the latter, the estimated proportion linked to *BRCA1* in families with six or more breast cancers was higher at 29% as compared with 19%.

Predictive testing for *BRCA1* and *BRCA2*

It is generally agreed that none of the currently available cancer susceptibility mutation tests is appropriate for the screening of asymptomatic persons in the general population, although the population-specific mutations described among Ashkenazi Jews and Icelanders, for example, may achieve that status in the future. The testing of unaffected members of a family known to carry a *BRCA1* or *BRCA2* mutation or another cancer-predisposing gene (known as a predictive genetic test) is probably best done at specialist clinics. Counselling is discussed in greater detail in Chapters 9, 11 and 18.

'BRCAX'

Studies indicate that 10–20% of families at high risk of breast cancer are not linked to either *BRCA1* or *BRCA2*. Studies continue to look for evidence of linkage in families with multiple affected individuals. A recent study of the histopathology of *BRCA1/2*-associated familial cancers has shown evidence of features specific to *BRCA1*- and *BRCA2*-associated tumours. The characteristics of tumours in familial forms not linked to *BRCA1/2* may provide phenotypic discriminatory information to assist in future gene identification. Similarly, other features, e.g. sensitivity of fibroblasts from individuals with breast cancer to ionizing radiation, may extend the phenotype (Bishop, 1994; Lakhani et al., 2000).

Several recent studies indicate that the majority of families with five or fewer cases of breast cancer and no cases of ovarian cancer are not linked to *BRCA1* or *BRCA2*. It has been proposed that a further breast cancer susceptibility gene that may account for some of these families is located on chromosome 8p12–22 (Imbert et al., 1996). Thirty-one site-specific breast cancer families have been identified that have a greater than 80% posterior probability of being due to genes other than *BRCA1* or *BRCA2*. These families have been examined for linkage to 8p12–22 using markers flanking the putative location of the gene. The data obtained do not lend support to the hypothesis that chromosome 8p12–22 harbours a familial breast cancer susceptibility gene (Rahman et al., 2000).

Li–Fraumeni syndrome

This syndrome was first described in 1969 (Li and Fraumeni, 1969; Birch, 1994) and is associated with early-onset and bilateral breast cancer in young women and with other tumours such as soft-tissue sarcomas, osteosarcomas, brain tumours, leukaemia and adrenocortical carcinoma. There is a high lifetime penetrance and up to 50% of female mutation carriers will have had breast cancer by 50 years of age. The Li–Fraumeni syndrome is associated with germline *TP53* mutations in the majority of families, but mutations have not been found in all classic Li–Fraumeni families (Malkin et al., 1990; Birch et al., 1994). Investigation of cancer incidence in 34 Li–Fraumeni families, according to their constitutional *TP53* mutation status, showed that families with germline missense mutations in the core DNA binding domain showed a more highly penetrant cancer phenotype than families with other *TP53* mutations or no mutation. Cancer phenotype in families carrying such mutations was characterized by a higher cancer incidence and earlier ages at diagnosis, especially of breast cancer and brain tumours, compared with families carrying protein-truncating or other inactivating mutations. Proband cancers showed significantly younger ages at diagnosis in those with missense mutations in the DNA binding domain than in those with protein-inactivating mutations. In women with sporadic breast cancer, less than 1% have a *p53* mutation and hence germline *p53*-associated breast cancer is found mainly in families with Li–Fraumeni syndrome.

Recently, mutations have been described in the hChk2 gene in Li–Fraumeni families (Varley et al., 1997; Birch et al., 1998). The hChk2 gene encodes the human homologue of the yeast *Cds1* and *RAD53 G2* checkpoint kinases, whose activation in response to DNA damage prevents cellular entry into mitosis. Heterozygous germline mutations in hChk2 occur in Li–Fraumeni syndrome. These observations suggest that hChk2 is a tumour suppressor gene conferring predisposition to sarcoma, breast cancer and brain tumours, and they also provide a link between the central role of p53 inactivation in human cancer and the well-defined G2 checkpoint in yeast.

Chk2 is a DNA damage-activated protein kinase that lies downstream of *ATM* in the DNA damage response pathway. Two of the reported Chk2 mutations identified in Li–Fraumeni syndrome result in loss of Chk2 kinase activity. While one mutation within the Chk2 forkhead homology-associated (FHA) domain, R145W, retains some basal kinase activity, this mutant cannot be phosphorylated at Thr-68, an *ATM*-dependent phosphorylation site, and cannot be activated following gamma radiation. The other FHA domain mutant, I157T, behaves as wild-type Chk2 in all the assays utilized. Since the FHA domain is involved in protein–protein interactions, this mutation may affect associations of Chk2 with other proteins. Additionally, it was shown that Chk2 could be inactivated by down-regulation of its expression in cancer cells. Thus, Chk2 may be inactivated by multiple mechanisms in the cell (Bell et al., 1999; Wu et al., 2001).

Low penetrance/modifier genes

Candidate genes with a function known to be consistent with a potential role in carcinogenesis have been studied to determine whether they influence the risk of breast cancer in both the general population and, more recently, in individuals carrying *BRCA1* and *BRCA2* gene mutations. The polymorphisms in these genes are usually common in the general population and may be associated with a small increased risk. They may only be seen to have an effect in carriers of other known gene mutations or in certain environmental circumstances.

The androgen receptor (AR) gene located on chromosome Xq11.2–12 has a 'CAG' (cytosine–adenine–guanine) repeat in exon 1. AR alleles containing longer CAG repeat are associated with a decreased ability to activate AR-responsive genes. In women carrying a *BRCA1* mutation, it has been found that the age at breast cancer diagnosis was earlier in women who had one copy of the CAG repeat that was very long. These results suggest that the pathway involving androgen signalling may affect the risk of *BRCA1*-associated breast cancer. In addition, germline mutations of this gene may contribute to male breast cancer. However, the majority of male breast cancers are not X-linked, and other genetic alterations must be considered in the pathogenesis (Rebbeck et al., 1999).

CYP1A1 is a P450 gene and encodes aryl hydrocarbon hydroxylase, which catalyses the conversion of oestradiol to hydroxylated oestrogen. Some small studies have suggested that polymorphisms in this gene may be associated with an increased risk of breast cancer in some populations. In experimental systems, polychlorinated biphenyls (PCBs) can induce *CYP1A1*. In postmenopausal women, women heterozygous for an exon 7 point mutation and who had an increased exposure to PCBs were at an increased risk of breast cancer (Crofts et al., 1994; Moysich et al., 1999; Taioli et al., 1999).

Glutathione *S*-transferases are a family of genes encoding enzymes that catalyse the conjugation of reactive metabolic intermediates to soluble glutathione conjugates and hence facilitate clearance (Forrester et al., 1990). Of the four classes of polymorphisms, three are expressed in the breast. Two – *GSTμ* and *GSTθ* genes – have null polymorphisms, which, in homozygotes, results in a total lack of enzyme. Studies have suggested that these alleles influence the age at first cancer diagnosis in *BRCA1* carriers with a 22% difference across the observed age range (25–40 years) by the GSTT1 genotype but may not affect the risk in the general population (Rebbeck et al., 1995; Lancaster et al., 1996; Miki et al., 1996; Rebbeck, 1997; Ambrosone et al., 1999).

The H-*ras*-1 variable number of tandem repeats (VNTR) polymorphism site lies one kilobase downstream from the H-*ras*-1 proto-oncogene on chromosome 11p15.5. Individuals who have rare alleles of the VNTR have an increased risk of certain types of cancers, including breast cancer (Phelan et al., 1996). These alleles are found in up to 6% of the general population, and as a result, up to 9% of all breast cancer may be attributable to this genetic polymorphism. The risk of breast cancer is increased in patients with one or two rare alleles and, in addition, analyses of somatic alterations in tumour DNA have shown the loss of one allele, in general the longest, in 6.7% of informative cases and an instability to H-*ras* locus in 6.5% of tumours that appeared as a size increase of one of the two alleles. These results demonstrated an association of rare H-*ras* alleles with breast cancer.

Phelan et al. (1996) investigated this polymorphism in 307 female *BRCA1* carriers. The risk for ovarian cancer in this group was 2.11 times greater for *BRCA1* carriers with one or two rare H-*ras*-1 alleles, compared with carriers with only common alleles. Susceptibility to breast cancer did not appear to be affected by the presence of rare H-*ras*-1 alleles (Gosse-Brun et al., 1999).

Polymorphisms in the *N*-acetyltransferase (*NAT2*) gene are associated with an altered rate of metabolism of carcinogens, with wild-type alleles producing a rapid acetylator phenotype and homozygosity for combinations of variant alleles resulting in a slow phenotype. It has been shown that there is a statistically significant interaction between acetylator status among *BRCA1* carriers and the number of packs of cigarettes they smoke per week, duration of time they had smoked, or age at which they started smoking. This suggests that *BRCA1* carriers who smoke are at increased risk of breast cancer if they are slow acetylators (Ambrosone et al., 1996; Rebbeck et al., 1997; Ambrosone et al., 1998).

Conclusions

It is important to note that only a minority of breast cancers (5–6%) are due to highly penetrant inherited genes, and that the majority are likely to be due to adverse environmental influences, although there may be genetic susceptibilities to such influences.

There is still a great deal to be learnt about *BRCA* mutation carriers. In addition, at least eight genes have been identified that may contribute to inherited breast cancer susceptibility, and others are likely to be found. *BRCA1* and *BRCA2* are currently the most important of these genes, and predictive genetic testing to identify mutations at these loci is under way.

Families in which a mutation in *BRCA1/2* is associated with predisposition to cancer are relatively uncommon. Specific *BRCA1/2* mutations may be of special importance in selected populations. The relatively rare but highly penetrant genes, for example *BRCA1*, *BRCA2* and *TP53*, produce dramatic familial aggregations of breast cancer. The ultimate outcome of the ongoing work will be the identification of the molecular mechanisms by which inherited breast cancers develop, thereby allowing primary prevention to be accomplished as the pathogenic genetic lesions are being repaired.

It is important to remember that the incidence of sporadic cancer is very high in the general population, and so even if an individual is found *not* to be a carrier for a gene mutation, they still have a residual risk of developing a similar cancer, and therefore need to be counselled accordingly.

REFERENCES

Abbott DW, Thompson ME, Robinson-Benion C, et al. (1999). BRCA1 expression restores radiation resistance in BRCA1-defective cancer cells through enhancement of transcription-coupled DNA repair. *J Biol Chem* **274**: 18 808–12.

Ambrosone CB, Freudenheim JL, Graham S, et al. (1996). Cigarette smoking, N-acetyltransferase 2 genetic polymorphisms, and breast cancer risk. *JAMA* **276**: 1494–501.

Ambrosone CB, Freudenheim JL, Sinha R, et al. (1998). Breast cancer risk, meat consumption and N-acetyltransferase (NAT2) genetic polymorphisms. *Int J Cancer* **75**: 825–30.

Ambrosone CB, Coles BF, Freudenheim JL and Shields PG (1999). Glutathione-S-transferase (GSTM1) genetic polymorphisms do not affect human breast cancer risk, regardless of dietary antioxidants. *J Nutr* **129** (Suppl. 2S): S565–S568.

Bar-Sade RB, Kruglikova A, Modan B, et al. (1998). The 185delAG BRCA1 mutation originated before the dispersion of Jews in the diaspora and is not limited to Ashkenazim. *Hum Mol Genet* **7**: 801–5.

Bell DW, Varley JM, Szydlo TE, et al. (1999). Heterozygous germ line hCHK2 mutations in Li–Fraumeni syndrome. *Science* **286**(5449): 2528–31.

Bertwistle D, Swift S, Marston NJ, et al. (1997). Nuclear location and cell cycle regulation of the BRCA2 protein. *Cancer Res* **57**: 5485–8.

Birch JM (1994). Li–Fraumeni syndrome. *Eur J Cancer* **30A**: 1935–41.

Birch JM, Hartley AL, Ticker KJ, et al. (1994). Prevalence and diversity of constitutional mutations in the p53 gene among 21 Li–Fraumeni families. *Cancer Res* **54**: 1298–304.

Birch JM, Blair V, Kelsey AM, et al. (1998). Cancer phenotype correlates with constitutional TP53 genotype in families with the Li–Fraumeni syndrome. *Oncogene* **17**(9): 1061–8.

Bishop DT (1994). BRCA1, BRCA2, BRCA3 . . . a myriad of breast cancer genes. *Eur J Cancer* **30A**: 1738–9.

Bork P, Hofmann K, Bucher P, et al. (1997). A superfamily of conserved domains in DNA damage-responsive cell cycle checkpoint proteins. *FASEB J* **11**: 68–76.

Breast Cancer Linkage Consortium (1999). Cancer risks in BRCA2 mutation carriers. *J Natl Cancer Inst* **91**: 1310–6.

Callebaut I and Mornon JP (1997). From BRCA1 to RAP1: a widespread BRCT module closely associated with DNA repair. *FEBS Lett* **400**: 25–30.

Chen JJ, Silver D, Cantor S, Livingston DM and Scully R (1999). BRCA1, BRCA2, and Rad51 operate in a common DNA damage response pathway. *Cancer Res* **59**(7): 1752–6S.

Claus EB, Risch N and Thompson WD (1991). Genetic analysis of breast cancer in the Cancer and Steroid Hormone study. *Am J Hum Genet* **48**: 232–42.

Claus EB, Schildkraut JM, Thompson WD and Risch NJ (1996). The genetic attributable risk of breast and ovarian cancer. *Cancer* **77**: 2318–24.

Crofts F, Taioli E, Trachman J, et al. (1994). Functional significance of different human CYP1A1 genotypes. *Carcinogenesis* **15**: 2961–3.

Easton D and Peto J (1990). The contribution of inherited predisposition to cancer incidence. *Cancer Surv* **9**(3): 395–416.

Easton DF, Ford D, Bishop DT and Breast Cancer Linkage Consortium (1995). Breast and ovarian cancer incidence in BRCA1-mutation carriers. *Am J Hum Genet.* **56**: 265–71.

FitzGerald MG, MacDonald DJ, Krainer M, et al. (1996). Germ-line mutations in Jewish and non-Jewish women with early-onset breast cancer. *N Engl J Med* **334**: 143–9.

Fodor FH, Weston A, Bleiweiss IJ, et al. (1998). Frequency and carrier risk associated with common BRCA1 and BRCA2 mutations in Ashkenazi Jewish breast cancer patients. *Am J Hum Genet* **63**: 45–51.

Ford D, Easton DF, Bishop DT, et al. (1994). Risks of cancer in BRCA1-mutation carriers. *Lancet* **343**: 692–5.

Ford D, Easton DF, Stratton MR, et al. (1998). Genetic heterogeneity and penetrance analysis of the *BRCA1* and *BRCA2* genes in breast cancer families. *Am J Hum Genet* **62**: 676–89.

Forrester LM, Hayes JD, Millis R, et al. (1990). Expression of glutathione S-transferases and cytochrome P450 in normal and tumor breast tissue. *Carcinogenesis* **11**: 2163–70.

Futreal PA, Liu Q, Shattuck-Eidens D, et al. (1994). BRCA1 mutations in primary breast and ovarian carcinomas. *Science* **266**: 120–2.

Gayther SA, Warren W, Mazoyer S, et al. (1995). Germline mutations of the BRCA1 gene in breast and ovarian cancer families provide evidence for a genotype–phenotype correlation. *Nat Genet* **11**: 428–33.

Gosse-Brun S, Sauvaigo S, Daver A, et al. (1999). Specific H-Ras minisatellite alleles in breast cancer susceptibility. *Anticancer Res* **19**(6B): 5191–6.

Hall JM, Lee MK, Newman B, et al. (1990). Linkage of early-onset breast cancer to chromosome 17q21. *Science* **250**: 1684–9.

Hsu LC and White RL (1998). BRCA1 is associated with the centrosome during mitosis. *Proc Natl Acad Sci USA* **95**: 12 983–8.

Imbert A, Chaffanet M, Essioux L, et al. (1996). Integrated map of the chromosome 8p12–p21 region, a region involved in human cancers and Werner syndrome. *Genomics* **32**(1): 29–38.

Johannesdottir G, Gudmundsson J, Bergthorsson JT, et al. (1996). High prevalence of the 999del5 mutation in icelandic breast and ovarian cancer patients. *Cancer Res* **56**: 3663–5.

Koonin EV, Altschul SF and Bork P (1996). BRCA1 protein products: functional motifs. *Nat Genet* **13**(3): 266–8.

Lakhani SR, Gusterson BA, Jacquemier J, et al. (2000). The pathology of familial breast cancer: histological features of cancers in families not attributable to mutations in BRCA1 or BRCA2. *Clin Cancer Res* **6**(3): 782–9.

Lancaster JM, Wooster R, Mangion J, et al. (1996). BRCA2 mutations in primary breast and ovarian cancers. *Nat Genet* **13**: 238–40.

Langston AA, Malone KE, Thompson JD, Darling JR and Ostrander EA (1996). *BRCA1* mutations in a population-based sample of young women with breast cancer. *N Engl J Med* **334**: 137–42.

Li FP and Fraumeni JF Jr (1969). Soft tissue sarcomas, breast cancer, and other neoplasms. A familial syndrome? *Ann Intern Med* **71**: 747–52.

Liede A, Cohen B, Black D, et al. (1999). Evidence of a founder mutation in Scotland [abstract]. *Am J Hum Genet* **65**: A135.

Malkin D, Li FP, Strong LC, et al. (1990). Germ line p53 mutations in a familial syndrome of breast cancer, sarcomas, and other neoplasms. *Science* **250**: 1233–8.

McPherson K, Steel CM and Dixon JM (2000). Breast cancer – epidemiology, risk factors and genetics. *BMJ* **321**: 624–8.

Miki Y, Swensen J, Shattuck-Eidens D, et al. (1994). A strong candidate for the breast and ovarian cancer susceptibility gene BRCA1. *Science* **266**: 66–71.

Miki Y, Katagiri T, Kasumi F, Yoshimoto T and Nakamura Y (1996). Mutation analysis in the BRCA2 gene in primary breast cancers. *Nat Genet* **13**: 245–7.

Moysich KB, Shields PG, Freudenheim JL, et al. (1999). Polychlorinated biphenyls, cytochrome P4501A1 polymorphism, and postmenopausal breast cancer risk. *Cancer Epidemiol Biomarkers Prev* **8**: 41–4.

Muderspach LI (1994). In *Practical Oncology*, ed. R.B. Cameron. London: Prentice-Hall International.

Narod SA, Ford D, Devilee P, et al. (1995). An evaluation of genetic heterogeneity in 145 breast–ovarian cancer families. Breast Cancer Linkage Consortium. *Am J Hum Genet* **56**: 254–64.

Oddoux C, Struewing JP, Clayton CM, et al. (1996). The carrier frequency of the BRCA2 6174delT mutation among Ashkenazi Jewish individuals is approximately 1%. *Nat Genet* **14**: 188–90.

Peelen T, van Vliet M, Petrij-Bosch A, et al. (1997). A high proportion of novel mutations in BRCA1 with strong founder effects among Dutch and Belgian hereditary breast and ovarian cancer families. *Am J Hum Genet* **60**: 1041–9.

Peto PJ, Collins N, Barfoot R, et al. (1999). Prevalence of BRCA1 and BRCA2 gene mutations in patients with early-onset breast cancer. *J Natl Cancer Inst* **91**(11): 943–9.

Petrij-Bosch A, Peelen T, van Vliet M, et al. (1997). BRCA1 genomic deletions are major founder mutations in Dutch breast cancer patients. *Nat Genet* **17**: 341–5.

Phelan CM, Rebbeck TR, Weber BL, et al. (1996). Ovarian cancer risk in BRCA1 carriers is modified by the HRAS1 variable number of tandem repeat (VNTR) locus. *Nat Genet* **12**(3): 309–11.

Puget N, Stoppa-Lyonnet D, Sinilnikova OM, et al. (1999a). Screening for germ line rearrangements and regulatory mutations in BRCA1 led to the identification of four new deletions

Cancer Res **59**: 455–61.

Puget N, Sinilnikova OM, Stoppa-Lyonnet D, et al. (1999b). An Alu-mediated 6-kb duplication in the BRCA1 gene: a new founder mutation? *Am J Hum Genet* **64**: 300–2.

Rahman N and Stratton MR (1998). The genetics of breast cancer susceptibility. *Annu Rev Genet* **32**: 95–121.

Rahman N, Teare MD, Seal S, et al. (2000). Absence of evidence for a familial breast cancer susceptibility gene at chromosome 8p12–p22. *Oncogene* **19**(36): 4170–3.

Rebbeck TR (1997). Molecular epidemiology of the human glutathione S-transferase genotypes GSTM1 and GSTT1 in cancer susceptibility. *Cancer Epidemiol Biomarkers Prev* **6**: 733–43.

Rebbeck T, Walker A, Hoskins K, et al. (1995). Modifications of familial breast cancer penetrance by glutathione-S-transferase genotypes [abstract]. *Am J Hum Genet* **57**: A4.

Rebbeck T, Blackwood M, Walker A, et al. (1997). Association of breast cancer incidence with NAT2 genotype and smoking in BRCA1 mutation carriers (abstract). *Am J Hum Genet* **61**: A46.

Rebbeck TR, Kantoff PW, Krithivas K, et al. (1999). Modification of BRCA1-associated breast cancer risk by the polymorphic androgen-receptor CAG repeat. *Am J Hum Genet* **64**: 1371–7.

Struewing JP, Hartge P, Wacholder S, et al. (1997). The risk of cancer associated with specific mutations of BRCA1 and BRCA2 among Ashkenazi Jews. *N Engl J Med* **336**(20): 1401–8.

Szabo CI and King MC (1997). Population genetics of BRCA1 and BRCA2 [editorial]. *Am J Hum Genet* **60**: 1013–20.

Taioli E, Bradlow HL, Garbers SV, et al. (1999). Role of estradiol metabolism and CYP1A1 polymorphisms in breast cancer risk. *Cancer Detect Prev* **23**: 232–7.

Takahashi H, Chiu H-C, Bandera CA, et al. (1996). Mutations of the BRCA2 gene in ovarian carcinomas. *Cancer Res* **56**: 2738–41.

Tavtigian SV, Simard J, Rommens J, et al. (1996). The complete BRCA2 gene and mutations in chromosome 13q-linked kindreds. *Nat Genet* **12**: 333–7.

Varley JM, McGown G, Thorncroft M, et al. (1997). Germ-line mutations of TP53 in Li–Fraumeni families: an extended study of 39 families. *Cancer Res* **57**(15): 3245–52.

Wooster R, Neuhausen SL, Mangion J, et al. (1994). Localization of a breast cancer susceptibility gene, BRCA2, to chromosome 13q12–13. *Science* **265**: 2088–90.

Wooster R, Bignell G, Lancaster J, et al. (1995). Identification of the breast cancer susceptibility gene BRCA2. *Nature* **378**: 789–92 [published erratum appears in *Nature* (1996) **379**: 749].

Wu X, Webster SR and Chen J (2001). Characterization of tumor-associated Chk2 mutations. *J Biol Chem* **276**(4): 2971–4.

3

Cowden syndrome and related disorders

Charis Eng

Ohio State University, Columbus, OH, USA; University of Cambridge, UK

Introduction

The differential diagnosis of familial breast and ovarian cancer must always include Cowden syndrome (CS, Mendelian Inheritance in Man Catalogue Number (MIM) 158350). CS, also known as multiple hamartoma syndrome, is named after Rachel Cowden (Lloyd and Denis, 1963), who died of bilateral breast cancer in her early thirties (Brownstein et al., 1978). It is an under-diagnosed, under-recognized, autosomal dominant inherited cancer syndrome characterized by hamartomas, which can develop from derivatives of any of the three germ-cell layers, and carries a high risk of breast, thyroid and possibly endometrial cancers (Eng, 2000b). Germline mutations of *PTEN*, a tumour suppressor gene localized to 10q23.3, are associated with the great majority of CS cases (Nelen et al., 1996; Li et al., 1997; Liaw et al., 1997; Marsh et al., 1998b). Other syndromes, such as Bannayan–Riley–Ruvalcaba syndrome (BRR, MIM 153480) and a previously unclassified Proteus-like syndrome, which previously were not suspected of having an increased risk of cancer, have also been found to be partly accounted for by *PTEN* mutations (Marsh et al., 1997a, 1999; Zhou et al., 2000b).

Clinical aspects

Epidemiology

Because the diagnosis of CS is difficult, the true incidence is unknown. Prior to gene identification, a population-based estimate in Amsterdam was one in a million (Starink et al., 1986; Nelen et al., 1996). However, after identification of the susceptibility gene, the same population base yielded an incidence of one in 200 000 (Nelen et al., 1997, 1999), although the latter is still likely to be an under-estimate. Nonetheless, CS has been reported from many countries from around the world, including those in North America, Europe and Asia. Little is known about the epidemiology of BRR.

Table 3.1. Common manifestations of Cowden syndrome

Mucocutaneous lesions (90–100%)
Trichilemmomas
Acral keratoses
Verucoid or papillomatous papules

Thyroid abnormalities (50–67%)
Goitre
Adenoma
Cancer (3–10%)

Breast lesions
Fibroadenomas/fibrocystic disease (76% of affected females)
Adenocarcinoma (25–50% of affected females)

Gastrointestinal lesions (40%)
Hamartomatous polyps
Macrocephaly (38%)

Genitourinary abnormalities (44% of females)
Uterine leiomyoma (multiple, early onset)

Because CS is under-recognized, it is difficult to obtain a true count of the proportion that is familial and that which is isolated. From the literature, the experience of a major CS centre in North America and a series of CS probands ascertained for research purposes, perhaps 10–50% are familial and the remainder isolated cases. Similarly, it would appear that many BRR cases are isolated, and that no more than 50% are familial (Marsh et al., 1999).

Diagnosis

Cowden syndrome

CS usually presents by the late twenties. It is believed that more than 90% of affected individuals manifest a phenotype by their twenties (Nelen et al., 1996; Eng, 2000b). By the third decade, 99% of affected individuals would have developed the mucocutaneous stigmata, although any of the features could be present already (Tables 3.1 and 3.2). Because the clinical literature on CS consists mostly of reports of the most obvious or most unusual families, or case reports by sub-specialists interested in their respective organ systems, the true spectrum of component signs is unknown. Despite this, the most commonly reported manifestations are: mucocutaneous lesions; thyroid abnormalities; fibrocystic disease and carcinoma of the breast; gastrointestinal hamartomas; multiple, early-onset

Table 3.2. International Cowden syndrome Consortium operational criteria for the diagnosis of Cowden syndrome (version 2000)*

Pathognomonic criteria
Mucocutaneous lesions:
 Trichilemmomas, facial
 Acral keratoses
 Papillomatous papules
 Mucosal lesions

Major criteria
Breast carcinoma
Thyroid carcinoma (non-medullary), especially follicular thyroid carcinoma
Macrocephaly (megalencephaly) (say, ≥ 97 percentile)
Lhermitte–Duclos disease (LDD)
Endometrial carcinoma

Minor criteria
Other thyroid lesions (e.g. adenoma or multinodular goitre)
Mental retardation (say, IQ ≤ 75)
Gastrointestinal hamartomas
Fibrocystic disease of the breast
Lipomas
Fibromas
Gastrointestinal tumours (e.g., renal cell carcinoma, uterine fibroids) or malformation

Operational diagnosis in an individual
1. Mucocutaneous lesions alone if:
    (a) there are six or more facial papules, of which three or more must be trichilemmoma, or
    (b) cutaneous facial papules and oral mucosal papillomatosis, or
    (c) oral mucosal papillomatosis and acral keratoses, or
    (d) palmo-plantar keratoses, 6 or more
2. Two major criteria but one must include macrocephaly or LDD
3. One major and three minor criteria
4. Four minor criteria

Operational diagnosis in a family where one individual is diagnostic for CS
1. The pathognomonic criterion/criteria
2. Any one major criterion with or without minor criteria
3. Two minor criteria

---

*Operational diagnostic criteria are reviewed and revised on a continuous basis as new clinical and genetic information becomes available. The 1995 and 2000 versions have been accepted by the US-based National Comprehensive Cancer Network Genetics/High Risk Panel.

uterine leiomyoma; macrocephaly (specifically, megalencephaly) and mental retardation (Table 3.1) (Starink et al., 1986; Hanssen and Fryns, 1995; Mallory,
1995; Longy and Lacombe, 1996; Eng, 2000b). Pathognomonic mucocutaneous
lesions are trichilemmomas and papillomatous papules (Table 3.2). Because of the
lack of uniform diagnostic criteria for CS prior to 1995, a group of individuals –
the International Cowden Consortium – who were interested in systematically
studying this syndrome to localize the susceptibility gene arrived at a set of
consensus operational diagnostic criteria (Nelen et al., 1996; Eng, 1998). These
criteria have been revised recently in the context of new data and are reflected in
the practice guidelines of the US-based National Comprehensive Cancer Network
Genetics/High Risk Panel (Table 3.2) (NCCN, 1999; Eng, 2000b).

   The two documented component cancers in CS are carcinoma of the breast and
of the thyroid (Starink et al., 1986). By contrast, in the general population, lifetime
risks for breast and thyroid cancers are approximately 11% (in women) and 1%,
respectively. In women with CS, lifetime risk estimates for the development of
breast cancer range from 25% to 50% (Starink et al., 1986; Hanssen and Fryns,
1995; Longy and Lacombe, 1996; Eng, 1997). The mean age at diagnosis of CS
breast cancer is likely to be 10 years earlier than that of breast cancer occurring in
the general population (Starink et al., 1986; Longy and Lacombe, 1996). Although
Rachel Cowden died of breast cancer at the age of 31 years (Lloyd and Denis, 1963;
Brownstein et al., 1978) and the earliest recorded age of diagnosis of breast cancer
is 14 years (Starink et al., 1986), the majority of CS breast cancers are diagnosed
after the age of 30–35 years (range 14–65) (Longy and Lacombe, 1996). Until
genotype–phenotype analyses were performed with the discovery of the susceptibility gene, it was thought that male breast cancer was not a component of CS.
However, male breast cancer does occur in *PTEN*-mutation-positive CS but with
unknown frequency (Marsh et al., 1998b; Fackenthal et al., 2001).

   The lifetime risk for non-medullary thyroid cancer can be as high as 10% in
males and females with CS. Because of small numbers, it is unclear if the age of
onset is truly earlier than that of the general population. Histologically, the thyroid
cancer is predominantly follicular carcinoma, although papillary histology has
also been observed rarely (Starink et al., 1986; Hanssen and Fryns, 1995; Longy
and Lacombe, 1996; Eng, unpublished observations). Medullary thyroid carcinoma has yet to be observed in patients with CS.

   Benign tumours are also common in CS (Tables 3.1 and 3.4). Apart from those
of the skin, benign tumours or disorders of breast and thyroid are the most
frequently noted, and likely represent true component features of this syndrome
(Table 3.1). Fibroadenomas and fibrocystic disease of the breast are common signs
in CS, as are follicular adenomas and multinodular goitre of the thyroid. An
unusual central nervous system tumour – cerebellar dysplastic gangliocytoma – or

Table 3.3. Reported malignancies in patients with Cowden syndrome

Central nervous system
Glioblastoma multiforme

Mucocutaneous
Squamous cell carcinoma
Basal cell carcinoma
Malignant melanoma
Merkel cell carcinoma

Breast
Adenocarcinoma

Endocrine
Non-medullary thyroid carcinoma (classically of follicular histology)

Pulmonary
Non-small-cell carcinoma

Gastrointestinal
Colorectal carcinoma
Hepatocellular carcinoma
Pancreatic carcinoma

Genitourinary
Uterine carcinoma
Ovarian carcinoma
Transitional cell carcinoma of the bladder
Renal cell carcinoma

Other
Liposarcoma

Lhermitte–Duclos disease, has only recently been associated with CS (Padberg et al., 1991; Eng et al., 1994).

Other malignancies and benign tumours have been reported in patients or families with CS (Tables 3.3 and 3.4). Given the availability of new data with the discovery of the gene, exponents of this field believe that endometrial carcinoma might also be a component tumour of CS as well (Table 3.2 and see below; Eng, 2000b). Whether malignant tumours, other than those in the breast, thyroid and endometrium, are true components of CS or whether some are coincidental findings is as yet unknown.

Table 3.4. Non-cutaneous benign lesions reported in Cowden syndrome

Nervous system	*Genitourinary*
Lhermitte–Duclos disease	Female:
Megalencephaly	Leiomyomas
Glioma	Ovarian cysts
Meningioma	Vaginal and vulvar cysts
Neuroma	Various developmental anomalies (e.g.
Neurofibroma	duplicated collecting system)
Bridged sella turcica	Male:
Mental retardation	Hydrocele
	Varicocele
Breast	Hypoplastic testes
Fibrocystic disease	
Fibroadenoma	*Skeletal*
Hamartoma	Craniomegaly
Gynaecomastia of the male breast	Adenoid facies
	High arched palate
Thyroid	Hypoplastic zygoma
Goitre	Kyphoscoliosis
Adenoma	Pectus excavatum
Thyroiditis	Bone cysts
Thyroglossal duct cyst	Rudimentary sixth digit
Hyperthyroidism	
Hypothyroidism	*Other*
	Hypoplastic vulva
Gastrointestinal	Atrial septal defect
Hamartomatous polyposis of the entire tract	Ateriovenous malformations
Diverticuli of the colon and sigmoid	Eye cataracts
Ganglioneuroma	Retinal angioid streaks
Leiomyoma	
Hepatic hamartomas	

Bannayan–Riley–Ruvalcaba syndrome

BRR, also known as Bannayan–Zonana syndrome, Ruvalcaba–Riley–Smith syndrome and Myhre–Smith syndrome, is diagnosed by the classic criteria. In general, macrocephaly secondary to megalencephaly, lipomatosis, haemangiomatosis and speckled penis are the hallmark features (Bannayan, 1971; Zonana et al., 1976; Higginbottom and Schultz, 1982; Halal and Silver, 1989; Gorlin et al., 1992).

Genetics

CS is inherited as an autosomal dominant condition with age-related penetrance. The major susceptibility gene, or at least a major susceptibility gene, has been mapped to 10q22–23 (Nelen et al., 1996). Fine-structure genetic analysis, somatic genetics on sporadic component tumours and candidate gene analysis identified *PTEN*, encoding a dual-specificity phosphatase as the CS susceptibility gene (Liaw et al., 1997). That *PTEN* is the CS gene has been confirmed by other groups (Lynch et al., 1997; Nelen et al., 1997; Tsou et al., 1997).

Germline *PTEN* mutations in families with BRR have also been found (Marsh et al., 1997a). Thus, at least a subset of BRR and CS may be considered allelic. Recently, an individual with an unclassified Proteus-like syndrome, who did not meet the criteria for diagnosis of either BRR or Proteus syndrome, was found to harbour a germline *PTEN* mutation as well as a germline mosaic *PTEN* mutation (Zhou et al., 2000b). What proportion of Proteus-like, or even classic Proteus, patients actually have *PTEN* mutations is currently unknown and is the topic of ongoing investigation.

Genotype–phenotype associations
Cowden syndrome

A series of 37 unrelated CS probands was ascertained by the strict operational diagnostic criteria of the International Cowden Consortium (1995 version) (Eng, 1998) for purposes of genotype–phenotype analyses (Marsh et al., 1998b). Of the 37 CS probands, 30 (81%) were found to carry germline *PTEN* mutations (Marsh et al., 1998b). Among the 30 mutation-positive probands were two males with breast cancer. Approximately two out of three of all mutations were found in exons 5, 7 or 8. Although exon 5, which encodes the phosphatase core motif, represents 20% of the coding sequence, it harbours 40% of all *PTEN* mutations in CS. Association analyses revealed that CS families with germline *PTEN* mutations are more likely to develop malignant breast disease when compared with *PTEN*-mutation-negative families (Marsh et al., 1998b). Furthermore, non-truncating mutations and those within the phosphatase core motif and 5' region of it appeared to be associated with the involvement of five or more organs, a surrogate phenotype for severity of disease (Marsh et al., 1998b). Another group examined families for germline *PTEN* mutations and found mutations in only 13 probands (Nelen et al., 1999). They could not find any clear genotype–phenotype associations, most likely owing to their small sample size.

Bannayan–Riley–Ruvalcaba syndrome

When germline *PTEN* mutations were found in BRR, it suggested that CS and BRR are allelic (Marsh et al., 1997a). A series of 43 unrelated BRR probands were ascertained in order to examine their mutation spectrum in the context of the CS spectrum and to examine genotype–phenotype association in BRR (Marsh et al., 1999). In contrast to CS, 60% of BRR cases were found to have germline *PTEN* mutations. Furthermore, two of these mutations included one with a cytogeneti-cally detectable deletion of 10q23, encompassing *PTEN*, and another with a translocation involving 10q23. The mutational spectra of BRR and CS seemed to overlap, thus lending formal proof that CS and BRR, at least a subset, are allelic (Marsh et al., 1999). There was no difference in mutation frequencies between isolated BRR and familial BRR. Of interest, more than 90% of CS–BRR overlap families were found to have germline *PTEN* mutations. The presence of *PTEN* mutation in BRR was found to be associated with the development of any cancer as well as tumours of the breast and lipomas. Therefore, the presence of *PTEN* mutations in BRR may have implications for cancer surveillance in this syndrome previously not believed to be associated with malignancy. In view of the genetic and molecular epidemiological data to date, some clinical cancer geneticists have found it more useful to consider, and thus medically manage, individuals with germline *PTEN* mutations not by clinical syndromic names but under the rubric of 'PTEN Hamartoma Tumour Syndrome' (PHTS) (Marsh et al., 1999).

Cryptic PHTS

Because the spectrum of PHTS may be broader than was previously believed, it would be important to recognize cryptic cases. Since CS, in and of itself, is difficult to diagnose clinically, *PTEN* mutation frequencies in series of 'CS' individuals ranged from a low of 10% (Tsou et al., 1997) to a high of 81% (Marsh et al., 1998b). The highest mutation frequencies are obtained when CS is strictly defined by the operational diagnostic criteria of the International Cowden syndrome Consortium (Table 3.2) (Liaw et al., 1997; Marsh et al., 1998b). A study was performed that ascertained CS-like probands in which the subjects were not required to meet the Consortium criteria but were required to have a minimum of breast cancer and thyroid disease in a single individual or in two first-degree relatives (Marsh et al., 1998a). Sixty-four unrelated probands were enrolled, and one germline mutation was found, in a family with follicular thyroid cancer, bilateral breast cancer and endometrial cancer. This study concluded that the Consortium criteria were robust, even at the molecular level, and that endometrial carcinoma might be an important component cancer of CS. In another recent study, a nested cohort of 103 eligible women with multiple primary cancers within the 32 826-member Nurses' Health Study were examined for the occult presence of germline *PTEN* mutations (De Vivo et al., 2000). Among 103 cases, five (5%) were found to have germline missense mutations, all of which have been shown to cause some loss of function. Of these five, two individuals themselves had en-dometrial cancer. This study therefore suggests that occult germline mutations of *PTEN* and, by extrapolation, CS occur with a higher frequency than was previously believed. Further, these data confirm the previous observations (Marsh et al., 1998a) that endometrial carcinoma is an important component cancer of CS, and perhaps its presence in a case or family that is reminiscent of CS but does not quite meet Consortium criteria might actually help to increase the prior probability of finding *PTEN* mutations (Eng, 2000b).

When 62 unrelated women with breast cancer diagnosed under the age of 40 years old were examined for the occult presence of germline *PTEN* mutations, two (3.2%) were found to have missense mutations (FitzGerald et al., 1998). Despite all these studies, site-specific breast cancer families without CS features not linked to *BRCA1/2* were found not to be linked to 10q23 (Shugart et al., 1999) and not to have germline *PTEN* mutations (Chen et al., 1998). Interestingly, there have been no cases of occult germline *PTEN* mutations uncovered in series of non-familial, non-medullary, thyroid cancer cases or endometrial cancer cases (Dahia et al., 1997; Kong et al., 1997; Risinger et al., 1997; Tashiro et al., 1997; Halachmi et al., 1998; Mutter et al., 2000).

Differential diagnosis

CS has variable expression, and thus, this disorder may be considered as a great imitator of many syndromes. BRR could be considered in the differential diagnosis although, with the identification of *PTEN* mutations in this syndrome, most believe that CS and at least a subset of BRR should be considered as a single genetic entity with the proposed name of 'PTEN Hamartoma Tumour Syndrome' or 'PHTS' (Marsh et al., 1999). The PHTS entity is particularly germane because there are currently more than 14 families with an overlap of both CS and BRR features (Marsh et al., 1999; Eng, unpublished observations). Now, at least one Proteus-like individual has been found to have germline *PTEN* mutation (Zhou et al., 2000b).

Natural differential diagnoses to consider include other hamartoma syndromes, especially juvenile polyposis syndrome (JPS, MIM 174900) and Peutz–Jeghers syndrome (PJS, MIM 174900). JPS is an autosomal dominant disorder characterized by hamartomatous polyps in the gastrointestinal tract and a high risk of colorectal cancer and, in a sense, may be viewed as a clinical diagnosis of exclusion. A single report claimed that germline *PTEN* mutations can occur in JPS (Olschwang et al., 1998). However, closer inspection of these probands revealed that it is likely that one has CS and the other was too young to clinically exclude CS, given that the penetrance under the age of 20 years for classic CS is less than 10%. When Kurose et al. ascertained a series of patients with the diagnosis of juvenile polyposis, he found one with germline *PTEN* mutation, and unlike the previous series, these investigators were able to recall that patient for re-examination, and discovered clinical stigmata of CS (Kurose et al., 1999). Thus, finding a germline *PTEN* mutation in a presumed JPS case alters the diagnosis to CS (Eng and Ji,

1998). Subsequently, a major JPS locus was identified on 18q, and germline mutations in *SMAD4* have been found in a subset of JPS (Houlston et al., 1998; Howe et al., 1998a, 1998b). PJS, which carries a high risk of intestinal carcinomas and breast cancers, should be clinically quite distinct. The pigmentation of the peri-oral region in this autosomal dominant hamartoma syndrome is pathognomonic (Eng and Blackstone, 1988; Rustgi, 1994). The hamartomatous polyp in PJS has a diagnostic appearance as well, and is referred to as the 'Peutz–Jeghers polyp'. They are unlike the hamartomatous polyps seen in CS and JPS. Clinically, while Peutz–Jeghers polyps are often symptomatic (intussusceptions, rectal bleeding), CS polyps are rarely so. Germline mutations in *LKB1/STK11*, on 19p, have been found in isolated and familial PJS cases (Hemminki et al., 1997; Hemminki et al., 1998; Jenne et al., 1998), although some believe that there is a minor susceptibility gene on 19q as well (Mehenni et al., 1997).

Proteus syndrome (MIM 176920) could be considered in the differential diagnosis of CS because of the common theme of overgrowth, e.g. hemihypertrophy, macrocephaly, connective tissue naevi and lipomatosis (Gorlin, 1984). Like CS, Proteus syndrome can have a broad spectrum of phenotypic expression, and so its diagnosis is also made by consensus operational criteria (Biesecker et al., 1999). Mandatory diagnostic criteria include mosaic distribution of lesions, progressive course and sporadic occurrence (Biesecker et al., 1999). Connective tissue naevi are pathognomonic for this syndrome. In a small pilot study to determine whether Proteus syndrome is part of PHTS, an apparently isolated case of a Proteus-like syndrome, comprising hemihypertrophy, macrocephaly, lipomas, connective tissue naevi and multiple arteriovenous malformations, was found to have a germline *PTEN* mutation R335X (Zhou et al., 2000b). Interestingly, a naevus, a lipomatous region and arteriovenous malformation tissue were found to harbour a second-hit non-germline *PTEN* mutation R130X, possibly representing a germline mosaic. Both of these mutations have been previously described in classic CS and BRR. Thus, this Proteus-like case may be classified as PHTS at the molecular level, with all its implications for development of malignancies characteristic of CS/BRR. What proportion of clinical Proteus syndrome or Proteus-like cases will be reclassified as PHTS at the molecular level is being investigated.

Minor differential diagnoses to consider are neurofibromatosis type 1 (NF-1) and basal cell naevus (Gorlin) syndrome, although the latter should not be confused clinically with CS or BRR. In NF-1, the only two consistent features are café-au-lait macules and neurofibromas of the skin. Plexiform neuromas are highly suggestive of NF-1. The susceptibility gene for this syndrome has been isolated as NF-1 on 17q (Viskochil et al., 1990; Wallace et al., 1990). Because of the large size of the gene, direct mutation analysis is still not practical. In informative families, linkage analysis is feasible for predictive testing purposes and is 98%

accurate (Ward et al., 1990). Basal cell naevus syndrome is an autosomal dominant condition characterized by basal cell naevi, basal cell carcinoma and diverse developmental abnormalities. In addition, affected individuals can develop other tumours and cancers, such as fibromas, hamartomatous gastric polyps and medulloblastomas. However, the dermatological findings and developmental features in CS and basal cell naevus syndrome are markedly different. For instance, the palmar pits, together with the characteristic facies of the latter, are never seen in CS. The major susceptibility gene for basal cell naevus syndrome is also distinct from CS/BRR, and is the human homologue of the *Drosophila patched* gene, *PTC*, on 9q22–31 (Johnson et al., 1996). Linkage analysis and mutation analysis are technically possible. However, since it is not known what proportion of patients with this syndrome will actually turn out to have mutations in *PTC*, predictive testing based on mutation analysis alone should be deferred until more data become available.

Clinical cancer genetic management

The key to proper genetic counselling in CS is recognition of the syndrome. Families with CS should be counselled as for any autosomal dominant trait with high penetrance. What is unclear, however, is the variability of expression between and within families. We suspect that there are CS families who have nothing but trichilemmomas and who, therefore, never come for medical attention. Based on the current data, it might also be prudent to treat all PHTS cases like CS, regardless of their apparent clinical syndrome.

The two most serious, and established, component tumours in CS are breast cancer and non-medullary thyroid cancer for affected females and males. Endometrial cancer is now believed to be a component of CS as well. Patients with CS or those who are at risk of CS should undergo surveillance for these three cancers. Beginning in their teens, these individuals should undergo annual physical examinations, paying particular attention to the thyroid examination. Beginning in their mid-twenties, women with CS or those at risk of it should be encouraged to perform monthly breast self-examinations and to have careful breast examinations during their annual check-ups. The value of annual imaging studies is unclear as no objective data are available. Nonetheless, we usually recommend annual mammography and/or breast ultrasounds performed by skilled individuals in at-risk women, beginning at age 30 years or 5 years younger than the earliest breast cancer case in the family, whichever is earlier. Some women with CS develop severe, sometimes disfiguring, fibroadenomas of the breasts well before the age of 30 years. This situation should be treated individually. For example, if the fibroadenomas cause pain or if they make breast cancer surveillance impossible, then some have advocated prophylactic mastectomies (Brownstein et al.,

1978). Careful annual physical examination of the thyroid and neck region, beginning at age 18 or 5 years younger than the earliest diagnosis of thyroid cancer in the family (whichever is earlier), should be sufficient although a single baseline thyroid ultrasound in the early twenties might be considered as well. Surveillance for endometrial carcinoma (see Chapter 14) is recommended, perhaps beginning at the age of 35–40 years (no data for age at onset) or 5 years younger than the earliest onset case in the family. For premenopausal women, annual blind repel (suction) biopsies of the endometrium should be performed. In the post-menopausal years, uterine ultrasound should suffice.

Whether other tumours are true components of CS is unknown. It is believed, however, that skin cancers, for instance, might be features of CS. For now, therefore, surveillance of other organs should follow the American Cancer Society guidelines, although proponents of CS will advise routine skin surveillance as well. Some clinical cancer geneticists recommend surveillance for the development of renal cell carcinoma as well, including urinalysis for occult blood and perhaps renal ultrasound.

A preliminary study has demonstrated that the presence of germline *PTEN* mutation in BRR is associated with cancer development (Marsh et al., 1999). Until additional data become available, it might be conservative to manage all BRR individuals and families, especially those harbouring germline *PTEN* mutations, like CS cases with respect to cancer formation and surveillance. Given the data that have accumulated regarding *PTEN* mutations and PHTS, it would seem that routine clinical laboratory testing for *PTEN* mutations, both as a molecular diagnostic tool and as a predictive tool, might become commonplace. In the US, at least one academic centre offers clinical *PTEN* testing, with the molecular diagnostics laboratory working very closely with the Clinical Cancer Genetics Program.

The key to successful management of CS and all PHTS patients and their families is a multidisciplinary team. There should always be a primary care provider, usually a general internist, who orchestrates the care of such patients, some of whom will need the care of surgeons, gynaecologists, dermatologists, oncologists and geneticists at some point.

Somatic *PTEN* alterations in sporadic tumours

It is not uncommon to find a high frequency of somatic mutations in a gene, X, in sporadic counterpart tumours that are components of an inherited cancer syndrome whose susceptibility gene is X. For example, germline mutations in the *RET* proto-oncogene cause multiple endocrine neoplasia type 2, which is characterized by medullary thyroid carcinoma, phaeochromocytoma and hyperparathyroidism (reviewed by Eng, 2000a). Somatic *RET* mutations have been found in 20–80% of sporadic medullary thyroid carcinoma (reviewed in Eng, 1999). The three

sporadic counterpart tumours of CS are breast, thyroid and endometrial carcinomas. While a broad range of cancer cell lines harbour a high frequency of
intragenic *PTEN* mutations and homozygous *PTEN* deletions (Li et al., 1997; Teng
et al., 1997), this does not hold for non-cultured neoplasias. While breast cancer
can occur in up to 50% of females affected by CS, somatic intragenic *PTEN*
mutations in non-cultured primary adenocarcinomas of the breast are very rare
(Rhei et al., 1997; Singh et al., 1998; Feilotter et al., 1999). In one study of 54
unselected primary breast carcinomas, only one true somatic mutation was noted
(Rhei et al., 1997). Even when selected for 10q23 hemizygous deletion, only 1 out
of 14 samples had a somatic intragenic mutation (Bose et al., 1998). However, the
10q region has not previously shown prominent loss of heterozygosity in breast
cancers. Yet, deletions in the region of *PTEN* occur in 30–40% of primary breast
carcinomas (Bose et al., 1998; Singh et al., 1998; Feilotter et al., 1999). In one
study, hemizygous deletion of *PTEN* and the 10q23 region occurred with any
frequency only in invasive carcinomas of the breast but not in *in situ* cancers, and
appeared to be associated with loss of oestrogen receptor (Bose et al., 1998). In
order to gather evidence of mechanisms of *PTEN* inactivation other than a genetic
mechanism, 33 well-characterized primary invasive breast adenocarcinomas without intragenic *PTEN* mutations (Feilotter et al., 1999) were examined for *PTEN*
deletion and *PTEN* expression by immunohistochemistry (Perren et al., 1999). Of
these cancers, 11 had hemizygous deletion of *PTEN*. Five of these 11 with
hemizygous deletion had complete *PTEN* silencing, while the remainder had
markedly decreased *PTEN* expression. These observations argue that the second
hit in breast cancers is epigenetic.

Thyroid cancers develop in up to 10% of individuals with CS. Yet, again,
somatic intragenic *PTEN* mutations are vanishingly rare in non-cultured primary
thyroid cancers. Three studies have demonstrated that hemizygous deletion of
PTEN occurs with a higher frequency in follicular adenomas (20–25%) compared
with follicular carcinomas (5–10%) (Dahia et al., 1997; Marsh et al., 1997b; Yeh et
al., 1999) although a fourth study did not make these findings (Halachmi et al.,
1998). The only intragenic point mutation was a somatic frameshift mutation in a
single papillary thyroid carcinoma (Dahia et al., 1997). This observation suggests
that the pathogenesis of adenomas and carcinomas may proceed along two
different pathways, and that the adenoma–carcinoma sequence is not the rule in
epithelial thyroid neoplasia (Yeh et al., 1999). The data were initially surprising in
view of the clinical phenotype evident in CS; one would expect a larger proportion
of sporadic thyroid carcinomas to be associated with somatic *PTEN* mutations.
However, a recent expression and genetic analysis of 139 benign and malignant
non-medullary thyroid tumours yielded some interesting data, which may begin
to address this apparent paradox (Gimm et al., 2000b). In this series, follicular

adenomas, follicular carcinomas and papillary thyroid carcinomas all had a 20–30% frequency of hemizygous deletion, while almost 60% of undifferentiated carcinomas had hemizygous *PTEN* deletion. Of note, hemizygous deletion and decreased *PTEN* expression were associated. Decreasing *PTEN* expression was observed with a declining degree of differentiation. Decreasing nuclear *PTEN* expression seemed to precede that in the cytoplasm. The thyroid data suggest that in addition to structural deletion, inappropriate subcellular compartmentalization might also contribute to *PTEN* inactivation. These observations are corroborated by the observations in endocrine pancreatic tumours where 10q loss is not associated with immunostaining intensity (Perren et al., 2000). Instead, 10q loss was associated with malignant status. More interestingly, *PTEN* expression was predominantly cytoplasmic in the endocrine pancreatic tumours, whereas expression was predominantly nuclear in normal islet cells (Perren et al., 2000).

To date, three early series have demonstrated somatic *PTEN* mutation in 34–50% of apparently sporadic endometrial carcinoma (Kong et al., 1997; Risinger et al., 1997; Tashiro et al., 1997). From these, it was noted that the frequency of intragenic mutation was much higher (86%) in those of endometrioid histology with microsatellite instability (Tashiro et al., 1997). Recently, however, 83% of endometrioid endometrial carcinomas were shown to have somatic intragenic mutations, and the frequency was equivalently high irrespective of microsatellite stability status (Mutter et al., 2000). Interestingly, only 33% had deletions or mutations involving both *PTEN* alleles, yet 61% expressed no protein (Mutter et al., 2000). In matched pre-cancers, 55% had intragenic mutation while 75% had no expression. Hence, *PTEN* mutation is an early event that initiates endometrial pre-cancers, and epigenetic *PTEN* silencing can precede genetic alteration in the earliest pre-cancers.

Many other types of sporadic cancers have also been examined. For example, sporadic glioblastoma multiforme carries a relatively high frequency of somatic *PTEN* mutations as well as 'second hit' intragenic mutations or deletions (Rasheed et al., 1997; Wang et al., 1997; Dürr et al., 1998; Maier et al., 1998). However, lower-grade gliomas were not found to be associated with *PTEN* mutations. It has now become obvious that *PTEN* may be inactivated by several different mechanisms, and not just somatic intragenic mutations. Several mechanisms of inactivation can occur in a single tumour type, although the sense is that one particular mechanism predominates in any one tissue type. For example, in the endometrial neoplasia system, either two genetic hits, or one genetic hit and one epigenetic silencing hit, can occur, although the latter predominates. In malignant melanoma, both inactivating hits for *PTEN* are epigenetic (Zhou et al., 2000a). In contrast, *PTEN* might also be inactivated by differential subcellular compartmentalization, as illustrated by thyroid neoplasia and endocrine pancreatic tumours.

This mechanism is somewhat puzzling, as *PTEN* has no obvious nuclear localization signal. The precise mechanisms of epigenetic inactivation have to be explored in further detail.

PTEN function

The phenotype of CS easily lent clues as to the function of PTEN. From the salient features alone, it was predicted that the susceptibility gene for CS would be important in normal development and would affect the cell cycle and/or apoptosis (Nelen et al., 1996). All of these predictions have been borne out, including *PTEN*'s role in normal human development (Di Cristofano et al., 1998; Suzuki et al., 1998; Podsypanina et al., 1999; Gimm et al., 2000a), cell cycle arrest (Furnari et al., 1997; Furnari et al., 1998; Li and Sun, 1998) and apoptosis (Li et al., 1998; Weng et al., 1999).

PTEN is the major 3-phosphatase for phosphoinositide-3,4,5-triphosphate (Maehama and Dixon, 1998; Myers et al., 1998; Stambolic et al., 1998) and signals down the Akt/PKB apoptotic pathway (Furnari et al., 1998; Li et al., 1998; Myers et al., 1998; Stambolic et al., 1998; Dahia et al., 1999). Accordingly, when *PTEN* was transiently ectopically expressed in PTEN-null breast cancer lines, only apoptosis occurred (Li et al., 1998). When *PTEN* was expressed in endogenously wild-type breast cancer lines, no differences were observed (Li et al., 1998). In contrast, when *PTEN* was transiently expressed in glioma lines, only G1 cell cycle arrest was observed (Furnari et al., 1997; Furnari et al., 1998; Li and Sun, 1998). However, when wild-type *PTEN* was stably expressed in endogenous wild-type *PTEN* breast cancer lines, a time-dependent G1 arrest followed by apoptosis was observed (Weng et al., 1999). Further, when wild-type *PTEN* was transiently expressed in a panel of non-medullary thyroid cancer lines, whether they underwent both apoptosis and G1 arrest, or G1 arrest alone, appeared to be cell type dependent (Weng et al., 2001b). The lines derived from well-differentiated papillary thyroid carcinomas underwent G1 arrest only. From the existing data, it is believed, probably somewhat naïvely, that apoptosis occurs through PTEN's lipid phosphatase activity via Akt because downstream of Akt lies BAD, Bcl, 14-3-3 sigma and FKRLH, which presumably could act as the transcription factor for the death factor FAS (Di Cristofano et al., 1999). However, there is now evidence that PTEN-mediated apoptosis can occur via Akt/PI3 kinase-dependent and independent pathways (Weng et al., 2001a). The full panoply of the mediators of PTEN-mediated G1 arrest is unknown but might include cyclin D1 and p27. Whether it is RB-dependent or -independent remains controversial.

Acknowledgements

I am grateful to the many patients and their families with CS, BRR and Proteus-like syndromes who have participated in our studies over the years. I would like to acknowledge the members of my laboratory – Jessica Brown, Patricia Dahia, Heather Dziema, Oliver Gimm, Jennifer Kum, Keisuke Kurose, Debbie Marsh, Margaret Ginn Pease, Aurel Perren, Wendy M. Smith, Liang-Ping Weng and Xiao-Ping Zhou – who, over the course of the last 5 years, have contributed to some of the work described in this chapter. No comprehensive human genetics studies would have been possible without the assistance of the many cancer genetic counsellors, especially Heather Hampel and Kathy Schneider, and numerous collaborators and clinicians, especially George Mutter and Monica Peacocke, with whom I have worked. Work in my laboratory is funded by the American Cancer Society, the US Army Breast Cancer Research Program, the Susan G. Komen Breast Cancer Research Foundation, the Mary Kay Ash Charitable Foundation and the National Institutes of Health.

Note added in proof

Two of five individuals with classic Proteus syndrome have been found to carry germline *PTEN* mutations (Zhou et al., 2001).

REFERENCES

Bannayan GA (1971). Lipomatosis, angiomatosis, and macrencephalia: a previously undescribed congenital syndrome. *Arch Pathol Lab Med* **92**: 1–5.

Biesecker LG, Happle R, Mulliken JB, et al. (1999). Proteus syndrome: diagnostic criteria, differential diagnosis and patient evaluation. *Am J Med Genet* **84**: 389–95.

Bose S, Wang SI, Terry MB, Hibshoosh H and Parsons R (1998). Allelic loss of chromosome 10q23 is associated with tumor progression in breast carcinomas. *Oncogene* **17**: 123–7.

Brownstein MH, Wolf M and Bilowski JB (1978). Cowden's disease. *Cancer* **41**: 2393–8.

Chen J, Lindblom P and Lindblom A (1998). A study of the *PTEN/MMAC1* gene in 136 breast cancer families. *Hum Genet* **102**: 124–5.

Dahia PLM, Marsh DJ, Zheng Z, et al. (1997). Somatic deletions and mutations in the Cowden disease gene, *PTEN*, in sporadic thyroid tumors. *Cancer Res* **57**: 4710–13.

Dahia PLM, Aguiar RCT, Alberta J, et al. (1999). PTEN is inversely correlated with the cell survival factor PKB/Akt and is inactivated by diverse mechanisms in haematologic malignancies. *Hum Mol Genet* **8**: 185–93.

De Vivo I, Gertig D, Nagase S, et al. (2000). Novel germline mutations in the *PTEN* tumour suppressor gene found in women with multiple cancers. *J Med Genet* **37**: 336–41.

Di Cristofano A, Pesce B, Cordon-Cardo C and Pandolfi PP (1998). *Pten* is essential for embryonic development and tumour suppression. *Nat Genet* **19**: 348–55.

Di Cristofano A, Kotsi P, Peng YF, Cordon-Cardo C, Elkon KB and Pandolfi PP (1999). Impaired Fas response and autoimmunity in *Pten* +/− mice. *Science* **285**: 2122–5.

Dürr E-M, Rollbrocker B, Hayashi Y, et al. (1998). *PTEN* mutations in gliomas and glioneuronal tumours. *Oncogene* **16**: 2259–64.

Eng C (1997). Cowden syndrome. *J Genet Counsel* **6**: 181–91.

Eng C (1998). Genetics of Cowden syndrome – through the looking glass of oncology. *Int J Oncol* **12**: 701–10.

Eng C (1999). *RET* proto-oncogene in the development of human cancer. *J Clin Oncol* **17**: 380–93.

Eng C (2000a). Multiple endocrine neoplasia type 2 and the practice of molecular medicine. *Rev Endocrinol Metab Dis* **1**: 283–90.

Eng C (2000b). Will the real Cowden syndrome please stand up: revised diagnostic criteria. *J Med Genet* **37**: 828–30.

Eng C and Blackstone MO (1988). Peutz–Jeghers syndrome. *Med Rounds* **1**: 165–71.

Eng C and Ji H (1998). Molecular classification of the inherited hamartoma polyposis syndromes: clearing the muddied waters. *Am J Hum Genet* **62**: 1020–2.

Eng C, Murday V, Seal S, et al. (1994). Cowden syndrome and Lhermitte–Duclos disease in a family: a single genetic syndrome with pleiotropy? *J Med Genet* **31**: 458–61.

Fackenthal J, Marsh DJ, Richardson AL, et al. (2001). Male breast cancer in Cowden syndrome patients with germline *PTEN* mutations. *J Med Genet* **38**: 159–64.

Feilotter HE, Coulon V, McVeigh JL, et al. (1999). Analysis of the 10q23 chromosomal region and the *PTEN* gene in human sporadic breast carcinoma. *Br J Cancer* **79**: 718–23.

FitzGerald MG, Marsh DJ, Wahrer D, et al. (1998). Germline mutations in *PTEN* are an infrequent cause of genetic predisposition to breast cancer. *Oncogene* **17**: 727–31.

Furnari FB, Lin H, Huang H-JS and Cavanee WK (1997). Growth suppression of glioma cells by PTEN requires a functional catalytic domain. *Proc Natl Acad Sci USA* **94**: 12 479–84.

Furnari FB, SuHuang H-J and Cavanee WK (1998). The phosphoinositol phosphatase activity of *PTEN* mediates a serum-sensitive G1 growth arrest in glioma cells. *Cancer Res* **58**: 5002–8.

Gimm O, Attié-Bitach T, Lees JA, Vekemens M and Eng C (2000a). Expression of *PTEN* in human embryonic development. *Hum Mol Genet* **9**: 1633–9.

Gimm O, Perren A, Weng LP, et al. (2000b). Differential nuclear and cytoplasmic expression of PTEN in normal thyroid tissue, and benign and malignant epithelial thyroid tumors. *Am J Pathol* **156**: 1693–1700.

Gorlin RJ (1984). Proteus syndrome. *J Dysmorphol* **2**: 8–9.

Gorlin RJ, Cohen MM, Condon LM and Burke BA (1992). Bannayan–Riley–Ruvalcaba syndrome. *Am J Med Genet* **44**: 307–14.

Halachmi N, Halachmi S, Evron E, Parsons R and Sidransky D (1998). Somatic mutations of the

PTEN tumor suppressor gene in sporadic follicular thyroid tumors. *Genes Chromosomes Cancer* **23**: 239–43.

Halal F and Silver K (1989). Slowly progressive macrocephaly with hamartomas: a new syndrome? *Am J Med Genet* **33**: 182–5.

Hanssen AMN and Fryns JP (1995). Cowden syndrome. *J Med Genet* **32**: 117–19.

Hemminki A, Tomlinson I, Markie D, et al. (1997). Localisation of a susceptibility locus for Peutz–Jeghers syndrome to 19p using comparative genomic hybridization and targeted linkage analysis. *Nature Genet* **15**: 87–90.

Hemminki A, Markie D, Tomlinson I, et al. (1998). A serine/threonine kinase gene defective in Peutz–Jeghers syndrome. *Nature* **391**: 184–7.

Higginbottom MC and Schultz P (1982). The Bannayan syndrome: an autosomal dominant disorder consisting of macrocephaly, lipomas and hemangiomas, and risk for intracranial tumours. *Pediatrics* **69**: 632–4.

Houlston R, Bevan S, Williams A, et al. (1998). Mutations in *DPC4* (*SMAD4*) cause juvenile polyposis syndrome, but only account for a minority of cases. *Hum Mol Genet* **7**: 1907–12.

Howe JR, Ringold JC, Summers RW, Mitros FA, Nishimura DY and Stone EM (1998a). A gene for familial juvenile polyposis maps to chromosome 18q21.1. *Am J Hum Genet* **62**: 1129–36.

Howe JR, Roth S, Ringold JC, et al. (1998b). Mutations in the *SMAD4/DPC4* gene in juvenile polyposis. *Science* **280**: 1086–8.

Jenne DE, Reimann H, Nezu J-I, et al. (1998). Peutz–Jeghers syndrome is caused by mutations in a novel serine threonine kinase. *Nat Genet* **18**: 38–44.

Johnson RL, Rothman AL, Xie J, et al. (1996). Human homolog of *patched*, a candidate gene for the basal cell nevus syndrome. *Science* **272**: 1668–71.

Kong D, Suzuki A, Zou T-T, et al. (1997). *PTEN1* is frequently mutated in primary endometrial carcinomas. *Nat Genet* **17**: 143–4.

Kurose K, Araki T, Matsunaka T, Takada Y and Emi M (1999). Variant manifestation of Cowden disease in Japan: hamartomatous polyposis of the digestive tract with mutation of the *PTEN* gene. *Am J Hum Genet* **64**: 308–10.

Li DM and Sun H (1998). PTEN/MMAC1/TEP1 suppresses the tumorigenicity and induces G1 cell cycle arrest in human glioblastoma cells. *Proc Natl Acad Sci USA* **95**: 15 406–11.

Li J, Yen C, Liaw D, et al. (1997). *PTEN*, a putative protein tyrosine phosphatase gene mutated in human brain, breast and prostate cancer. *Science* **275**: 1943–7.

Li J, Simpson L, Takahashi M, et al. (1998). The *PTEN/MMAC1* tumor suppressor induces cell death that is rescued by the AKT/protein kinase B oncogene. *Cancer Res* **58**: 5667–72.

Liaw D, Marsh DJ, Li J, et al. (1997). Germline mutations of the *PTEN* gene in Cowden disease, an inherited breast and thyroid cancer syndrome. *Nat Genet* **16**: 64–7.

Lloyd KM and Denis M (1963). Cowden's disease: a possible new symptom complex with multiple system involvement. *Ann Intern Med* **58**: 136–42.

Longy M and Lacombe D (1996). Cowden disease. Report of a family and review. *Ann Genet* **39**: 35–42.

Lynch ED, Ostermeyer EA, Lee MK, et al. (1997). Inherited mutations in *PTEN* that are associated with breast cancer, Cowden syndrome and juvenile polyposis. *Am J Hum Genet* **61**: 1254–60.

Maehama T and Dixon JE (1998). The tumor suppressor, PTEN/MMAC1, dephosphorylates the lipid second messenger phosphoinositol 3,4,5-triphosphate. *J Biol Chem* **273**: 13 375–8.

Maier D, Zhang ZW, Taylor E, et al. (1998). Somatic deletion mapping on chromosome 10 and sequence analysis of *PTEN/MMAC1* point to the 10q25–26 region as the primary target in low-grade and high-grade gliomas. *Oncogene* **16**: 3331–5.

Mallory SB (1995). Cowden syndrome (multiple hamartoma syndrome). *Dermatol Clin* **13**: 27–31.

Marsh DJ, Dahia PLM, Zheng Z, et al. (1997a). Germline mutations in *PTEN* are present in Bannayan–Zonana syndrome. *Nat Genet* **16**: 333–4.

Marsh DJ, Zheng Z, Zedenius J, et al. (1997b). Differential loss of heterozygosity in the region of the Cowden locus within 10q22–23 in follicular thyroid adenomas and carcinomas. *Cancer Res* **57**: 500–3.

Marsh DJ, Caron S, Dahia PLM, et al. (1998a). Germline *PTEN* mutations in Cowden syndrome-like families. *J Med Genet* **35**: 881–5.

Marsh DJ, Coulon V, Lunetta KL, et al. (1998b). Mutation spectrum and genotype–phenotype analyses in Cowden disease and Bannayan–Zonana syndrome, two hamartoma syndromes with germline *PTEN* mutation. *Hum Mol Genet* **7**: 507–15.

Marsh DJ, Kum JB, Lunetta KL, et al. (1999). *PTEN* mutation spectrum and genotype–phenotype correlations in Bannayan–Riley–Ruvalcaba syndrome suggest a single entity with Cowden syndrome. *Hum Mol Genet* **8**: 1461–72.

Mehenni H, Blouin JL, Radhakrishna U, et al. (1997). Peutz–Jeghers syndrome: confirmation of linkage to chromosome 19p13.3 and identification of a potential second locus on 19q13.4. *Am J Hum Genet* **61**: 1327–34.

Mutter GL, Lin M-C, Fitzgerald JT, et al. (2000). Altered PTEN expression as a diagnostic marker for the earliest endometrial precancers. *J Natl Cancer Inst* **92**: 924–31.

Myers MP, Pass I, Batty IH, et al. (1998). The lipid phosphatase activity of PTEN is critical for its tumor suppressor function. *Proc Natl Acad Sci USA* **95**: 13 513–18.

NCCN (1999). NCCN practice guidelines: genetics/familial high risk cancer. *Oncology* **13**(11A): 161–86.

Nelen MR, Padberg GW, Peeters EAJ, et al. (1996). Localization of the gene for Cowden disease to 10q22–23. *Nat Genet* **13**: 114–16.

Nelen MR, van Staveren CG, Peeters EAJ, et al. (1997). Germline mutations in the *PTEN/MMAC1* gene in patients with Cowden disease. *Hum Mol Genet* **6**: 1383–7.

Nelen MR, Kremer H, Konings IBM, et al. (1999). Novel *PTEN* mutations in patients with Cowden disease: absence of clear genotype–phenotype correlations. *Eur J Hum Genet* **7**: 267–73.

Olschwang S, Serova-Sinilnikova OM, Lenoir GM and Thomas G (1998). *PTEN* germline mutations in juvenile polyposis coli. *Nat Genet* **18**: 12–14.

Padberg GW, Schot JDL, Vielvoye GJ, Bots GTAM and de Beer FC (1991). Lhermitte–Duclos disease and Cowden syndrome: a single phakomatosis. *Ann Neurol* **29**: 517–23.

Perren A, Weng LP, Boag AH, et al. (1999). Immunohistochemical evidence of loss of PTEN expression in primary ductal adenocarcinomas of the breast. *Am J Pathol* **155**: 1253–60.

Perren A, Komminoth P, Saremaslani P, et al. (2000). Mutation and expression analyses reveal differential subcellular compartmentalization of PTEN in endocrine pancreatic tumors compared to normal islet cells. *Am J Pathol* **157**: 1097–103.

Podsypanina K, Ellenson LH, Nemes A, et al. (1999). Mutation of Pten/Mmac1 in mice causes neoplasia in multiple organ systems. *Proc Natl Acad Sci USA* **96**: 1563–8.

Rasheed BKA, Stenzel TT, McLendon RE, et al. (1997). *PTEN* gene mutations are seen in high-grade but not in low-grade gliomas. *Cancer Res* **37**: 4187–90.

Rhei E, Kang L, Bogomoliniy F, Federici MG, Borgen PI and Boyd J (1997). Mutation analysis of the putative tumor suppressor gene *PTEN/MMAC1* in primary breast carcinomas. *Cancer Res* **57**: 3657–9.

Risinger JI, Hayes AK, Berchuck A and Barrett JC (1997). *PTEN/MMAC1* mutations in endometrial cancers. *Cancer Res* **57**: 4736–8.

Rustgi AK (1994). Medical progress – hereditary gastrointestinal polyposis and nonpolyposis syndromes. *N Engl J Med* **331**: 1694–1702.

Shugart YY, Cour C, Renard H, et al. (1999). Linkage analysis of 56 multiplex families excludes the Cowden disease gene PTEN as a major contributor to familial breast cancer. *J Med Genet* **36**: 720–1.

Singh B, Ittman MM and Krolewski JJ (1998). Sporadic breast cancers exhibit loss of heterozygosity on chromosome segment 10q23 close to the Cowden disease locus. *Genes Chromosomes Cancer* **21**: 166–71.

Stambolic V, Suzuki A, de la Pompa JL, et al. (1998). Negative regulation of PKB/Akt-dependent cell survival by the tumor suppressor PTEN. *Cell* **95**: 1–20.

Starink TM, van der Veen JPW, Arwert F, et al. (1986). The Cowden syndrome: a clinical and genetic study in 21 patients. *Clin Genet* **29**: 222–33.

Suzuki A, de la Pompa JL, Stambolic V, et al. (1998). High cancer susceptibility and embryonic lethality associated with mutation of the *PTEN* tumor suppressor gene in mice. *Curr Biol* **8**: 1169–78.

Tashiro H, Blazes MS, Wu R, et al. (1997). Mutations in *PTEN* are frequent in endometrial carcinoma but rare in other common gynecological malignancies. *Cancer Res* **57**: 3935–40.

Teng DH-F, Hu R, Lin H, et al. (1997). *MMAC1/PTEN* mutations in primary tumor specimens and tumor cell lines. *Cancer Res* **57**: 5221–5.

Tsou HC, Teng D, Ping XL, et al. (1997). Role of *MMAC1* mutations in early onset breast cancer: causative in association with Cowden's syndrome and excluded in *BRCA1*-negative cases. *Am J Hum Genet* **61**: 1036–43.

Viskochil D, Buchberg AM, Xu G, et al. (1990). Deletions and translocation interrupt a cloned gene at the neurofibromatosis type 1 locus. *Cell* **62**: 187–92.

Wallace MR, Marchuk DA, Anderson LB, et al. (1990). Type 1 neurofibromatosis gene: identification of a large transcript disrupted in three NF 1 patients. *Science* **249**: 181–6.

Wang SI, Puc J, Li J, et al. (1997). Somatic mutations of *PTEN* in glioblastoma multiforme. *Cancer Res* **57**: 4183–6.

Ward K, O'Connell P, Carey J, et al. (1990). Diagnosis of neurofibromatosis 1 by using tightly linked, flanking DNA markers. *Am J Hum Genet* **46**: 943–9.

Weng LP, Smith WM, Dahia PLM, et al. (1999). PTEN suppresses breast cancer cell growth by phosphatase function-dependent G1 arrest followed by apoptosis. *Cancer Res* **59**: 5808–14.

Weng LP, Brown JL and Eng C (2001a). PTEN induces apoptosis and cell cycle arrest through phosphoinositol-3-kinase/Akt-dependent and independent pathways. *Hum Mol Genet* **10**: 237–42.

Weng LP, Gimm O, Kum JB, et al. (2001b). Transient ectopic expression of *PTEN* in thyroid cancer cell lines induces cell cycle arrest and cell type-dependent cell death. *Hum Mol Genet* **10**: 251–8.

Yeh JJ, Marsh DJ, Zedenius J, et al. (1999). Fine structure deletion analysis of 10q22–24 demonstrates novel regions of loss and suggests that sporadic follicular thyroid adenomas and follicular thyroid carcinomas develop along distinct parallel neoplastic pathways. *Gene Chromosomes Cancer* **26**: 322–8.

Zhou XP, Gimm O, Hampel H, Niemann T, Walker MJ and Eng C (2000a). Epigenetic PTEN silencing in malignant melanomas without *PTEN* mutation. *Am J Pathol* **157**: 1123–8.

Zhou XP, Marsh DJ, Hampel H, Mulliken JB, Gimm O and Eng C (2000b). Germline and germline mosaic mutations associated with a Proteus-like syndrome of hemihypertrophy, lower limb asymmetry, arterio-venous malformations and lipomatosis. *Hum Mol Genet* **9**: 765–8.

Zhou XP, Hampel H, Thiele H, et al. (2001). Association of germline mutation in the PTEN tumour suppressor gene and a subset of Proteus and Proteus-like syndromes. *Lancet* **358**: 210–11.

Zonana J, Rimoin DL and Davis DC (1976). Macrocephaly with multiple lipomas and hemangiomas. *J Pediatr* **89**: 600–3.

4

Overview of the clinical genetics of ovarian cancer

Pierre O. Chappuis[1] and William D. Foulkes[1,2,3]

[1]McGill University Health Centre, Montreal, QC, Canada
[2]Sir M. B. Davis-Jewish General Hospital, McGill University, Montreal, QC, Canada
[3]McGill University, Montreal, QC, Canada

Summary

Ovarian cancer is the fifth most common cause of cancer death in women in Western countries and family history of the disease is one of the strongest known risk factors. In most populations, 5–10% of all ovarian cancer cases are caused by the inheritance of cancer-predisposing genes with an autosomal dominant pattern of transmission. In the Ashkenazi Jewish population, this figure is very higher (20–30%). Hereditary ovarian cancer usually occurs in the context of hereditary breast cancer and is attributable to mutations in *BRCA1* or *BRCA2*. Rarely, it occurs in a site-specific form, again usually due to these two genes. Mutations in mismatch repair genes are also associated with an increased risk of ovarian cancer. The age of onset of hereditary ovarian cancer varies according to which gene carries the mutation. Thus far, the clinicopathological features of *BRCA1/2*-related ovarian cancer do not differ markedly from the non-hereditary form. Nevertheless, the identification of the genes responsible for most hereditary ovarian cancers has opened a new area of early detection methods and preventive procedures specifically dedicated to women identified as carrying ovarian cancer predisposing genes.

Introduction

Ovarian cancer is the fifth most common malignancy and the fifth leading cause of cancer deaths among North American and northern European women. More women will die of ovarian cancer than from cancer arising in all other female reproductive organs combined. Ovarian cancer is mostly a disease of peri-menopausal and postmenopausal women. Like breast cancer, there is a steady increase in ovarian cancer incidence with age, and ovarian cancer before the age of

40 years is rare. Besides age, the other risk factors associated with the disease are a family history of ovarian or breast cancer, infertility, nulliparity, early menarche and late menopause (Hildreth et al., 1981; Parazzini et al., 1991; Whittemore et al., 1992; Amos and Struewing, 1993; Godard et al., 1998). Other factors, including dietary intake of calcium, lactose, fibre, alcohol and coffee, have been associated less consistently with an increased risk of the disease (Mori et al., 1988; Whittemore et al., 1988; Cramer et al., 1989; Parazzini et al., 1992; Godard et al., 1998). High parity, oral contraceptive use, tubal ligation and hysterectomy have been associated with a reduction in risk (Casagrande et al., 1979; Hildreth et al., 1981; Cramer et al., 1983; Franceschi et al., 1991; Whittemore et al., 1992; Hankinson et al., 1993; Adami et al., 1994; Rosenberg et al., 1994; Kerber and Slattery, 1995; Purdie et al., 1995). After age, the factor most strongly associated with ovarian cancer risk is a family history of ovarian cancer (Whittemore et al., 1992; Amos and Struewing, 1993).

The increase in ovarian cancer cases in women with a family history of the disease has led to a search for inherited genetic causes of ovarian cancer. From epidemiological studies and mutation surveys, it is now estimated that between 5% and 13% of all epithelial ovarian cancers result from the inheritance of germline mutations in cancer-predisposing genes (Houlston et al., 1991; Narod et al., 1994a, 1995; Claus et al., 1996; Whittemore et al., 1997; Godard et al., 1998). This estimate varies substantially by ethnicity, being approximately 5% in non-Ashkenazi-Jewish populations and about 20% in Ashkenazim (Modan et al., 1996; Muto et al., 1996; Gotlieb et al., 1998; Moslehi et al., 2000). Among common adult malignancies, ovarian cancer was predicted to have the highest proportions attributable to susceptibility genes (Kerber and Slattery, 1995). Nevertheless, less than 5 in 10 000 women in the United States were estimated to be at increased risk of developing ovarian cancer owing to a strong genetic predisposition (Claus and Schwartz, 1995).

Risks of ovarian cancer and their assessment

Population risk

Approximately 140 000 new cases of ovarian cancer occur worldwide yearly (Parazzini et al., 1991). This number represents 4% of all female cancers, and the disease is more prevalent in developed countries. The highest age-adjusted incidence rates are observed in eastern and northern Europe, North America and among Jews born in America or Europe (range 7.0–15.1 per 100 000) (Parkin et al., 1997). The lowest age-adjusted incidence rates occur in northern and western Africa, and Asia, including Japan (range 0.7–6.7 per 100 000). Worldwide, one of the highest rates of ovarian cancer in the world occurs in Israeli Jews born in North

America or Europe (age standardized incidence rate, 13.5 per 100 000). There are clearly ethnic-specific variations in incidence. For example, the prevalence of mutations in the major breast/ovarian cancer susceptibility genes *BRCA1* and *BRCA2* is very high in the Ashkenazi Jewish population.

In the United States, it was estimated that in the year 2000, 23 100 women would develop ovarian cancer and 14 000 would die of the disease (Greenlee et al., 2000). The lifetime probability of developing ovarian cancer in the North American population is approximately 1.4%. Of note, even in the absence of a family history of ovarian cancer, this estimation is substantially influenced by the other risk factors. Based on pooled data from seven case-control studies and the SEER (US Surveillance, Epidemiology and End Results program) incidence data, the lifetime risk of developing ovarian cancer ranges from 0.6% for women with three or more term pregnancies and 4 or more years of oral contraceptive use to 3.4% among nulliparous women with no oral contraceptive use (Hartge et al., 1994).

Familial ovarian cancer

Familial aggregation of ovarian cancer has been variably defined as occurring when: (1) two first-degree relatives have ovarian cancer, or (2) the proband has ovarian cancer as well as one or more of her first- or second-degree relatives (Lynch and Lynch, 1992). Case-control studies designed to estimate the relative risk of developing ovarian cancer associated with a family history of the disease are summarized in Table 4.1. In a meta-analysis of case-control and cohort studies on family history and risk of ovarian cancer, the relative risk for all first-degree relatives was 3.1 (95% CI, 2.6–3.7), 1.1 (95% CI, 0.8–1.6) for mothers of cases, 3.8 (95% CI, 2.9–5.1) for sisters and 6.0 (95% CI, 3.0–11.9) for daughters, respectively (Stratton et al., 1998). In another study, the risk increased with the number of first-degree relatives affected (Kerber and Slattery, 1995).

Initial work suggested that women who have one first-degree relative affected by, or who died of, ovarian cancer were at greater risk of developing ovarian cancer, but not at an age earlier than the general population (Schildkraut and Thompson, 1988a; Schildkraut et al., 1989; Greggi et al., 1990; Amos et al., 1992; Easton et al., 1996). However, an inverse relationship between age at onset of the ovarian cancer and risk for close relatives has been reported in some studies (Houlston et al., 1993; Lynch et al., 1993; Hemminki et al., 1998; Vaittinen and Hemminki, 1999; Moslehi et al., 2000). Houlston et al. analysed 391 ovarian cancer pedigrees and found that the risk of developing ovarian cancer among the relatives of ovarian cancer case patients diagnosed before age 45 years, between 45 and 54 years, and after 55 years were 14.2, 5.2 and 3.7, respectively (Houlston et al., 1993). In a Swedish population-based study, the familial hazard ratio of ovarian cancer in daughters, adjusted for age and decade of birth, was 4.2 (95% CI,

Table 4.1. Relative risk of developing ovarian cancer associated with a family history of the disease

Relatives studied	Country	Age (years)	No. of cases studied	No. of controls	Relative risk of developing OC (95% CI)	Reference
Any	USA	All	150	300	'No positive association'	Wynder et al., 1969
First- and second-degree	USA	<50	150	150	15.7 (0.9–278)	Casagrande et al., 1979
First-degree	USA	45–74	62	1068	18.2 (4.8–69)	Hildreth et al., 1981
First-degree	USA	18–80	215	215	11.3 (0.6–211)	Cramer et al., 1983
First-degree	Greece	All	146	243	∞ (3.4–∞)	Tzonou et al., 1984
First-degree	Japan	N/A	110	220	∞ (0.1–∞)	Mori et al., 1988
First-degree	USA	20–54	493	2465	3.6 (1.8–7.1)	Schildkraut and Thompson, 1988a
Second-degree					2.9 (1.6–5.3)	
First-degree	USA	20–79	296	343	3.3 (1.1–9.4)	Hartge et al., 1989
First-degree and aunts	Canada	All	197	210	2.5 (0.7–11.1)	Koch et al., 1989
First-degree	Italy	25–74	755	2023	1.9 (1.1–3.6)	Parazzini et al., 1992
First-degree	USA	N/A	883	Population incidence rate	2.1 (1.0–3.4)	Goldgar et al., 1994
First-degree	USA	<65	441	2065	8.2 (3.0–23)	Rosenberg et al., 1994
First-degree	USA	All	662	2647	4.3 (2.4–7.9)	Kerber and Slattery, 1995
Second-degree					2.1 (1.2–3.8)	
Third-degree					1.5 (1.0–2.2)	
First-degree	Australia	18–79	824	860	3.9 (1.6–9.7)	Purdie et al., 1995
First-degree	Finland	<76	559	Population incidence rate	2.8 (1.8–4.2)	Auranen et al., 1996a
First-degree	UK	<60	1188	Population incidence rate	SMR = 223 (155–310)	Easton et al., 1996

Relationship	Country	Age	Cases	Comparison	RR (95% CI)	Reference
Any	Canada	20–84	170	170	1.9 (0.8–4.4)	Godard et al., 1998
Daughters (≤53 years)	Sweden	—	N/A	Population incidence rate	2.7 (1.9–3.7)	Hemminki et al., 1998
First-degree	USA Israel	All	213	386	3.2 (1.5–6.8)	Moslehi et al., 2000
First-degree	UK		≥2 OC cases in 316 families	Population incidence rate	7.2 (3.8–12.3)	Sutcliffe et al., 2000

Three studies (Auranen et al., 1996a; Easton et al., 1996; Sutcliffe et al., 2000) have a population-based cohort design; the others are case-control studies.

CI, confidence intervals; N/A, not available; OC, ovarian cancer; SMR, standardized mortality ratio.

2.2–8.2) when mothers with ovarian cancer were younger than 50 years at diagnosis, compared with 2.3 (95% CI, 1.6–3.4) when mothers were diagnosed at or after 50 years (Hemminki et al., 1998). A higher risk of early-onset ovarian cancer is also recognized in the small proportion of women who have several affected relatives (Amos et al., 1992).

Besides ovarian cancer, case-control studies have also shown that relatives of women with ovarian cancer have a significantly increased risk of developing breast cancers (Mori et al., 1988; Schildkraut et al., 1989; Parazzini et al., 1992; Jishi et al., 1995; Moslehi et al., 2000), colon cancers (Cramer et al., 1983; Godard et al., 1998), pancreatic cancers (Goldgar et al., 1994; Kerber and Slattery 1995; Moslehi et al., 2000), prostate cancers (Cramer et al., 1983; Jishi et al., 1995; Moslehi et al., 2000), uterine cancers (Jishi et al., 1995) and leukaemia (Godard et al., 1998). The significantly elevated risk for breast and ovarian cancer noted among relatives of ovarian cancer patients is usually greater for ovarian cancer than for breast cancer (Schildkraut et al., 1989; Vaittinen and Hemminki, 1999). Interestingly, an increased risk of ovarian cancers in the family members of women with borderline ovarian cancers was not reported (Schildkraut and Thompson, 1988a; Auranen et al., 1996b). Nevertheless, one study did not show a difference in ovarian cancer risk among first-degree relatives of 254 patients with invasive ovarian cancer and 61 patients with borderline ovarian tumours (Rader et al., 1998). The inverse relationship has also been reported, i.e. an increased risk of developing ovarian cancer that has been associated with family histories of breast, uterine, colon and pancreatic cancers (Prior and Waterhouse, 1981; Schildkraut and Thompson, 1988b; Parazzini et al., 1992; Tulinius et al., 1994; Kerber and Slattery, 1995; Olsen et al., 1999).

Several investigators have evaluated the risks associated with more than one affected relative and showed a substantially increased risk for the relatives, but with wide confidence intervals (Schildkraut and Thompson, 1988a; Amos et al., 1992; Easton et al., 1996). A combined analysis of these data estimated the relative risk of developing ovarian cancer to be 11.7 (95% CI, 5.3–25.9) for these women (Stratton et al., 1998). Ovarian and breast cancer relative risks were estimated from the UKCCCR (UK Coordinating Committee for Cancer Research) Familial Ovarian Cancer Study Group prospective cohort of 316 families with two or more confirmed cases of epithelial ovarian cancer in first-degree relatives. In contrast to the prediction of a model based on related data (Antoniou et al., 2000), when the analyses were restricted to families that were not carrying a BRCA1/2 germline mutation, the ovarian cancer risk was 11.6 (95% CI, 3.1–29.7) – similar to the risk estimated for the BRCA1/2-related ovarian cancer families (11.9, 95% CI, 3.8–27.7) (Sutcliffe et al., 2000). It is important to recognize that there is a possibility that at least some of these 'BRCA1/BRCA2-negative' families do indeed carry mutations in *BRCA1/BRCA2* that were not detected by the screening methods used.

Inherited genetic syndromes and ovarian cancer

Some characteristics of the autosomal dominantly inherited syndromes associated with an increased risk of developing ovarian cancer are summarized in Table 4.2. In a population-based series of 450 unselected epithelial ovarian cancers studied in southern Ontario, Canada, Narod et al. estimated the proportion of hereditary ovarian cancer in the Ontario population to be 2.9–6.9% of cases of ovarian cancer (Narod et al., 1994a). From other population-based studies, the fraction of hereditary ovarian cancer cases has been estimated as between 5% and 13% (Houlston et al., 1991; Claus et al., 1996; Auranen and Iselius, 1998). The key feature of hereditary ovarian cancer is the vertical transmission of cancer susceptibility consistent with an autosomal dominantly inherited factor (Lynch and Lynch, 1992).

Hereditary breast/ovarian cancer

The association between breast and ovarian cancer is well known. Over the last 50 years (Liber, 1950), there have been numerous reports of familial aggregation of ovarian cancer. In most cases, breast cancer was also present in these pedigrees. Segregation analysis performed on breast/ovarian cancer families identified by Lynch et al. led them to conclude that the clustering of breast and ovarian cancer could result from the inheritance of a single dominant gene (Go et al., 1983). In 1990, evidence was found for linkage of 15 early-onset breast cancer pedigrees to a single locus on the chromosome 17q21 (Hall et al., 1990). It was subsequently confirmed in a series of five breast/ovarian cancer families, where three were linked to the same locus (Narod et al., 1991). After intensive search, the *BRCA1* gene was finally identified in 1994 (Miki et al., 1994). In the same year, a second breast/ovarian cancer susceptibility locus was located on chromosome 13q (Wooster et al., 1994). The *BRCA2* gene was characterized in 1995 (Wooster et al., 1995). Most early-onset breast/ovarian cancer families are linked to *BRCA1* (Easton et al., 1993; Narod et al., 1995; Ford et al., 1998; Frank et al., 1998). In fact, the presence of ovarian cancer is strongly predictive of *BRCA1* germline mutation, even in small breast/ovarian cancer families (Tonin et al., 1996; Ligtenberg et al., 1999).

The frequency of *BRCA1/2* mutations in the general population is estimated to be about 1 in 800 for *BRCA1* and somewhat less for *BRCA2*, but it can vary significantly among some ethnic groups or geographical regions. Thus, the prevalence of the three *BRCA1/2* founder mutations among the Ashkenazim is approximately 1 in 50 (Struewing et al., 1995a; Oddoux et al., 1996; Roa et al., 1996). The

Table 4.2. Ovarian cancer as a feature of hereditary genetic syndromes

Syndrome	Gene (chromosome)	Percentage of hereditary ovarian cancer	Risk of ovarian cancer by age 70 years (%)	Type of ovarian cancer	Other clinical features
Hereditary breast/ovarian cancer	BRCA1 (17q)	65	20–50	Epithelial (serous)	Breast, fallopian tube cancer
	BRCA2 (13q)	10	10–30	Epithelial (serous)	Breast, prostate, pancreas, head and neck cancer
Site-specific ovarian cancer	BRCA1 (17q)	10–15	20–50	Epithelial (serous)	—
Hereditary non-polyposis colorectal cancer	MLH1 (3p) MSH2 (2p) MSH6 (2p) PMS1 (2q) PMS2 (7p)	5–10	≤10	Epithelial	Colorectal, endometrial, stomach, urinary tract and small bowel cancer
Peutz–Jeghers syndrome	STK11 (19p)	<1	<5[a]	Sex cord-stromal tumour with annular tubules	Mucocutaneous melanin spots; GI hamartomatous polyps; adenoma malignum of uterine cervix; breast, GI and pancreas cancer
Cowden disease	PTEN (10q)	<1	<5[a]	N/S	Multiple hamartomas; neurological signs; breast and thyroid cancer
Nevoid basal cell carcinoma (Gorlin's) syndrome	PTCH (9q)	<1	<5[a]	Fibrosarcoma, carcinoma	Basal cell naevi/carcinoma; palmoplantar pits; skeletal abnormalities; odontogenic keratocysts; medulloblastoma
Multiple enchondromatosis (Ollier's disease)	?	≪1	<5[a]	Juvenile granulosa cell tumour	Osteochondromatosis; haemangiomata
Epidermolytic palmoplantar keratoderma	KRT9 (17q)	≪1	<5[a]	N/S	Epidermolytic hyperkeratosis

GI, gastrointestinal; N/S, not specified.

[a] No prospective data in the literature.

Icelandic population carries the founder *BRCA2* 999del5 mutation at a frequency of 0.4% (Johannesdottir et al., 1996). The frequency of *BRCA1* and *BRCA2* mutations in unselected series of women with ovarian carcinoma has been extensively studied, particularly in so-called 'founder populations'. A founder effect can occur when a relatively small group is genetically isolated from the rest of the population, because of geographical conditions or religious belief. If an individual in that isolated population carries a rare genetic alteration, the frequency of this allele in the next generations could increase in the absence of selection. Specific *BRCA1/2* mutations have been identified in diverse populations, such as in Ashkenazi Jewish, Icelandic, Swedish, Norwegian, Austrian, Dutch, British, Belgian, Russian, Hungarian and French-Canadian families (Gayther et al., 1995; Shattuck-Eidens et al., 1995; Andersen et al., 1996; Johannesdottir et al., 1996; Johannsson et al., 1996; Wagner et al., 1996; Dorum et al., 1997; Gayther et al., 1997a; Peelen et al., 1997; Ramus et al., 1997; Shattuck-Eidens et al., 1997; Tonin et al., 1998). The knowledge of well-characterized founder mutations in individuals of particular ethnic origins can simplify genetic counselling and testing, as the initial mutation screening can be limited to specific panels of mutations.

Three founder mutations (185delAG and 5382insC in *BRCA1*; 6174delT in *BRCA2*) have been identified in the Ashkenazi Jewish families of Eastern European ancestry (Friedman et al., 1995; Berman et al., 1996; Neuhausen et al., 1996; Tonin et al., 1996). These mutations are carried by about 2.5% of the Ashkenazi Jewish population (Struewing et al., 1995a; Oddoux et al., 1996; Roa et al., 1996). These founder mutations are particularly common in Ashkenazi Jewish women with ovarian cancer, even without a family history of breast/ovarian cancer. Table 4.3 summarizes the published literature on the prevalence of these mutations in non-Ashenazi-Jewish women, whereas Table 4.4 includes studies carried out in Ashkenazim only. From Table 4.3 it can be seen that germline mutations in *BRCA1* and *BRCA2* contribute to only a minority of cases of unselected ovarian carcinoma. Additionally, among otherwise unselected very early onset cases, mutations have not been observed (Stratton et al., 1999a). These results show that among women with ovarian cancer, *BRCA1* and *BRCA2* mutations are at least three times more likely to be found in Ashkenazi Jewish women than in non-Ashkenazi women.

A different way of looking at the contribution of *BRCA1/2* mutations to ovarian cancer incidence is to estimate the risk of ovarian cancer in known gene carriers. These data are summarized in Table 4.5. In summary, the point estimate for risk of ovarian cancer conferred by mutations in *BRCA1* varies between 12% and 68% up to the age of 70 years, and the confidence intervals for all studies are wide. In addition, virtually all studies show that the incidence of ovarian cancer increases

Table 4.3. Prevalence of *BRCA1* and *BRCA2* germline mutation in ovarian cancer: population- or hospital-based studies

Population studied	BRCA1/2 screening	Results (%, 95% CI)	Reference
76 OC Japan	*BRCA1*: SSCA	4/76 (5%, 1.5–13)	Matsushima et al., 1995
115 OC USA	*BRCA1*: SSCA	7/115 (6%, 2.5–12)	Takahashi et al., 1995
50 OC Australia, UK, USA	*BRCA2*: HA, PTT	2/50 (4%, 0.5–14)	Foster et al., 1996
38 OC Iceland	*BRCA2*: 999del5	3/38 (8%, 1.7–21)	Johannesdottir et al., 1996
55 OC UK, USA	*BRCA2*: SSCA, PTT	0/55	Lancaster et al., 1996
130 OC USA	*BRCA2*: SSCA	4/130 (3%, 0.8–7)	Takahashi et al., 1996
374 OC <70 years UK	*BRCA1*: HA	13/374 (3.5%, 2–6)	Stratton et al., 1997
103 OC USA	*BRCA1*: sequencing	4/103 (4%, 1–10)	Berchuck et al., 1998
116 OC USA	*BRCA1*: SSCA *BRCA2*: SSCA	10/116 (9%, 4–15) 1/116 (0.9%, 0–5)	Rubin et al., 1998
25 OC families The Netherlands	*BRCA1*: PTT + 185delAG *BRCA2*: PTT	9/25 (36%, 18–57) 1/25 (4%, 0.1–20)	Zweemer et al., 1998
615 OC Sweden	*BRCA1*: 1675delA *BRCA1*: 1135insA	13/615 (2%, 1–4) 5/615 (0.8%, 0.3–2)	Dorum et al., 1999
107 OC USA	*BRCA1*: CA	2/107 (2%, 0.2–7)	Janezic et al., 1999
101 OC <30 years UK	*BRCA1*: HA *BRCA2*: PTT	0/101 0/101	Stratton et al., 1999a
113 OC French Canadians	7 French Canadian founder mutations[a]	8/113 (7%, 3–13)	Tonin et al., 1999
116 OC Japan	*BRCA1*: YSCA	7/116 (6%, 2.5–12)	Yamashita et al., 1999
90 OC Hungary	*BRCA1*: 185delAG, 300T → G, 5382insC *BRCA2*: 617delT, 9326insA	10/90 (11%, 6–19) 0/90	Van der Looij et al., 2000

[a]French Canadian founder mutations: *BRCA1* – C4446T, 2953del3 + C, 3768insA; *BRCA2* – 2816insA, G6085T, 6503delTT, 8765delAG.

CA, cleavage assay; CI, confidence intervals; HA, heteroduplex assay; SSCA, single-strand conformation assay; OC, ovarian cancers; PTT, protein truncation test; YSCA, yeast stop codon assay.

Table 4.4. Prevalence of *BRCA1/2* germline mutation in ovarian cancer: studies among Ashkenazi Jewish (AJ) patients

Population studied	*BRCA1/2* screening	Results (%, 95% CI)	Reference
79 OC Israel	*BRCA1*: 185delAG	15/79 (19%, 11–29)	Modan et al., 1996
31 OC USA	*BRCA1*: 185delAG	6/31 (19%, 7–37)	Muto et al., 1996
21 OC Israel	AJ panel[a]	185delAG: 7/21 (33%, 15–57) 5382insC: 0/21 6174delT: 6/21 (29%, 11–52)	Abeliovich et al., 1997
29 OC Israel	AJ panel[a]	185delAG: 8/29 (28%, 13–47) 5382insC: 4/29 (14%, 4–32) 6174delT: 5/29 (17%, 6–36)	Beller et al., 1997
22 OC Israel	AJ panel[a]	185delAG: 5/22 (23%, 8–45) 5382insC: 2/22 (9%, 1–29) 6174delT: 3/22 (14%, 3–35)	Levy-Lahad et al., 1997
59 OC Israel	*BRCA1*: 185delAG *BRCA2*: 6174delT	17/59 (29%, 18–42) 2/59 (3%, 0.4–12)	Gotlieb et al., 1998
15 OC UK	AJ panel[a] +*BRCA1*: 188del11	185delAG: 1/15(7%, 0.2–32) 5382insC: 1/15 (7%, 0.2–32) 6174delT: 1/15 (7%, 0.2–32) *BRCA1*: 188del11: 0/15	Hodgson et al., 1999
32 OC USA	AJ panel[a]	185delAG: 8/32 (25%, 11–43) 5382insC: 0/32 6174delT: 6/32 (19%, 7–36)	Lu et al., 1999
208 OC North America, Israel	AJ panel[a] + PTT	185delAG: 43/208 (21%, 15–27) 5382insC: 14/208 (7%, 4–11) 6174delT: 29/208 (14%, 9–19)	Moslehi et al., 2000

[a]AJ panel: *BRCA1* – 185delAG, 5382insC; *BRCA2* – 6174delT.

strikingly only after the age of 40 years (Ford et al., 1994). Compared with *BRCA1*, mutations in *BRCA2* may confer a lower risk of ovarian cancer (11%–27%).

Hereditary site-specific ovarian cancer syndrome

A woman with two affected first-degree relatives has a risk of developing ovarian cancer that is substantially higher than having one affected first-degree relative (Schildkraut and Thompson, 1988a; Amos et al., 1992; Easton et al., 1996; Stratton et al., 1998; Sutcliffe et al., 2000). Thus, the occurrence of ovarian cancer in a

Table 4.5. *BRCA1/2* mutation and ovarian cancer penetrance

Population studied	*BRCA1/2* screening	Penetrance by age 70–75 years (%) (95% CI)	Reference
33 early-onset BC (<60 years) and OC families	*BRCA1* linkage	*BRCA1*: 44% (28–56)	Ford et al., 1994
33 early-onset BC (<60 years) and OC families	*BRCA1* linkage	*BRCA1*: 63%	Easton et al., 1995
237 early-onset BOC families	Linkage or sequencing	*BRCA1*: 42% *BRCA2*: 27% (0–47)	Narod et al., 1995 Ford et al., 1998
14 AJ BOC families	Risk estimate for mutation carrier relatives	*BRCA1* 185delAG: 41% *BRCA1* 5382insC: 0% *BRCA2* 6174delT: 30%	Abeliovich et al., 1997
2 BOC families	*BRCA2* linkage	*BRCA2*: 10% (at age 60 years)	Easton et al., 1997
25 AJ BOC families	3 AJ founder mutations[a]	*BRCA1* (185delAG and 5382insC): 57% *BRCA2* 6174delT: 49%	Levy-Lahad et al., 1997
5318 AJ patients (population-based)	3 AJ founder mutations[a]	*BRCA1/2*: 16% (6–28)	Struewing et al., 1997
922 incident OC (population-based)	Segregation analysis	*BRCA1*: 22% (5–60)	Whittemore et al., 1997
412 AJ BC patients	3 AJ founder mutations[a]	*BRCA1/2*: 12%	Warner et al., 1999
(a) 112 families with ≥ two relatives with OC, +/– BC (<60 years)	PTT, SSCA, sequencing	*BRCA1*: 53% *BRCA2*: 31%	Antoniou et al., 2000
(b) 374 OC (<70 years)		*BRCA1/2*: 68% (36–94)	
191 AJ OC patients (<75 years)	3 AJ founder mutations[a]	*BRCA1* 185delAG: 37% *BRCA1* 5382insC: 21% *BRCA2* 6174delT: 14%	Moslehi et al., 2000
Relatives of 861 AJ BC patients	3 AJ founder mutations[a]	*BRCA1* (185delAG and 5382insC): 55% (47–62) *BRCA2* 6174delT: 28% (14–41)	The New York Breast Cancer Study[b]

[a] AJ founder mutations: *BRCA1* – 185delAG, 5382insC; *BRCA2* – 6174delT.

[b] Oral communication by M-C King at the American Society of Human Genetics meeting, Philadelphia, October 3–7, 2000.

AJ, Ashkenazi Jewish; BC, breast cancer; BOC, breast/ovarian cancer; OC, ovarian cancer; PTT, protein truncation test; SSCA, single-strand conformation analysis; RR, relative risk.

family with two or more first-degree relatives is likely to be explained by the inheritance of a mutated gene (Easton et al., 1996; Richards et al., 1999). A family with three or more cases of invasive epithelial ovarian cancer at any age and no case of breast cancer diagnosed before age 50 years qualifies as a site-specific ovarian cancer family (Lynch and Lynch, 1992; Steichen-Gersdorf et al., 1994). Nearly all site-specific hereditary ovarian cancer is a result of *BRCA1*, or less frequently *BRCA2*, mutations (Steichen-Gersdorf et al., 1994; Shattuck-Eidens et al., 1995; Liede et al., 1998; Roth et al., 1998; Gayther et al., 1999; Santarosa et al., 1999; Antoniou et al., 2000). Gayther et al. studied 112 families, identified through the Familial Ovarian Cancer Register of the UKCCCR, that were characterized by the presence of at least two first- or second-degree relatives with epithelial ovarian cancer (Gayther et al., 1999). *BRCA1* germline mutations were identified in 40 (36%) families and eight (7%) *BRCA2* mutations were identified. Antoniou et al. modelled ovarian cancer using the same set of families (Antoniou et al., 2000). When a third high-risk ovarian cancer susceptibility gene was allowed for in the genetic models, none of the models fitted gave significant evidence of a third gene. The authors concluded that the majority of familial ovarian cancer may be explained by mutations in *BRCA1/2*, and families without mutations can be explained by insensitivity of mutation testing and chance clustering of sporadic cases. Nevertheless, the existence of other rare or low-risk susceptibility alleles cannot be excluded at this time.

In summary, hereditary site-specific ovarian cancer syndrome should be considered as a variant of the hereditary breast/ovarian cancer syndrome, in which early-onset breast cancer has not yet appeared (Steichen-Gersdorf et al., 1994). Thus, it is currently prudent to counsel women who belong to families with three or more cases of ovarian cancer that they are at increased risk of developing breast cancer (Liede et al., 1998).

Hereditary non-polyposis colorectal cancer syndrome

The hereditary non-polyposis colorectal cancer (HNPCC) is one of the most common autosomal conditions predisposing to cancer, accounting for 5–8% of all colorectal cancers. The genetic susceptibility to the disease is transmitted in a dominant fashion, generally with high penetrance. The diagnosis of HNPCC relies on the observation of familial clustering of colorectal cancers, meeting a set of obligate criteria referred to as the 'Amsterdam criteria', defined in 1991 (Vasen et al., 1991). In fact, this syndrome is associated with an increased risk of developing cancers in several other sites. Colorectal cancers represent about two-thirds of the malignancies in HNPCC families, whereas up to 40% of the malignancies are extracolonic cancers of epithelial origin. The second most frequently affected organ is the endometrium; thereafter, a higher frequency of other target organs has been reported, including the stomach, small intestine, upper renal tract and ovary. It should be noted that mutations in *MLH1* and *MSH2* are rare in ovarian cancers not selected on the basis of family history of cancer (Rubin et al., 1998). Ovarian cancer in the context of HNPCC is discussed in detail in Chapter 5.

Other syndromes

Very few cases of ovarian cancer have been reported in association with other inherited genetic syndromes (Table 4.2). Only two case reports have found clear germline *TP53* mutations in women with ovarian cancer in a strongly familial setting (Børresen, 1992; Jolly et al., 1994) and ovarian cancer is not considered to be a feature of the Li–Fraumeni syndrome (Buller et al., 1995; Kleihues et al., 1997; Birch et al., 1998). Familial aggregation of ovarian germ-cell cancer has been reported (Stettner et al., 1999), but must be very rare.

Risk prediction models

Detailed pedigree drawing is an essential step in cancer risk evaluation. Relying on family history information to identify cases of ovarian cancer in relatives is permissible (Koch et al., 1989; Douglas et al., 1999). Nevertheless, it is important to get pathological reports or death certificates to confirm the family history whenever possible, particularly to adequately evaluate cancer risks and discuss the option of genetic testing.

Risk estimation models have been developed for breast cancer. These have been designed to estimate the risk during a given period of follow-up time of developing the disease, based on the family history (number of breast cancer cases, age of diagnosis) (Ottman et al., 1983; Anderson and Badzioch, 1985; Claus et al., 1994) or additional variables (current age, age of menarche, age at first childbirth, number of breast biopsies) (Gail et al., 1989). However, these statistical models, based on large population-based epidemiological studies, do not integrate ovarian cancer diagnosed in relatives and are not appropriate for use in families that manifest an autosomal dominant pattern of breast cancer cases (Weitzel, 1999). Tables that do allow one to estimate the probability that an individual or a family carries a *BRCA1/2* mutation have been derived from analyses of genotype–phenotype correlation among individuals identified as *BRCA1/2* carriers (Couch et al., 1997; Frank et al., 1998). Key clinical factors are age of onset of breast and ovarian cancer. The recent BRCAPRO computer program uses a Bayesian calculation to estimate the probability that either a *BRCA1* or a *BRCA2* mutation is present in a family based on first- and second-degree family history of breast and ovarian cancer (Parmigiani et al., 1998). Variables include the prevalence of mutations and age-specific penetrance estimate. BRCAPRO tends to underestimate the likelihood of a *BRCA1/2* mutation when only ovarian cancer is present in the pedigree, particularly if the cases do not occur at a young age. Risk prediction models are discussed in more detail in Chapter 8.

Clinical, pathological and outcome characteristics of *BRCA*-related ovarian cancer

Clinicopathological characteristics of ovarian tumour have been evaluated in familial aggregation of ovarian cancers or among patients with *BRCA1/2* germline mutation (hereditary ovarian cancer). Few data are available for ovarian cancer associated with other inherited genetic syndromes and will not be discussed further here. This whole topic is discussed in detail in Chapter 7.

Age of onset

Early age of onset is often considered to be a hallmark of most of the hereditary cancers. As discussed above, in some studies the average age of onset for familial or hereditary ovarian cancer was significantly lower (about 5 years) than that of ovarian cancer in the general population (Bewtra et al., 1992; Lynch et al., 1993; Piver et al., 1993a; Muto et al., 1996; Rubin et al., 1996; Zweemer et al., 1998; Boyd et al., 2000). This significant difference in age of onset has not been found consistently (Narod et al., 1994a; Chang et al., 1995; Auranen et al., 1997; Stratton et al., 1997; Johannsson et al., 1998; Gayther et al., 1999; Yamashita et al., 1999). Interestingly, among *BRCA1/2*-related ovarian cancer, some evidence suggests an earlier age of onset restricted to women carrying the *BRCA1* mutations, but an older or a similar age of onset for women with *BRCA2* mutations (Takahashi et al., 1996; Levy-Lahad et al., 1997; Tonin et al., 1999; Boyd et al., 2000; Moslehi et al., 2000).

Histopathological type

Papillary serous adenocarcinoma is the predominant histological type and a lower proportion of mucinous and borderline tumours were found among familial/hereditary ovarian cancer cases when compared with sporadic cases (Greggi et al., 1990; Bewtra et al., 1992; Piver et al., 1993a; Narod et al., 1994a, 1994b; Chang et al., 1995; Matsushima et al., 1995; Takahashi et al., 1995; Rubin et al., 1996; Stratton et al., 1997; Takano et al., 1997; Aida et al., 1998; Berchuck et al., 1998; Pharoah et al., 1999; Sagawa et al., 1999; Tonin et al., 1999). In a study from the Gilda Radner Familial Ovarian Cancer Registry, the most important difference between familial and sporadic ovarian cancer was that mucinous adenocarcinomas were rarely seen in familial cases (1.4% versus 12.7% in unselected ovarian cancers from the SEER database) (Piver et al., 1993a). In a hospital-based series, 83% of patients with familial ovarian cancer and only 49% of matched controls had a serous cystadenocarcinoma ($P=0.0025$) (Chang et al., 1995). However, the difference in histological subtype distribution between familial/ hereditary ovarian cancers and the sporadic cases has not always been observed (Auranen et al., 1997; Johannsson et al., 1997; Boyd et al., 2000). For example, in a large retrospective cohort study of Ashkenazi Jewish women with invasive epithelial ovarian cancer, no differences were noted regarding histological type, grade and stage between hereditary and sporadic cases (Boyd et al., 2000). However, no well-differentiated tumours were observed in the *BRCA1/2* group and no mucinous subtypes were described. Based on various epidemiological and mutation-based studies, it appears that the cancer risk to relatives of cases of mucinous or borderline ovarian tumours is less than for other forms (Schildkraut and Thompson, 1988a; Piver et al., 1993a; Narod et al., 1994a; Gotlieb et al., 1998; Lu et al., 1999). In one study, rare granulosa cell tumours were associated with the highest familial risks of any histological subtype (Kerber and Slattery, 1995). This finding must be treated with caution, as granulosa cell tumours have only been associated with the rare, hereditary Peutz–Jeghers syndrome. Familial occurrence of small-cell ovarian carcinoma has been anecdotally reported (Lamovec et al., 1995; Longy et al., 1996).

Grade and stage

No difference in grade was found between site-specific familial ovarian cancer or *BRCA1/2*-associated ovarian cancer and sporadic ovarian tumours (Buller et al., 1993; Rubin et al., 1996; Pharoah et al., 1999; Boyd et al., 2000; Moslehi et al., 2000). Four studies showed significantly more FIGO (Fédération Internationale de Gynécologie et d'Obstétrique) stages III and IV for familial/hereditary ovarian cases, when compared with a national cancer registry or population controls (Zweemer et al., 1998; Pharoah et al., 1999; Sagawa et al., 1999; Yamashita et al., 1999).

Genotype–phenotype associations

Mutations in the 3' portion of the *BRCA1* gene (exons 13–24) were initially associated with a higher frequency of breast cancer relative to ovarian cancer in a series of 32 European families (Gayther et al., 1995). This observation has not been confirmed by most larger studies (Phelan et al., 1996; Tonin et al., 1996; Levy-Lahad et al., 1997; Shattuck-Eidens et al., 1997; Stoppa-Lyonnet et al., 1997; Ford et al., 1998), although one study provided non-significant evidence in favour of the original finding (Moslehi et al., 2000). In a series of 25 English breast/ovarian cancer families, ovarian cancer was more prevalent than breast cancer when *BRCA2* truncating mutations were located in a region of approximately 3.3 kb in exon 11 (the ovarian cancer cluster region, OCCR, nucleotides 3035–6629).

Additional data from 45 *BRCA2* families ascertained outside the United Kingdom provided support for this clustering (Gayther et al., 1997b). The analysis of 164 families with *BRCA2* mutations, 67 of whom had mutations in the OCCR, has been reported recently (Thompson et al., 1999). The odds ratio for ovarian versus breast cancer in families with mutations in the OCCR, relative to non-OCCR mutations, was 3.9 ($P<0.0001$), but the association was not seen in the more recently ascertained families, questioning the true importance of the OCCR. The OCCR corresponds to the coding region for a sequence of internal repeats in the *BRCA2* protein that have been shown to interact with the DNA repair protein RAD51.

Pre-malignant and early invasive lesions

The existence of pre-malignant lesion for epithelial ovarian cancer is uncertain (Scully, 2000). Careful histopathological analysis of prophylactic oophorectomy specimens among high-risk women, either because they have been identified as *BRCA1/2* mutation carriers or based on their family history, gave conflicting results regarding the presence of histological alterations that were susceptible to evolving into invasive carcinoma (Tobacman et al., 1982; Deligdisch et al., 1999; Stratton et al., 1999b; Werness et al., 1999; Casey et al., 2000). Interestingly, there has been a recent report of a tiny carcinoma *in situ* identified in an otherwise normal prophylactic oophorectomy specimen from women with a *BRCA1* mutation (Werness et al., 2000). Carcinoma *in situ* is very rarely seen in ovarian tissue, and this finding will prompt extensive re-analysis of available samples.

Peritoneal cancer

The incidence of primary serous carcinoma of the peritoneum among *BRCA1/2* carriers, before or after oophorectomy, is not known, but it is likely to be substantially higher than in the general population. This cancer is indistinguishable histologically or macroscopically from ovarian cancer occurring among *BRCA1/2* mutation carriers and represents a major challenge in terms of prevention of cancer in mutation carriers (Tobacman et al., 1982; Piver et al., 1993b; Struewing et al., 1995b; Salazar et al., 1996; Bandera et al., 1998; Berchuck et al., 1999; Karlan et al., 1999; Morice et al., 1999). The potential increased risk of malignant transformation of the entire peritoneal surface is thought to reflect the common origin of the ovarian epithelium and peritoneum from embryonic mesoderm. However, the peritoneum on the surface of the ovary may be particularly vulnerable to malignant transformation as a result of repeated injury following ovulation and/or high levels of local oestrogen exposure (Fathalla, 1971; Eisen and Weber, 1998). Preliminary evidence suggests that some peritoneal carcinomas may arise multifocally, particularly in the context of *BRCA1* mutations (Schorge et al., 1998), and a recent publication provided evidence for a unique molecular pathogenesis of *BRCA1*-related papillary serous carcinoma of the peritoneum (Schorge et al., 2000).

The natural history of *BRCA1/2*-related ovarian cancer

Fifty-three ovarian carcinoma patients with germline *BRCA1* mutations were enrolled into a study to determine the clinicopathological features of *BRCA1*-related hereditary ovarian carcinoma (Rubin et al., 1996). Forty-three (81%) were serous adenocarcinomas, and 38 (72%) were stage III at presentation. The actuarial median survival for the 43 cases with advanced-stage disease was 77 months, compared with 29 months for the age, stage and histological type-matched control group who were believed not to have mutations in *BRCA1* on the basis of family history ($P < 0.001$). This good prognosis was attributed partly to the relative youth of the patients (mean age 48 years) but was also thought to be directly related to the presence of a *BRCA1* mutation. This study was criticized on methodological grounds, but a second study from the senior author using a historical cohort approach (which is not susceptible to ascertainment bias) gave similar results (Boyd et al., 2000). Interestingly, the better survival in hereditary cases was particularly noted for those women receiving platinum-containing chemotherapy. A Japanese study also found a better outcome for hereditary ovarian cancer (Aida et al., 1998), although this study is open to criticism on the grounds of ascertainment bias. Moreover, data from the population-based US SEER program gave indirect support to an improved ovarian cancer survival in potential *BRCA1/2* mutation carriers (McGuire et al, 2000). The 824 women from the SEER series with ovarian cancer and a previous history of breast cancer had a significantly better survival compared with women without such a history, even after adjustment for age and stage at ovarian cancer diagnosis. It has been previously estimated that up to 88% of women with both breast and ovarian cancer are *BRCA1* mutation carriers (Frank et al., 1998).

In contrast, four other studies found that the survival after hereditary ovarian carcinoma did not differ from its sporadic counterpart. In a briefly described Canadian study (Brunet et al., 1997) among 44 women from *BRCA1*-positive families who were diagnosed with ovarian carcinoma, the actuarial median survival was 2.6 years, and the 5-year survival was 32.6%, a figure similar to that observed in the control groups of two previous studies (Aida et al., 1998; Johannsson et al., 1998). The Swedish group did not find a difference in outcome between 38 *BRCA1*-related cases and 97 apparently sporadic cases (Johannsson et al., 1998). The *BRCA1*-associated ovarian cancer patients were matched for age, stage of the disease and year of diagnosis. A study from the UK also found that the overall survival for *BRCA1*-related ovarian cancer was 21%, for *BRCA2*-related ovarian cancer it was 25%, and for those with no identified mutation it was 19% ($P=0.91$) (Pharoah et al., 1999). Interestingly, when all familial cases were combined (whether or not a mutation was either identified or looked for), the survival was significantly worse for familial cases compared with non-familial cases. The authors did not control for stage, as previous studies had done. It is debatable whether controlling for stage is appropriate, as if BRCA1/2-related tumours are per se more likely to present with late-stage disease then controlling for this will remove an effect that is specifically due to the presence of the mutation. Indeed, when the authors did control for stage the worse survival observed for familial cases disappeared. Finally, Lee et al. compared ovarian cancer survival among 10 first-degree relatives of Ashkenazi Jewish BRCA1 or BRCA2 mutation carriers with that of 116 ovarian cancer patients who were first-degree relatives of Ashkenazi Jewish BRCA1/2 non-carriers (Lee et al., 1999). They found no difference in survival in these groups of relatives.

Conclusion

The prevention of hereditary ovarian cancer is one of the great challenges of clinical cancer genetics. It is important to identify individuals at risk of ovarian cancer for whom genetic testing may be informative. This can be most easily achieved by establishing an extensive verified family history. Based on an accurate personal and family history of cancer, including ethnicity and pathological confirmation of the cancer cases, empirical cancer risk estimates and mathematical models can usually adequately assess the ovarian cancer risk and the probability of a germline alteration in cancer susceptibility genes implicated in hereditary ovarian cancer. Ovarian cancer genetic susceptibility testing is now widely available under both clinical and research protocols. However, because the benefits of genetic testing remain hypothetical, women should receive adequate counselling explaining the postulated risks and benefits of the genetic testing, including the ethical, legal and social implications of this type of analysis.

Acknowledgements

This chapter is based in part on two previously published works of the authors: 'Hereditary ovarian cancer' by Kasprzak et al. (1999) and 'Risk assessment and genetic testing' by Chappuis and Foulkes (2002).

POC is funded by grants from the Ligue Genevoise contre le Cancer et Cancer et Solidarité Fondation, Geneva, Switzerland. WDF is a Boursier Chercheur Clinicien J2 of the Fonds de la Recherche en Santé du Québec.

REFERENCES

Abeliovich D, Kaduri L, Lerer I, et al. (1997). The founder mutations 185delAG and 5382insC in BRCA1 and 6174delT in BRCA2 appear in 60 percent of ovarian cancer and 30 percent of early-onset breast cancer patients among Ashkenazi women. *Am J Hum Genet* **60**: 505–14.

Adami HO, Hsieh CC, Lambe M, et al. (1994). Parity, age at first childbirth, and risk of ovarian cancer. *Lancet* **344**: 1250–4.

Aida H, Takakuwa K, Nagata H, et al. (1998). Clinical features of ovarian cancer in Japanese women with germ-line mutations of BRCA1. *Clin Cancer Res* **4**: 235–40.

Amos CI and Struewing JP (1993). Genetic epidemiology of epithelial ovarian cancer. *Cancer* **71**: 566–72.

Amos CI, Shaw GL, Tucker MA and Hartge P (1992). Age at onset for familial epithelial ovarian cancer. *JAMA* **268**: 1896–9.

Andersen TI, Borresen AL and Moller P (1996). A common BRCA1 mutation in Norwegian breast and ovarian cancer families? *Am J Hum Genet* **59**: 486–7.

Anderson DE and Badzioch MD (1985). Risk of familial breast cancer. *Cancer* **56**: 383–7.

Antoniou AC, Gayther SA, Stratton JF, Ponder BA and Easton DF (2000). Risk models for familial ovarian and breast cancer. *Genet Epidemiol* **18**: 173–90.

Auranen A and Iselius L (1998). Segregation analysis of epithelial ovarian cancer in Finland. *Br J Cancer* **77**: 1537–41.

Auranen A, Pukkala E, Makinen J, Sankila R, Grenman S and Salmi T (1996a). Cancer incidence in the first-degree relatives of ovarian cancer patients. *Br J Cancer* **74**: 280–4.

Auranen A, Grenman S, Makinen J, Pukkala E, Sankila R and Salmi T (1996b). Borderline ovarian tumors in Finland: epidemiology and familial occurrence. *Am J Epidemiol* **144**: 548–53.

Auranen A, Grenman S and Kleml PJ (1997). Immunohistochemically detected p53 and HER-2/neu expression and nuclear DNA content in familial epithelial ovarian carcinomas. *Cancer* **79**: 2147–53.

Bandera CA, Muto MG, Schorge JO, Berkowitz RS, Rubin SC and Mok SC (1998). BRCA1 gene mutations in women with papillary serous carcinoma of the peritoneum. *Obstet Gynecol* **92**: 596–600.

Beller U, Halle D, Catane R, Kaufman B, Hornreich G and Levy-Lahad E (1997). High frequency of BRCA1 and BRCA2 germline mutations in Ashkenazi Jewish ovarian cancer patients, regardless of family history. *Gynecol Oncol* **67**: 123–6.

Berchuck A, Heron KA, Carney ME, et al. (1998). Frequency of germline and somatic BRCA1 mutations in ovarian cancer. *Clin Cancer Res* **4**: 2433–7.

Berchuck A, Schildkraut JM, Marks JR and Futreal PA (1999). Managing hereditary ovarian cancer risk. *Cancer* **86**: 1697–704.

Berman DB, Costalas J, Schultz DC, Grana G, Daly M and Godwin AK (1996). A common mutation in BRCA2 that predisposes to a variety of cancers is found in both Jewish Ashkenazi and non-Jewish individuals. *Cancer Res* **56**: 3409–14.

Bewtra C, Watson P, Conway T, Read-Hippee C and Lynch HT (1992). Hereditary ovarian cancer: a clinicopathological study. *Int J Gynecol Pathol* **11**: 180–7.

Birch JM, Blair V, Kelsey AM, et al. (1998). Cancer phenotype correlates with constitutional TP53 genotype in families with the Li–Fraumeni syndrome. *Oncogene* **17**: 1061–8.

Børresen AL (1992). Oncogenesis in ovarian cancer. *Acta Obstet Gynecol Scand Suppl* **155**: 25–30.

Boyd J, Sonoda Y, Federici MG, et al. (2000). Clinicopathologic features of BRCA-linked and sporadic ovarian cancer. *JAMA* **283**: 2260–5.

Brunet JS, Narod SA, Tonin P and Foulkes WD (1997). BRCA1 mutations and survival in women with ovarian cancer. *N Engl J Med* **336**: 1256.

Buller RE, Anderson B, Connor JP and Robinson R (1993). Familial ovarian cancer. *Gynecol Oncol* **51**: 160–6.

Buller RE, Skilling JS, Kaliszewski S, Niemann T and Anderson B (1995). Absence of significant germ-line p53 mutations in ovarian cancer patients. *Gynecol Oncol* **58**: 368–74.

Casagrande JT, Louie EW, Pike MC, Roy S, Ross RK and Henderson BE (1979). 'Incessant ovulation' and ovarian cancer. *Lancet* **2**: 170–3.

Casey MJ, Bewtra C, Hoehne LL, Tatpati AD, Lynch HT and Watson P (2000). Histology of prophylactically removed ovaries from BRCA1 and BRCA2 mutation carriers compared with non carriers in hereditary breast/ovarian cancer syndrome kindreds. *Gynecol Oncol* **78**: 278–87.

Chang J, Fryatt I, Ponder B, Fisher C and Gore ME (1995). A matched control study of familial epithelial ovarian cancer: patient characteristics, response to chemotherapy and outcome. *Ann Oncol* **6**: 80–2.

Chappuis PO and Foulkes WD (2002). Risk assessment and genetic testing. In *Ovarian Cancer*, ed. S Stack and DA Fishman. Norwell, MA: Kluwer Academic Publishers.

Claus EB and Schwartz PE (1995). Familial ovarian cancer. Update and clinical applications. *Cancer* **76**: 1998–2003.

Claus EB, Risch N and Thompson WD (1994). Autosomal dominant inheritance of early-onset breast cancer. Implications for risk prediction. *Cancer* **73**: 643–51.

Claus EB, Schildkraut JM, Thompson WD and Risch NJ (1996). The genetic attributable risk of breast and ovarian cancer. *Cancer* **77**: 2318–24.

Couch FJ, DeShano ML, Blackwood MA, et al. (1997). BRCA1 mutations in women attending clinics that evaluate the risk of breast cancer. *N Engl J Med* **336**: 1409–15.

Cramer DW, Hutchison GB, Welch WR, Scully RE and Ryan KJ (1983). Determinants of ovarian cancer risk. I. Reproductive experiences and family history. *J Natl Cancer Inst* **71**: 711–16.

Cramer DW, Harlow BL, Willett WC, et al. (1989). Galactose consumption and metabolism in relation to the risk of ovarian cancer. *Lancet* **2**: 66–71.

Deligdisch L, Gil J, Kerner H, Wu HS, Beck D and Gershoni-Baruch R (1999). Ovarian dysplasia in prophylactic oophorectomy specimens: cytogenetic and morphometric correlations. *Cancer* **86**: 1544–50.

Dorum A, Møller P, Kamsteeg EJ, et al. (1997). A BRCA1 founder mutation, identified with haplotype analysis, allowing genotype/phenotype determination and predictive testing. *Eur J Cancer* **33**: 2390–2.

Dorum A, Hovig E, Trope C, Inganas M and Møller P (1999). Three per cent of Norwegian ovarian cancers are caused by BRCA1 1675delA or 1135insA. *Eur J Cancer* **35**: 779–81.

Douglas FS, O'Dair LC, Robinson M, Evans DG and Lynch SA (1999). The accuracy of diagnoses as reported in families with cancer: a retrospective study. *J Med Genet* **36**: 309–12.

Easton DF, Bishop DT, Ford D and Crockford GP (1993). Genetic linkage analysis in familial breast and ovarian cancer: results from 214 families. Breast Cancer Linkage Consortium. *Am J Hum Genet* **52**: 678–701.

Easton DF, Ford D and Bishop DT (1995). Breast and ovarian cancer incidence in BRCA1-mutation carriers. Breast Cancer Linkage Consortium. *Am J Hum Genet* **56**: 265–71.

Easton DF, Matthews FE, Ford D, Swerdlow AJ and Peto J (1996). Cancer mortality in relatives of women with ovarian cancer – the OPCS study. *Int J Cancer* **65**: 284–94.

Easton DF, Steele L, Fields P, et al. (1997). Cancer risks in two large breast cancer families linked to BRCA2 on chromosome 13q12–13. *Am J Hum Genet* **61**: 120–8.

Eisen A and Weber BL (1998). Primary peritoneal carcinoma can have multifocal origins: implications for prophylactic oophorectomy. *J Natl Cancer Inst* **90**: 797–9.

Fathalla MF (1971). Incessant ovulation – a factor in ovarian neoplasia? *Lancet* **2**: 163.

Ford D, Easton DF, Bishop DT, Narod SA and Goldgar DE (1994). Risks of cancer in BRCA1-mutation carriers. Breast Cancer Linkage Consortium. *Lancet* **343**: 692–5.

Ford D, Easton DF, Stratton M, et al. (1998). Genetic heterogeneity and penetrance analysis of the BRCA1 and BRCA2 genes in breast cancer families. *Am J Hum Genet* **62**: 676–89.

Foster KA, Harrington P, Kerr J, et al. (1996). Somatic and germline mutations of the BRCA2 gene in sporadic ovarian cancer. *Cancer Res* **56**: 3622–5.

Franceschi S, Parazzini F, Negri E, et al. (1991). Pooled analysis of 3 European case-control studies of epithelial ovarian cancer. III. Oral contraceptive use. *Int J Cancer* **49**: 61–5.

Frank TS, Manley SA, Olopade OI, et al. (1998). Sequence analysis of BRCA1 and BRCA2: correlation of mutations with family history and ovarian cancer risk. *J Clin Oncol* **16**: 2417–25.

Friedman LS, Szabo CI, Ostermeyer EA, et al. (1995). Novel inherited mutations and variable expressivity of BRCA1 alleles, including the founder mutation 185delAG in Ashkenazi Jewish families. *Am J Hum Genet* **57**: 1284–97.

Gail MH, Brinton LA, Byar DP, et al. (1989). Projecting individualized probabilities of developing breast cancer for white females who are being examined annually. *J Natl Cancer Inst* **81**: 1879–86.

Gayther SA, Warren W, Mazoyer S, et al. (1995). Germline mutations of the BRCA1 gene in breast and ovarian cancer families provide evidence for a genotype–phenotype correlation. *Nat Genet* **11**: 428–33.

Gayther SA, Harrington P, Russell P, Kharkevich G, Garkavtseva RF and Ponder BA (1997a). Frequently occurring germ-line mutations of the BRCA1 gene in ovarian cancer families from Russia. *Am J Hum Genet* **60**: 1239–42.

Gayther SA, Mangion J, Russell P, et al. (1997b). Variation of risks of breast and ovarian cancer associated with different germline mutations of the BRCA2 gene. *Nat Genet* **15**: 103–5.

Gayther SA, Russell P, Harrington P, Antoniou AC, Easton DF and Ponder BAJ (1999). The contribution of germline BRCA1 and BRCA2 mutations to familial ovarian cancer: no evidence for other ovarian cancer-susceptibility genes. *Am J Hum Genet* **65**: 1021–9.

Go RC, King MC, Bailey-Wilson J, Elston RC and Lynch HT (1983). Genetic epidemiology of breast cancer and associated cancers in high-risk families. I. Segregation analysis. *J Natl Cancer Inst* **71**: 455–61.

Godard B, Foulkes WD, Provencher D, et al. (1998). Risk factors for familial and sporadic ovarian cancer among French Canadians: a case-control study. *Am J Obstet Gynecol* **179**: 403–10.

Goldgar DE, Easton DF, Cannon-Albright LA and Skolnick MH (1994). Systematic population-based assessment of cancer risk in first-degree relatives of cancer probands. *J Natl Cancer Inst* **86**: 1600–8.

Gotlieb WH, Friedman E, Bar-Sade RB, et al. (1998). Rates of Jewish ancestral mutations in BRCA1 and BRCA2 in borderline ovarian tumors. *J Natl Cancer Inst* **90**: 995–1000.

Greenlee RT, Murray T, Bolden S and Wingo PA (2000). Cancer statistics, 2000. *CA Cancer J Clin* **50**: 7–33.

Greggi S, Genuardi M, Benedetti-Panici P, et al. (1990). Analysis of 138 consecutive ovarian cancer patients: incidence and characteristics of familial cases. *Gynecol Oncol* **39**: 300–4.

Hall JM, Lee MK, Newman B, et al. (1990). Linkage of early-onset familial breast cancer to chromosome 17q21. *Science* **250**: 1684–9.

Hankinson SE, Hunter DJ, Colditz GA, et al. (1993). Tubal ligation, hysterectomy, and risk of ovarian cancer. A prospective study. *JAMA* **270**: 2813–18.

Hartge P, Schiffman MH, Hoover R, McGowan L, Lesher L and Norris HJ (1989). A case-control study of epithelial ovarian cancer. *Am J Obstet Gynecol* **161**: 10–16.

Hartge P, Whittemore AS, Itnyre J, McGowan L, Cramer D and the collaborative ovarian cancer group (1994). Rates and risks of ovarian cancer in subgroups of white women in the United States. *Obstet Gynecol* **84**: 760–4.

Hemminki K, Vaittinen P and Kyyronen P (1998). Age-specific familial risks in common cancers of the offspring. *Int J Cancer* **78**: 172–5.

Hildreth NG, Kelsey JL, LiVolsi VA, et al. (1981). An epidemiologic study of epithelial carcinoma of the ovary. *Am J Epidemiol* **114**: 398–405.

Hodgson SV, Heap E, Cameron J, et al. (1999). Risk factors for detecting germline BRCA1 and

BRCA2 founder mutations in Ashkenazi Jewish women with breast or ovarian cancer. *J Med Genet* **36**: 369–73.

Houlston RS, Collins A, Slack J, et al. (1991). Genetic epidemiology of ovarian cancer: segregation analysis. *Ann Hum Genet* **55**: 291–9.

Houlston RS, Bourne TH, Collins WP, Whitehead MI, Campbell S and Slack J (1993). Risk of ovarian cancer and genetic relationship to other cancers in families. *Hum Hered* **43**: 111–15.

Janezic SA, Ziogas A, Krumroy LM, et al. (1999). Germline BRCA1 alterations in a population-based series of ovarian cancer cases. *Hum Mol Genet* **8**: 889–97.

Jishi MF, Itnyre JH, Oakley-Girvan IA, Piver MS and Whittemore AS (1995). Risks of cancer among members of families in the Gilda Radner Familial Ovarian Cancer Registry. *Cancer* **76**: 1416–21.

Johannesdottir G, Gudmundsson J, Bergthorsson JT, et al. (1996). High prevalence of the 999del5 mutation in Icelandic breast and ovarian cancer patients. *Cancer Res* **56**: 3663–5.

Johannsson O, Ostermeyer EA, Hakansson S, et al. (1996). Founding BRCA1 mutations in hereditary breast and ovarian cancer in southern Sweden. *Am J Hum Genet* **58**: 441–50.

Johannsson OT, Idvall I, Anderson C, et al. (1997). Tumour biological features of BRCA1-induced breast and ovarian cancer. *Eur J Cancer* **33**: 362–71.

Johannsson OT, Ranstam J, Borg A and Olsson H (1998). Survival of BRCA1 breast and ovarian cancer patients: a population-based study from southern Sweden. *J Clin Oncol* **16**: 397–404.

Jolly KW, Malkin D, Douglass EC, Brown TF, Sinclair AE and Look AT (1994). Splice-site mutation of the p53 gene in a family with hereditary breast–ovarian cancer. *Oncogene* **9**: 97–102.

Karlan BY, Baldwin RL, Lopez-Luevanos E, et al. (1999). Peritoneal serous papillary carcinoma, a phenotypic variant of familial ovarian cancer: implications for ovarian cancer screening. *Am J Obstet Gynecol* **180**: 917–28.

Kasprzak L, Foulkes WD and Shelling AN (1999). Hereditary ovarian cancer. *Br Med J* **318**: 786–9.

Kerber RA and Slattery ML (1995). The impact of family history on ovarian cancer risk. The Utah Population Database. *Arch Intern Med* **155**: 905–12.

Kleihues P, Schauble B, zur Hausen A, Esteve J and Ohgaki H (1997). Tumors associated with p53 germline mutations: a synopsis of 91 families. *Am J Pathol* **150**: 1–13.

Koch M, Gaedke H and Jenkins H (1989). Family history of ovarian cancer patients: a case-control study. *Int J Epidemiol* **18**: 782–5.

Lamovec J, Bracko M and Cerar O (1995). Familial occurrence of small-cell carcinoma of the ovary. *Arch Pathol Lab Med* **119**: 523–7.

Lancaster JM, Wooster R, Mangion J, et al. (1996). BRCA2 mutations in primary breast and ovarian cancers. *Nat Genet* **13**: 238–40.

Lee JS, Wacholder S, Struewing JP, et al. (1999). Survival after breast cancer in Ashkenazi Jewish BRCA1 and BRCA2 mutation carriers. *J Natl Cancer Inst* **91**: 259–63.

Levy-Lahad E, Catane R, Eisenberg S, et al. (1997). Founder BRCA1 and BRCA2 mutations in

Ashkenazi Jews in Israel: frequency and differential penetrance in ovarian cancer and in breast–ovarian cancer families. *Am J Hum Genet* **60**: 1059–67.

Liber AF (1950). Ovarian cancer in a mother and five daughters. *Arch Pathol* **49**: 280–90.

Liede A, Tonin PN, Sun CC, et al. (1998). Is hereditary site-specific ovarian cancer a distinct genetic condition? *Am J Med Genet* **75**: 55–8.

Ligtenberg MJ, Hogervorst FB, Willems HW, et al. (1999). Characteristics of small breast and/or ovarian cancer families with germline mutations in BRCA1 and BRCA2. *Br J Cancer* **79**: 1475–8.

Longy M, Toulouse C, Mage P, Chauvergne J and Trojani M (1996). Familial cluster of ovarian small cell carcinoma: a new mendelian entity? *J Med Genet* **33**: 333–5.

Lu KH, Cramer DW, Muto MG, Li EY, Niloff J and Mok SC (1999). A population-based study of BRCA1 and BRCA2 mutations in Jewish women with epithelial ovarian cancer. *Obstet Gynecol* **93**: 34–7.

Lynch HT and Lynch JF (1992). Hereditary ovarian carcinoma. *Hematol Oncol Clin North Am* **6**: 783–811.

Lynch HT, Watson P, Lynch JF, Conway TA and Fili M (1993). Hereditary ovarian cancer. Heterogeneity in age at onset. *Cancer* **71**: 573–81.

Matsushima M, Kobayashi K, Emi M, et al. (1995). Mutation analysis of the BRCA1 gene in 76 Japanese ovarian cancer patients: four germline mutations, but no evidence of somatic mutation. *Hum Mol Genet* **4**: 1953–6.

McGuire V, Whittemore AS, Norris R and Oakley-Girvan I (2000). Survival in epithelial ovarian cancer patients with prior breast cancer. *Am J. Epidemiol* **152**: 528–32.

Miki Y, Swensen J, Shattuck-Eidens D, et al. (1994). A strong candidate for the breast and ovarian cancer susceptibility gene BRCA1. *Science* **266**: 66–71.

Modan B, Gak E, Sade-Bruchim RB, et al. (1996). High frequency of BRCA1 185delAG mutation in ovarian cancer in Israel. National Israel Study of Ovarian Cancer. *JAMA* **276**: 1823–5.

Mori M, Harabuchi I, Miyake H, Casagrande JT, Henderson BE and Ross RK (1988). Reproductive, genetic, and dietary risk factors for ovarian cancer. *Am J Epidemiol* **128**: 771–7.

Morice P, Pautier P, Mercier S, et al. (1999). Laparoscopic prophylactic oophorectomy in women with inherited risk of ovarian cancer. *Eur J Gynaecol Oncol* **20**: 202–4.

Moslehi R, Chu W, Karlan B, et al. (2000). BRCA1 and BRCA2 mutation analysis of 208 Ashkenazi Jewish women with ovarian cancer. *Am J Hum Genet* **66**: 1259–72.

Muto MG, Cramer DW, Tangir J, Berkowitz R and Mok S (1996). Frequency of the BRCA1 185delAG mutation among Jewish women with ovarian cancer and matched population controls. *Cancer Res* **56**: 1250–2.

Narod SA, Feunteun J, Lynch HT, et al. (1991). Familial breast–ovarian cancer locus on chromosome 17q12–q23. *Lancet* **338**: 82–3.

Narod SA, Madlensky L, Bradley L, et al. (1994a). Hereditary and familial ovarian cancer in southern Ontario. *Cancer* **74**: 2341–6.

Narod SA, Tonin P, Lynch H, Watson P, Feunteun J and Lenoir G (1994b). Histology of BRCA1-associated ovarian tumours. *Lancet* **343**: 236.

Narod SA, Ford D, Devilee P, et al. (1995). An evaluation of genetic heterogeneity in 145 breast–ovarian cancer families. Breast Cancer Linkage Consortium. *Am J Hum Genet* **56**: 254–64.

Neuhausen SL, Mazoyer S, Friedman L, et al. (1996). Haplotype and phenotype analysis of six recurrent BRCA1 mutations in 61 families: results of an international study. *Am J Hum Genet* **58**: 271–80.

Oddoux C, Struewing JP, Clayton CM, et al. (1996). The carrier frequency of the BRCA2 6174delT mutation among the Ashkenazi Jewish individuals is approximately 1 percent. *Nat Genet* **14**: 188–90.

Olsen JH, Seersholm N, Boice JDJ, Kruger KS and Fraumeni JF, Jr (1999). Cancer risk in close relatives of women with early-onset breast cancer – a population-based incidence study. *Br J Cancer* **79**: 673–9.

Ottman R, Pike MC, King MC and Henderson BE (1983). Practical guide for estimating risk for familial breast cancer. *Lancet* **2**: 556–8.

Parazzini F, Franceschi S, La Vecchia C and Fasoli M (1991). The epidemiology of ovarian cancer. *Gynecol Oncol* **43**: 9–23.

Parazzini F, Negri E, La Vecchia C, Restelli C and Franceschi S (1992). Family history of reproductive cancers and ovarian cancer risk: an Italian case-control study. *Am J Epidemiol* **135**: 35–40.

Parkin DM, Whelan SL, Ferlay J, Raymond L and Young J (1997). *Cancer Incidence in Five Continents*, Vol. VII. Lyon: IARC Scientific Publications.

Parmigiani G, Berry D and Aguilar O (1998). Determining carrier probabilities for breast cancer-susceptibility genes BRCA1 and BRCA2. *Am J Hum Genet* **62**: 145–58.

Peelen T, van Vliet M, Petrij-Bosch A, et al. (1997). A high proportion of novel mutations in BRCA1 with strong founder effects among Dutch and Belgian hereditary breast and ovarian cancer families. *Am J Hum Genet* **60**: 1041–9.

Pharoah PD, Easton DF, Stockton DL, Gayther S and Ponder BA (1999). Survival in familial, BRCA1-associated, and BRCA2-associated, epithelial ovarian cancer. United Kingdom Coordinating Committee for Cancer Research (UKCCCR) Familial Ovarian Cancer Study Group. *Cancer Res* **59**: 868–71.

Phelan CM, Rebbeck TR, Weber BL, et al. (1996). Ovarian cancer risk in BRCA1 carriers is modified by the HRAS1 variable number of tandem repeat (VNTR) locus. *Nat Genet* **12**: 309–11.

Piver MS, Baker TR, Jishi MF, et al. (1993a). Familial ovarian cancer. A report of 658 families from the Gilda Radner Familial Ovarian Cancer Registry 1981–1991. *Cancer* **71**: 582–8.

Piver MS, Jishi MF, Tsukada Y and Nava G (1993b). Primary peritoneal carcinoma after prophylactic oophorectomy in women with a family history of ovarian cancer. A report of the Gilda Radner Familial Ovarian Cancer Registry. *Cancer* **71**: 2751–5.

Prior P and Waterhouse JA (1981). Multiple primary cancers of the breast and ovary. *Br J Cancer* **44**: 628–36.

Purdie D, Green A, Bain C, et al. (1995). Reproductive and other factors and risk of epithelial ovarian cancer: an Australian case-control study. Survey of Women's Health Study Group. *Int J Cancer* **62**: 678–84.

Rader JS, Neuman RJ, Brady J, et al. (1998). Cancer among first-degree relatives of probands with invasive and borderline ovarian cancer. *Obstet Gynecol* **92**: 589–95.

Ramus SJ, Kote-Jarai Z, Friedman LS, et al. (1997). Analysis of BRCA1 and BRCA2 mutations in Hungarian families with breast or breast–ovarian cancer. *Am J Hum Genet* **60**: 1242–6.

Richards WE, Gallion HH, Schmittschmitt JP, Holladay DV and Smith SA (1999). BRCA1-related and sporadic ovarian cancer in the same family: implications for genetic testing. *Gynecol Oncol* **75**: 468–72.

Roa BB, Boyd AA, Volcik K and Richards CS (1996). Ashkenazi Jewish population frequencies for common mutations in *BRCA1* and *BRCA2. Nat Genet* **14**: 185–7.

Rosenberg L, Palmer JR, Zauber AG, et al. (1994). A case-control study of oral contraceptive use and invasive epithelial ovarian cancer. *Am J Epidemiol* **139**: 654–61.

Roth S, Kristo P, Auranen A, et al. (1998). A missense mutation in the BRCA2 gene in three siblings with ovarian cancer. *Br J Cancer* **77**: 1199–202.

Rubin SC, Benjamin I, Behbakht K, et al. (1996). Clinical and pathological features of ovarian cancer in women with germ-line mutations of BRCA1. *N Engl J Med* **335**: 1413–16.

Rubin SC, Blackwood MA, Bandera C, et al. (1998). BRCA1, BRCA2, and hereditary non-polyposis colorectal cancer gene mutations in an unselected ovarian cancer population: relationship to family history and implications for genetic testing. *Am J Obstet Gynecol* **178**: 670–7.

Sagawa T, Yamashita Y, Fujimoto T, et al. (1999). Clinicopathological comparisons of familial and sporadic cases in 219 consecutive Japanese epithelial ovarian cancer patients. *Jpn J Clin Oncol* **29**: 556–61.

Salazar H, Godwin AK, Daly MB, et al. (1996). Microscopic benign and invasive malignant neoplasms and a cancer-prone phenotype in prophylactic oophorectomies. J Natl Cancer Inst **88**: 1810–20.

Santarosa M, Dolcetti R, Magri MD, et al. (1999). BRCA1 and BRCA2 genes: role in hereditary breast and ovarian cancer in Italy. *Int J Cancer* **83**: 5–9.

Schildkraut JM and Thompson WD (1988a). Familial ovarian cancer: a population-based case-control study. *Am J Epidemiol* **128**: 456–66.

Schildkraut JM and Thompson WD (1988b). Relationship of epithelial ovarian cancer to other malignancies within families. *Genet Epidemiol* **5**: 355–67.

Schildkraut JM, Risch N and Thompson WD (1989). Evaluating genetic association among ovarian, breast, and endometrial cancer: evidence for a breast/ovarian cancer relationship. *Am J Hum Genet* **45**: 521–9.

Schorge JO, Muto MG, Welch WR, et al. (1998). Molecular evidence for multifocal papillary serous carcinoma of the peritoneum in patients with germline BRCA1 mutations. *J Natl Cancer Inst* **90**: 841–5.

Schorge JO, Muto MG, Lee SJ, et al. (2000). BRCA1-related papillary serous carcinoma of the peritoneum has a unique molecular pathogenesis. *Cancer Res* **60**: 1361–4.

Scully RE (2000). Influence of origin of ovarian cancer on efficacy of screening. *Lancet* **355**: 1028–9.

Shattuck-Eidens D, McClure M, Simard J, et al. (1995). A collaborative survey of 80 mutations in the BRCA1 breast and ovarian cancer susceptibility gene. Implications for presymptomatic testing and screening. *JAMA* **273**: 535–41.

Shattuck-Eidens D, Oliphant A, McClure M, et al. (1997). BRCA1 sequence analysis in women at high risk for susceptibility mutations – risk factor analysis and implications for genetic testing. *JAMA* **278**: 1242–50.

Steichen-Gersdorf E, Gallion HH, Ford D, et al. (1994). Familial site-specific ovarian cancer is linked to BRCA1 on 17q12–21. *Am J Hum Genet* **55**: 870–5.

Stettner AR, Hartenbach EM, Schink JC, et al. (1999). Familial ovarian germ cell cancer: report and review. *Am J Med Genet* **84**: 43–6.

Stoppa-Lyonnet D, Laurent-Puig P, Essioux L, et al. (1997). BRCA1 sequence variations in 160 individuals referred to a breast/ovarian family cancer clinic. *Am J Hum Genet* **60**: 1021–30.

Stratton JF, Gayther SA, Russell P, et al. (1997). Contribution of BRCA1 mutations to ovarian cancer. *N Engl J Med* **336**: 1125–30.

Stratton JF, Pharoah P, Smith SK, Easton D and Ponder BA (1998). A systematic review and meta-analysis of family history and risk of ovarian cancer. *Br J Obstet Gynaecol* **105**: 493–9.

Stratton JF, Thompson D, Bobrow L, et al. (1999a). The genetic epidemiology of early-onset epithelial ovarian cancer: a population-based study. *Am J Hum Genet* **65**: 1725–32.

Stratton JF, Buckley CH, Lowe D and Ponder BA (1999b). Comparison of prophylactic oophorectomy specimens from carriers and noncarriers of a BRCA1 or BRCA2 gene mutation. United Kingdom Coordinating Committee on Cancer Research (UKCCCR) Familial Ovarian Cancer Study Group. *J Natl Cancer Inst* **91**: 626–8.

Struewing JP, Abeliovich D, Peretz T, et al. (1995a). The carrier frequency of the BRCA1 185delAG mutation is approximately 1 percent in Ashkenazi Jewish individuals. *Nat Genet* **11**: 198–200.

Struewing JP, Watson P, Easton DF, Ponder BA, Lynch HT and Tucker MA (1995b). Prophylactic oophorectomy in inherited breast/ovarian cancer families. *J Natl Cancer Inst Monogr* **17**: 33–5.

Struewing JP, Hartge P, Wacholder S, et al. (1997). The risk of cancer associated with specific mutations of BRCA1 and BRCA2 among Ashkenazi Jews. *N Engl J Med* **336**: 1401–8.

Sutcliffe S, Pharoah PDP, Easton DF and Ponder BAJ (2000). Ovarian and breast cancer risks to women in families with two or more cases of ovarian cancer. *Int J Cancer* **87**: 110–17.

Takahashi H, Behbakht K, McGovern PE, et al. (1995). Mutation analysis of the BRCA1 gene in ovarian cancers. *Cancer Res* **55**: 2998–3002.

Takahashi H, Chiu HC, Bandera CA, et al. (1996). Mutations of the BRCA2 gene in ovarian carcinomas. *Cancer Res* **56**: 2738–41.

Takano M, Aida H, Tsuneki I, et al. (1997). Mutational analysis of BRCA1 gene in ovarian and breast–ovarian cancer families in Japan. *Jpn J Cancer Res* **88**: 407–13.

Thompson DJ, Easton DF and on behalf of the Breast Cancer Linkage Consortium (1999). Evidence for genotype–phenotype correlations in BRCA2 (abstract). *Am J Hum Genet* **65** (Suppl.): A327.

Tobacman JK, Greene MH, Tucker MA, Costa J, Kase R and Fraumeni JF, Jr (1982). Intra-abdominal carcinomatosis after prophylactic oophorectomy in ovarian-cancer-prone families. *Lancet* **2**: 795–7.

Tonin P, Weber B, Offit K, et al. (1996). Frequency of recurrent BRCA1 and BRCA2 mutations in Ashkenazi Jewish breast cancer families. *Nat Med* **2**: 1183–96.

Tonin PN, Mes-Masson AM, Futreal PA, et al. (1998). Founder BRCA1 and BRCA2 mutations in French Canadian breast and ovarian cancer families. *Am J Hum Genet* **63**: 1341–51.

Tonin PM, Mes-Masson AM, Narod SA, Ghadirian P and Provencher D (1999). Founder BRCA1 and BRCA2 mutations in French Canadian ovarian cancer cases unselected for family history. *Clin Genet* **55**: 318–24.

Tulinius H, Olafsdottir GH, Sigvaldason H, Tryggvadottir L and Bjarnadottir K (1994). Neoplastic diseases in families of breast cancer patients. *J Med Genet* **31**: 618–21.

Tzonou A, Day NE, Trichopoulos D, et al. (1984). The epidemiology of ovarian cancer in Greece: a case-control study. *Eur J Cancer Clin Oncol* **20**: 1045–52.

Vaittinen P and Hemminki K (1999). Familial cancer risks in offspring from discordant parental cancers. *Int J Cancer* **81**: 12–19.

Van der Looij M, Szabo C, Besznyak I, et al. (2000). Prevalence of founder BRCA1 and BRCA2 mutations among breast and ovarian cancer patients in Hungary. *Int J Cancer* **86**: 737–40.

Vasen HF, Mecklin JP, Khan PM and Lynch HT (1991). The International Collaborative Group on Hereditary Non-Polyposis Colorectal Cancer (ICG-HNPCC). *Dis Colon Rectum* **34**: 424–5.

Wagner TM, Moslinger R, Zielinski C, Scheiner O and Breiteneder H (1996). New Austrian mutation in BRCA1 gene detected in three unrelated HBOC families. *Lancet* **347**: 1263.

Warner E, Foulkes W, Goodwin P, et al. (1999). Prevalence and penetrance of BRCA1 and BRCA2 gene mutations in unselected Ashkenazi Jewish women with breast cancer. *J Natl Cancer Inst* **91**: 1241–7.

Weitzel JN (1999). Genetic cancer risk assessment: putting it all together. *Cancer* **86**: 1663–72.

Werness BA, Afify AM, Bielat KL, Eltabbakh GH, Piver MS and Paterson JM (1999). Altered surface and cyst epithelium of ovaries removed prophylactically from women with a family history of ovarian cancer. *Hum Pathol* **30**: 151–7.

Werness BA, Parvatiyar P, Ramus SJ, et al. (2000). Ovarian carcinoma in situ with germline BRCA1 mutation and loss of heterozygosity at BRCA1 and TP53. *J Natl Cancer Inst* **92**: 1088–91.

Whittemore AS, Wu ML, Paffenbarger RS, Jr, et al. (1988). Personal and environmental characteristics related to epithelial ovarian cancer. II. Exposures to talcum powder, tobacco, alcohol, and coffee. *Am J Epidemiol* **128**: 1228–40.

Whittemore AS, Harris R and Itnyre J (1992). Characteristics relating to ovarian cancer risk: collaborative analysis of 12 US case-control studies. II. Invasive epithelial ovarian cancers in white women. Collaborative Ovarian Cancer Group. *Am J Epidemiol* **136**: 1184–203.

Whittemore AS, Gong G and Itnyre J (1997). Prevalence and contribution of BRCA1 mutations in breast cancer and ovarian cancer: results from three U.S. population-based case-control studies of ovarian cancer. *Am J Hum Genet* **60**: 496–504.

Wooster R, Neuhausen SL, Mangion J, et al. (1994). Localization of a breast cancer susceptibility gene, BRCA2, to chromosome 13q12–13. *Science* **265**, 2088–90.

Wooster R, Bignell G, Lancaster J, et al. (1995). Identification of the breast cancer susceptibility gene BRCA2. *Nature* **378**: 789–92.

Wynder EL, Dodo H and Barber HR (1969). Epidemiology of cancer of the ovary. *Cancer* **23**: 352–70.

Yamashita Y, Sagawa T, Fujimoto T, et al. (1999). BRCA1 mutation testing for Japanese patients with ovarian cancer in breast cancer screening. *Breast Cancer Res Treat* **58**: 11–17.

Zweemer RP, Verheijen RH, Gille JJ, van Diest PJ, Pals G and Menko FH (1998). Clinical and genetic evaluation of thirty ovarian cancer families. *Am J Obstet Gynecol* **178**: 85–90.

5

Ovarian and breast cancer as part of hereditary non-polyposis colorectal cancer (HNPCC) and other hereditary colorectal cancer syndromes

H. F. A. Vasen and M. A. Nooy

Leiden University Medical Centre, the Netherlands

Introduction

Colorectal cancer is a common disease of Western populations. In the Netherlands (population: 15 million), 8000 new cases were diagnosed in 1996. In 5–10% of all colorectal cancer cases, genetic factors play a significant role. Two main groups of the hereditary form of colorectal cancer are commonly distinguished: polyposis types with multiple colorectal polyps, and non-polyposis types without multiple polyps. Non-polyposis colorectal cancer can be sub-classified into hereditary non-polyposis colorectal cancer (HNPCC), characterized by early-onset colorectal cancer and endometrial cancer, and families with clustering of colorectal cancer at an advanced age. Within the polyposis types, a further distinction is made between adenomatous, hamartomatous and hyperplastic polyposis, and polyposis with mixed pathology (Vasen, 2000).

During the last decade, great progress has been made in molecular genetics. The genes responsible for most of the inherited forms of colorectal cancer have been identified, and DNA testing has been implemented in clinical practice on a large scale. The identification of people at high risk of cancer is important as preventive measures may be taken in such cases, which may lead to a reduction in the cancer-related mortality.

Decisions on the protocol of surveillance recommended in the various forms of hereditary cancers are made on the basis of the level of risk of developing a specific cancer and the availability of sensitive and specific screening tests.

In this chapter we will address the question as to whether relatives from HNPCC families or families with other hereditary colorectal cancer syndromes have an increased risk of developing ovarian and/or breast cancer, and whether these family members need surveillance of these organs.

Hereditary non-polyposis colorectal cancer

Genetic basis

Hereditary non-polyposis colorectal cancer (HNPCC) is an autosomal dominant disorder associated with germline mutations in five mismatch repair genes: *MSH2*, *MLH1*, *PMS1*, *PMS2* and *MSH6* (Lynch and de la Chapelle, 1999). The protein products of HNPCC genes are key players in the correction of mismatches that arise during DNA replication. Mismatch repair (MMR) deficiency gives rise to microsatellite instability (MSI). MSI results from repetitive non-coding DNA sequences of unknown function found throughout the genome. Loss of MMR function may also result in mutations in the coding regions of genes involved in tumour initiation and progression, e.g. *APC*, *KRAS*, *TP53* and *TGFbRII*.

Clinical features

The so-called 'Amsterdam criteria' are often used to make a clinical diagnosis of HNPCC. According to the classical Amsterdam criteria (Amsterdam criteria I), there should be at least three relatives with colorectal cancer, one relative should be a first-degree relative of the other two, at least two successive generations should be affected, at least one of the cancers should be diagnosed before the age of 50 years, and familial adenomatous polyposis should be excluded in the patient(s) with colorectal cancer. Because many studies have provided evidence that several other extracolonic cancers are also associated with HNPCC, a new set of criteria (the Amsterdam criteria II) has been proposed, which includes these cancers (Table 5.1) (Vasen et al., 1999). In 50% of the families that meet these clinical criteria, a pathogenic mutation in one of the MMR genes can be detected.

Predisposed individuals from HNPCC families have a high lifetime risk of developing colorectal cancer (60–85%) and endometrial cancer (40–50%). Colorectal cancer is often diagnosed at an early age (mean age 45 years), is multiple in 35% of the cases, and is located in the proximal part of the colon in two-thirds of the cases (Vasen, 2000). Several studies have shown a better prognosis of patients with HNPCC-related colorectal cancer compared with non-hereditary colorectal cancer (Sankila et al., 1996). Also, other cancers are frequently observed in HNPCC, including cancer of the urinary tract (renal pelvis and ureter), small bowel, brain, skin (sebaceous tumours) and stomach.

Table 5.1. Classic ICG-HNPCC criteria

Amsterdam criteria I

There should be at least three relatives with colorectal cancer (CRC) and all of the following criteria should be present:

    (1) one should be a first-degree relative of the other two;

    (2) at least two successive generations should be affected;

    (3) at least one case should be diagnosed before the age of 50 years;

    (4) familial adenomatous polyposis should be excluded;

    (5) tumours should be verified by pathological examination.

Amsterdam criteria II

There should be at least three relatives with an HNPCC-associated cancer (CRC, or cancer of the endometrium, small bowel, ureter or renal pelvis) and all of the following criteria should be present:

    (1) one should be a first-degree relative of the other two;

    (2) at least two successive generations should be affected;

    (3) at least one case should be diagnosed before the age of 50 years;

    (4) familial adenomatous polyposis should be excluded in any CRC case(s);

    (5) tumours should be verified by pathological examination.

Do ovarian and breast cancer belong to the tumour spectrum of HNPCC?

Watson and Lynch (1993) evaluated the frequency of cancer in 1300 high-risk members of 23 extended kindreds with HNPCC. They reported 13 cases of ovarian cancers (mean age at diagnosis: 40 years) in these families, while 3.6 were expected on the basis of the general population incidence (observed/expected ratio: 3.5, $P<0.001$). Vasen compared the risk of developing ovarian cancer between carriers of an *MLH1* mutation ($n=124$) and carriers of an *MSH2* mutation ($n=86$) (Vasen et al., 1996). He reported relative risks of 6.35 (95% CI: 0.89–45.1) and 7.97 (95% CI: 1.1–56.6) for *MLH1* and *MSH2* mutation carriers, respectively. Aarnio assessed the incidence of cancer in a large series of mutation carriers (predominantly *MLH1* mutations) ($n=360$; 183 women, 177 men) known at the Finnish HNPCC registry (Aarnio et al., 1999). He reported a standardized incidence ratio (SIR) for ovarian cancer of 13 (95% CI: 5.3–25) and a cumulative ovarian cancer incidence of 12% by age 70 years. In conclusion, several studies indicated that ovarian cancer is part of the tumour spectrum of HNPCC.

  There is no agreement on whether breast cancer belongs to the tumour spectrum of HNPCC. Watson and Lynch (1993) reported 19 cases of breast cancer (mean age 51 years) in 23 HNPCC families (observed/expected ratio: 0.9, NS). Risinger performed molecular genetic studies in five cases of breast cancer from

HNPCC families, one with an identified mutation in *MLH1* (Risinger et al., 1996). In three out of the five tumours, widespread MSI was observed, and in the family with the known mutation, expression of only the mutant allele was observed in the breast cancer tissue. Aarnio reported a SIR for breast cancer in 183 mutation carriers of 1.4 (95% CI: 0.4–3.7) (Aarnio et al., 1999). Boyd described a male member of a large HNPCC family affected by breast and colorectal cancer (Boyd et al., 1999). This patient was found to harbour a germline mutation of the *MLH1* gene, and the breast tumour exhibited reduction to homozygosity for the *MLH1* mutation and MSI. Recently, Scott et al. evaluated the cancer incidence in 34 HNPCC families with a known mutation (12 with an *MSH2* mutation and 22 with an *MLH1* mutation) and in 61 HNPCC families without a mutation (Scott et al., 2001). Breast cancer was not over-represented in the *MSH2*-mutation-positive group (SIR 2.02; 95% CI: 0.3–12.7), but it was over-represented in both the *MLH1*-mutation-positive group (SIR 14.77; 95% CI: 6.2–35) and in the mutation-negative group, which was a highly significant difference. The SIR of breast cancer in the mutation-negative group was similar to that observed in the *MLH1*-mutation-positive group.

Recent data from the Dutch HNPCC registry

Currently, almost 200 families suspected of HNPCC are known at the Dutch registry, 138 of which meet the Amsterdam criteria or harbour an *MMR* gene germline mutation. In 79 families, a germline mutation has been detected: 34 mutations in *MLH1*, 40 in *MSH2* and 5 in *MSH6*. In these families, 24 cases of ovarian cancer were observed: 6 in families associated with an *MLH1* mutation, 13 in families with an *MSH2* mutation, none in the families with an *MSH6* mutation, and 5 in the families without an identified mutation. The mean age at diagnosis of ovarian cancer was 46 years (range: 19–75 years). The distribution of the ages at diagnosis is shown in Figure 5.1. The cumulative risk of developing ovarian cancer was higher in the *MSH2* mutation carriers (10.4%) than in the *MLH1* mutation carriers (3.4%).

A total of 34 cases of breast cancer were identified in the 138 families – 7 in families associated with an *MLH1* mutation and 12 in families with an *MSH2* mutation. The mean age at diagnosis of breast cancer was 50.6 years (range: 26–74 years). The distribution of the ages at diagnosis is depicted in Figure 5.2. The risk of developing breast cancer was equal to the risk in the general population in the Netherlands.

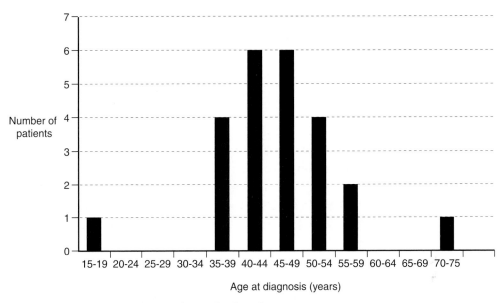

Figure 5.1   Distribution of ages at diagnosis of ovarian cancer.

Breast and ovarian cancer in other hereditary colorectal cancer syndromes

Cancer of the breast and ovaries has also been observed in two hereditary colorectal cancer syndromes associated with hamartomatous polyposis, i.e. the Peutz–Jeghers syndrome and Cowden syndrome.

Peutz–Jeghers syndrome

Peutz–Jeghers (PJ) syndrome is characterized by hamartomatous polyps in the small bowel and pigmented macules of the buccal mucosa and lips (Vasen, 2000). The syndrome is caused by germline mutations in *STK11/LKB1*, a serine–threonine kinase located on chromosome 19. The PJ syndrome is associated with an increased risk of developing cancer. The most frequently occurring cancers are cancer of the colon and breast. A retrospective study for determining cancer risk in PJ families assigned a relative risk (RR) for breast cancer or gynaecological cancer of 20.3 (Boardman et al., 2001). The mean age at diagnosis of breast cancer was 39 years. Recently, Giardello and others performed an individual patient meta-analysis to determine the relative risk (RR) of cancer in patients with PJ syndrome compared with the general population based on 210 individuals described in six publications (Giardiello et al., 2000). The RR for breast cancer was 15.2 (95% CI: 7.6–27) and the RR for ovarian cancer was 27 (95% CI: 7.3–68). The absolute risks of developing breast and ovarian cancer by the age of 64 years were 54% and 21%

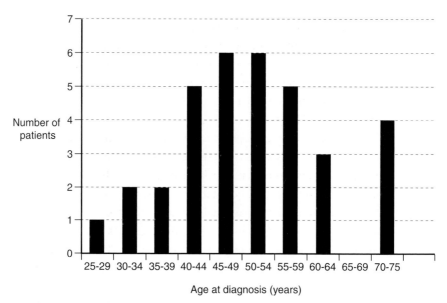

Figure 5.2   Distribution of ages at diagnosis of breast cancer.

respectively, which is comparable with families that carry a mutation in *BRCA1* and *BRCA2*.

In spite of the early onset of breast and ovarian cancer that can be seen in patients with the PJ syndrome, mutations in *STK11/LKB1* do not appear to play a role in sporadic breast cancer, based on the very low prevalence of mutations in the populations.

Cowden syndrome

Cowden syndrome is a rare autosomal predisposition characterized by multiple hamartomas and a high risk of breast, thyroid and, perhaps, other cancers (Eng, 2000). These hamartomas can arise in tissues derived from all three embryogenic germ-cell layers. The cardinal features of this syndrome include trichilemmomas, which are hamartomas of the infundibulum of the hair follicle, and mucocutaneous papillomatous papules. Breast cancer develops in 20–30% of female carriers. Other tumours seen among patients with Cowden syndrome include: adenomas and follicular cell carcinomas of the thyroid; polyps and adenocarcinomas of the gastrointestinal tract; and ovarian cysts and carcinoma. Cowden syndrome is caused by germline mutations in the *PTEN* gene.

Surveillance recommendations

In conclusion, several studies reported a substantially increased risk of developing ovarian cancer both in PJ syndrome and in HNPCC. Surveillance of the ovaries might lead to an earlier diagnosis and improvement of the prognosis. The protocol that is usually recommended comprises annual gynaecological examination, transvaginal ultrasound and estimation of CA125. Because the effectiveness of this protocol is uncertain, bilateral salpingo-oophorectomy is recommended in mutation carriers with a complete family. As almost all ovarian cancers observed in PJ syndrome and HNPCC were diagnosed in patients who were more than 30 years of age, the surveillance programme might start from this age.

There is also consensus that female members from families with PJ syndrome and Cowden syndrome have an increased risk of developing breast cancer. The surveillance protocol that is usually recommended in high-risk families includes annual mammography, biannual palpation of the breasts by a physician and monthly self-breast examination. As most studies do not indicate that breast cancer is part of the tumour spectrum of HNPCC, surveillance of the breasts appears not to be justified. On the other hand, clinicians managing HNPCC patients should always be alert when the patient exhibits unusual symptoms.

REFERENCES

Aarnio M, Sankila R, Pukkala E, et al. (1999). Cancer risk in mutation carriers of DNA-mismatch-repair genes. *Int J Cancer* **81**: 214–18.

Boardman LA, Thibodeau SN and Schaid DJ (2001). Increased risk for cancer in patients with the Peutz–Jeghers syndrome. *Ann Intern Med* **128**: 896–9.

Boyd J, Rhei E, Federici MG, et al. (1999). Male breast cancer in the hereditary nonpolyposis colorectal cancer syndrome. *Breast Cancer Res Treat* **53**: 87–91.

Eng C (2000). Will the real Cowden syndrome please stand up: revised diagnostic criteria. *J Med Genet* **37**: 828–30.

Giardiello FM, Brensinger JD, Tersmette AC, et al. (2000). Very high risk of cancer in familial Peutz–Jeghers syndrome. *Gastroenterology* **119**: 1447–53.

Lynch HT and de la Chapelle A (1999). Genetic susceptibility to non-polyposis colorectal cancer. *J Med Genet* **36**: 801–18.

Risinger JI, Barrett JC, Watson P, Lynch HT and Boyd J (1996). Molecular genetic evidence of the occurrence of breast cancer as an integral tumor in patients with the hereditary non-polyposis colorectal carcinoma syndrome. *Cancer* **77**: 1836–43.

Sankila R, Aaltonen LA, Jarvinen HJ and Mecklin JP (1996). Better survival rates in patients with MLH1-associated hereditary colorectal cancer. *Gastroenterology* **110**: 682–7.

Scott RJ, McPhillips M, Meldrum CJ, et al. (2001). Hereditary nonpolyposis colorectal cancer in 95 families: differences and similarities between mutation-positive and mutation-negative kindreds. *Am J Hum Genet* **68**: 118–27.

Vasen HF (2000). Clinical diagnosis and management of hereditary colorectal cancer syndromes. *J Clin Oncol* **18**: S81–92.

Vasen HF, Wijnen JT, Menko FH, et al. (1996). Cancer risk in families with hereditary nonpolyposis colorectal cancer diagnosed by mutation analysis. *Gastroenterology* **110**: 1020–7.

Vasen HF, Watson P, Mecklin JP and Lynch HT (1999). New clinical criteria for hereditary nonpolyposis colorectal cancer (HNPCC, Lynch syndrome) proposed by the International Collaborative group on HNPCC. *Gastroenterology* **116**: 453–6.

Watson P and Lynch HT (1993). Extracolonic cancer in hereditary nonpolyposis colorectal cancer. *Cancer* **71**: 677–85.

6

The natural history of hereditary breast cancer

Pierre O. Chappuis[1], Dominique Stoppa-Lyonnet[2], Bernard Asselain[2] and William D. Foulkes[1,3,4]

[1]McGill University Health Centre, Montreal, QC, Canada
[2]Institut Curie, Paris, France
[3]Sir M. B. Davis-Jewish General Hospital, McGill University, Montreal, QC, Canada
[4]McGill University, Montreal, QC, Canada

Summary

Determining the outcome following hereditary breast cancer is one of the key questions in clinical breast cancer genetics. There is increasing evidence that *BRCA1*- and *BRCA2*-related breast cancers are distinguishable from non-hereditary breast cancers: hereditary cancers demonstrate gene expression profiles and somatic genetic changes that are distinct from those seen in sporadic breast cancers and feature histopathological and immunohistochemical characteristics usually associated with a worse prognosis. Despite these findings, conflicting data exist as to whether the prognosis of hereditary breast cancer differs from that of sporadic cases. Some of the discrepancies may be explained by methodological differences or biases. However, no mutation-based studies have shown a survival advantage for *BRCA1/2* mutation carriers and several unrelated studies have recently found that the presence of a *BRCA1/2* mutation was an independent poor prognostic factor. Regarding the risk of further or recurrent breast cancer, it is established that the risk of contralateral breast cancer is significantly increased in breast cancer patients harbouring *BRCA1/2* germline mutations, but surprisingly, during the first 5 years after diagnosis, an increase in the rate of ipsilateral breast recurrences has not been found. These data suggest that radiation may protect against, or at least delay, ipsilateral recurrences.

Introduction

Up to five per cent of breast cancer cases are hereditary and germline mutations in the breast cancer predisposing genes *BRCA1* and *BRCA2* may account for 65–80%

of the hereditary cases (Ford et al., 1998; Rahman and Stratton, 1998). It is unclear whether the prognosis of hereditary breast cancer differs from that of sporadic cases. In hereditary non-polyposis colorectal cancer, patients with constitutional mutations in the *MLH1* or *MSH2* genes have been found to have a better prognosis than those without mutations (Sankila et al., 1996; Watson et al., 1998). Whether or not the same survival advantage is true for hereditary breast cancer is unclear.

Compared with its sporadic counterpart, distinct somatic genetic changes have been reported in hereditary breast cancer (Tirkkonen et al., 1997) and a recent study showed that gene-expression profiles are significantly different between both *BRCA1*- and *BRCA2*-related breast cancers and sporadic cases (Hedenfalk et al., 2001). Somatic mutations in *BRCA1* or *BRCA2* are extremely rare in sporadic breast cancer, supporting the hypothesis of a different carcinogenic mechanism in hereditary cases (Futreal et al., 1994). However, an extensive immunohistochemical study showed that most (non-hereditary) grade III breast cancers expressed low levels of BRCA1 (Wilson et al., 1999), suggesting an important role for *BRCA1* in most aggressive breast cancer, irrespective of the presence of a germline mutation. Pathological features also suggest that there are underlying differences in hereditary breast cancer compared with sporadic cases (see Chapter 7). For example, *BRCA1*-associated tumours are more often poorly differentiated, highly proliferating tumours, with a high frequency of oestrogen receptor negativity, and a higher rate of p53 mutations (Chappuis et al., 2000a; Phillips, 2000). Nevertheless, *BRCA1*-associated tumours also demonstrate intratumoural infiltrating lymphocytes, an increased proportion of medullary histological type, less frequent node involvement and a relatively low HER2/erb-b2/neu over-expression (Lakhani et al., 1997; Chappuis et al., 2000a). Similarly, cancers associated with *BRCA2* mutations exhibit significant differences when compared with age-matched sporadic cases, such as a reduction in tubule formation, a higher proportion of continuous pushing margins and a lower mitotic count (Lakhani et al., 1998).

Evaluation of the risks of development of ipsi- and contralateral breast cancers and survival rates may reveal further information on the biological differences between hereditary and sporadic tumours. Survival information is essential for decision-making regarding preventive and therapeutic strategies and thus for counselling women at increased risk of breast cancer.

Studies that examine differences in outcome between hereditary and sporadic cases of breast cancer can be grouped into three study categories: family-history-based, linkage-based and mutation-based. Family-history-based studies were particularly useful prior to the localization of the *BRCA1* and *BRCA2* genes. However, the definition of hereditary breast cancer has not been clearly established. Moreover, not all women with a family history of breast cancer have *BRCA1/2* mutations, and not all *BRCA1/2* affected carriers have a family history of breast cancer. It is known that familial clustering of postmenopausal breast cancer occurs, which has not been attributed to a genetic syndrome. Therefore, studies based on family history have the disadvantage of grouping true hereditary cases with those of familial clustering. Family-history-based studies have been previously reviewed (Chappuis et al., 1999) and will not be discussed further.

This chapter offers a review of the literature in an attempt to answer the question of whether *BRCA1/2* status – established either by linkage or by mutation-based studies – influences the risk of ipsilateral recurrence, contralateral new primary breast cancer and, ultimately, distant recurrence and death following breast cancer.

Ipsi- and contralateral breast cancer recurrences

Lumpectomy followed by radiation therapy, i.e. the conservative management of breast cancer, has been accepted as a standard of care for the majority of women with early breast cancer. Long-term follow-up data have consistently shown a risk of ipsilateral breast tumour recurrence (IBTR) of 0.5–2% per year (Recht et al., 1988; Fourquet et al., 1989; Kurtz et al., 1989; Fisher et al., 1991; Veronesi et al., 1995), but breast cancer survival was not significantly affected by IBTR when compared with patients undergoing a radical mastectomy (Haffty et al., 1991a; Fisher et al., 1995; Jacobson et al., 1995; Veronesi et al., 1995; Winchester et al., 1997). Early age of onset is associated with an increased risk of IBTR (Schnitt et al., 1984; Haffty et al., 1991b; de la Rochefordière et al., 1993), but an association was not consistently found when the patient reported a positive family history of breast cancer (Chabner et al., 1998; Harrold et al., 1998). Young age at primary breast cancer diagnosis, a family history of breast cancer, lobular histology type and radiation exposure at an early age are risk factors classically associated with the development of contralateral breast cancer (Dawson et al., 1998; Chen et al., 1999; Neugut et al., 1999). Although one large case-control study (Boice et al., 1992) found a slight increase (RR = 1.6) in contralateral breast cancer risk associated with radiotherapy in young women (< 45 years), most studies, including large randomized trials, that have evaluated adjuvant radiotherapy after breast conservative surgery for invasive or non-invasive breast carcinoma have not shown a significant increase in the number of contralateral cancers (Hankey et al., 1983; Fisher et al., 1985; Bernstein et al., 1992; Storm et al., 1992; Veronesi et al., 1994; Jacobson et al., 1995; Arriagada et al., 1996; Fisher et al., 1998a; Chen et al., 1999). Of note, the majority of the patients reported by Boice et al. were treated before 1960 with techniques and equipment that are no longer in use.

Studies that have evaluated the ipsi- and contralateral breast cancer recurrences among the patients either linked to *BRCA1* or *BRCA2* or identified as *BRCA1/2* germline mutation carriers are summarized in Tables 6.1 and 6.2, respectively. As expected, as all mammary cells are carrying a mutated *BRCA1* or *BRCA2* allele, a statistically significant excess of contralateral breast cancers has been noted in all studies. Unexpectedly, this has not been the case for ipsilateral breast cancer. A systematic evaluation of chest wall relapse rates after mastectomy has not been performed among patients with *BRCA1/2* mutations and all studies reported here have not discriminated between true local recurrence or new primary tumour (Smith et al., 2000) and counted recurrences and new primaries altogether. In spite of that, none of the studies showed an excess of ipsilateral recurrences. Only five groups have concomitantly evaluated the risk of IBTR and contralateral breast cancers in their series of *BRCA1/2* mutation carriers and non-carrier patients (Verhoog et al., 1998; Robson et al., 1999; Chappuis et al., 2000b; Pierce et al., 2000; Stoppa-Lyonnet et al., 2000). By combining data from two similarly design-ed historical cohorts, we determined the number of ipsi- and contralateral breast cancers found among 466 consecutive women who were diagnosed with primary invasive breast cancer at Memorial Sloan-Kettering Cancer Center, New York, and SMBD-Jewish General Hospital, Montreal (Foulkes et al., 2000a). All of these patients underwent conservative surgery plus adjuvant radiotherapy between 1980 and 1995 and were followed up for a median of nearly 9 years. All women were Ashkenazi Jewish and all were tested for the three common founder mutations: 185delAG and 5382insC in *BRCA1* and 6174delT in *BRCA2*. A total of 54 mutations were identified: 42 in *BRCA1* and 12 in *BRCA2*. There was no excess of ipsilateral breast cancer observed among mutation carriers, compared with non-carriers (hazard ratio, HR, 1.4; 95% CI 0.5–3.7; $P=0.48$), whereas the risk for contralateral breast cancer was markedly elevated (HR 4.7; 95% CI 2.0–9.1; $P=0.0003$). Of note, in the Offit and colleagues' study (Robson et al., 1999), the probability of IBTR was 22% at 10 years among Ashkenazi Jewish *BRCA1/2* mutation carriers compared with 7% among the non-carriers. This difference was not significant ($P=0.25$). Moreover, only five events were recorded among 35 *BRCA1/2* mutation carriers. In a retrospective cohort of 71 women with a *BRCA1/ 2* mutation and stage I and II breast cancer treated with breast-conserving therapy, there was no significant difference in rates of IBTR compared with matched sporadic controls after a median follow-up time of 5 years (Pierce et al., 2000). Interestingly, the median time to local recurrence was 8.2 years for the three patients in the genetic cohort compared with 3.1 years for the sporadic cohort. Turner et al. screened a cohort of 52 conservatively treated patients with IBTR for germline *BRCA1/2* mutations and a matched control group without IBTR (Turner et al., 1999). *BRCA1/2* mutations were significantly more frequent in the group of early-onset (<40 years) breast cancer patients who experienced IBTR ($P<0.03$).

Table 6.1. Contralateral breast cancer in *BRCA1/2* mutation carriers: *BRCA1/2* linkage-based studies

Study	Population	*BRCA*-related BC cases	Controls	Median follow-up	Results (cases vs controls)	P
Ford et al., 1994	BOC families linked to *BRCA1* (BCLC)	33 families mut. carriers	—	n/s	Cumulative risk: by age 50 yr: 48% by age 70 yr: 64%	—
Porter et al., 1994	*BRCA1*-linked families (Edinburgh, UK)	35 *BRCA1* mut. carriers	910 age-matched	n/s	13/35 (37%)	—
Easton et al., 1995	BOC families linked to *BRCA1* (BCLC)	33 families	—	n/s	Cumulative risk: by age 40 yr: 33% by age 50 yr: 50% by age 60 yr: 60% (95% CI, 41–73%) by age 70 yr: 65%	—
Marcus et al., 1996	HBOC families (≥3 BC) (Omaha, USA)	72 *BRCA1* mut. carriers 66 *BRCA2*/other mut. carriers	187	3.6 years (*BRCA1*) 5 years (*BRCA2*/other) 8.3 years (controls)	*BRCA1*: 20/72 (28%) vs 10/130 (8%) 10 yr: 38% (95% CI, 24–58%) *BRCA2*/other: 13/66 (20%) vs 10/130 (8%) 10 yr: 21% (95% CI, 10–39%)	0.0003 0.019

BC, breast cancer; BCLC, Breast Cancer Linkage Consortium; BOC, breast/ovarian cancer; CI, confidence intervals; HBOC, hereditary breast/ovarian cancer; n/s, not stated.

Note: None of the *BRCA1/2* linkage-based studies reported data on ipsilateral breast cancer recurrence.

Table 6.2. Ipsi- and contralateral breast cancer in *BRCA1/2* mutation carriers: *BRCA1/2* mutation-based studies

Study	Population	BRCA-related BC cases	Controls	Median follow-up	Ipsilateral BC results (cases vs controls)	P	Contralateral BC results (cases vs controls)	P
Ansquer et al., 1998	BC <36 yr (Paris, France)	15 *BRCA1*	108 *BRCA1* mutation-negative	3.6 yr	—	—	23% vs 4%[b]	<0.01
Frank et al., 1998	BC <50 yr or OC + positive FH (Myriad Genetic Lab, USA)	63 *BRCA1* 31 *BRCA2*	n/s	n/s	—	—	Rate/yr: *BRCA1/2*: 5.2% vs 2.8% *BRCA1*: 5.6% vs 2.8% *BRCA2*: 4.2% vs 2.8%	0.014
Gaffney et al., 1998	*BRCA1/2* mutation carriers with BC (Utah, USA)	30 *BRCA1* 20 *BRCA2* BCT: 7/56 (13%)	17 396 matched for age, yr of diagnosis, and tumour BCT: n/s	9.8 yr (*BRCA1*) 7.5 yr (*BRCA2*) 3.8 yr (BCT)	*BRCA1*: 1/4 (25%) *BRCA2*: 0/3 (0%)	—	*BRCA1*: 4/30 (13%) *BRCA2*: 2/20 (10%)	—
Johannsson et al., 1998	BC families (Lund, Sweden)	40 *BRCA1*	112 matched for age, yr of diagnosis, and stage	n/s	—	—	8/40 (20%) vs 7/112 (6%)	0.026
Robson et al., 1998	AJ patients with BC <42 yr (New York, USA)	30 AJ *BRCA1/2*[a] BCT: 9/28 (32%)	61 AJ *BRCA1/2* mutation[a]-negative BCT: 25/59 (42%)	BCT: 5.5 yr (cases) 3.7 yr (controls) 5.2 yr (contra)	1/9 (11%) vs 6/25 (24%)	0.65	5 yr: 31% vs 4%	0.0007
Verhoog et al., 1998	BC families (Rotterdam, the Netherlands)	49 *BRCA1* BCT: 18/48 (38%)	196 matched for age, yr of diagnosis, and stage BCT: 90/190 (47%)	n/s	5 yr: 14% vs 16%	0.84	Synchronous: 2/49 (4%) vs 1/196 (0.5%) Metachronous: 10/49 (20%) vs 11/196 (6%) 5 yr: 19% vs 5%	0.10 0.003 0.02

Study	Description	BRCA mutation / BCT	Controls	Follow-up	Local recurrence	p	Outcome	p
Wagner et al., 1998	BC families or BC ≤30 yr (Vienna, Austria)	34 BRCA1 BCT: n/s	328 N0 BCT: n/s	7.5 yr (cases) 6 yr (controls)	Local recurrence: 6/34 (18%) vs 8/68 (12%)	0.54	—	—
Breast Cancer Linkage Consortium, 1999	BOC families	173 families with BRCA2 mutation	—	—	—	—	Cumulative risk: by age 50 yr: 37% (95% CI, 26–47%) by age 70 yr: 52% (95% CI, 42–61%)	—
Noguchi et al., 1999	BC families (Osaka and Tokyo, Japan)	BRCA1: 19 BRCA2: 14	100 matched for age; no FH	n/s	—	—	BRCA1: 6/19 (32%) vs 6/100 (6%)[b] BRCA2: 4/14 (29%) vs 6/100 (6%)[b]	<0.01 <0.05
Robson et al., 1999	AJ BC patients with BCT (New York, USA)	22 AJ BRCA1[a] 7 AJ BRCA2[a]	277 AJ BRCA1/2 mutation[a]-negative	10.3 yr	5 yr: 15% vs 5% 10 yr: 22% vs 7% RR: 1.8 (0.6–5)	0.25	5 yr: 15% vs 4% 10 yr: 27% vs 10% RR: 3.5 (1.8–8.7)	0.002 0.001
Turner et al., 1999	BC + metachronous IBTR (New Haven, USA)	5 BRCA1 3 BRCA2	44 IBTR BRCA1/2 mutation-negative, matched for age, yr of diagnosis, stage and histological subtype	14.5 yr	—	—	5/8 (63%) vs 6/44 (14%)	0.007
Verhoog et al., 1999	BC families (Rotterdam, the Netherlands)	28 BRCA2 BCT: 10/28 (36%)	112 matched for age and yr of diagnosis BCT: 56/112 (50%)	n/s	—	—	Synchronous: 1/28 (4%) vs 3/111 (3%) Metachronous: 7/28 (25%) vs 5/111 (4%) 5 yr: 12% vs 2%	NS 0.003 0.02

Table 6.2. (cont.)

Study	Population	BRCA-related BC cases	Controls	Median follow-up	Ipsilateral BC results (cases vs controls)	P	Contralateral BC results (cases vs controls)	P
Chappuis et al., 2000b	AJ patients with BC <65 yr BCT: 189/202 (94%) (Montreal, Canada)	24 AJ BRCA1[a], 8 AJ BRCA2[a]	170 AJ BRCA1/2 mutation[a]-negative	6.4 yr	5 yr: 6% vs 7%	0.93	5 yr: 10% vs 2%	0.02
Foulkes et al., 2000a[c]	AJ BC patients with BCT (Montreal, Canada, and New York, USA)	42 AJ BRCA1[a], 12 AJ BRCA2[a]	413 AJ BRCA1/2 mutation[a]-negative	8.6 yr (BCT), 8.8 yr (contra)	5 yr: 13% vs 5%, 8.6 yr: 13% vs 5%, HR: 1.4 (0.5–3.7)	0.07, NS	5 yr: 14% vs 3%, 8.8 yr: 33% vs 7%, HR: 4.7 (2.4–9.1)	0.0001, 0.0003
Gershoni-Baruch et al., 2000a	AJ patients with BC ≤42 yr (Israel)	42 AJ BRCA1[a], 13 AJ BRCA2[a]	118 AJ BRCA1/2 mutation[a]-negative	6.3 yr (cases), 8.3 yr (controls)	—	—	15/54 (28%) vs 8/118 (7%)	<0.001
Haffty et al., 2000	BRCA1/2-related BC patients with BCT (New Haven, USA)	13 BRCA1, 7 BRCA2	—	13.6 yr	5 yr: 17%, 10 yr: 36%	—	5 yr: 16%, 10 yr: 28%	—
Hamann and Sinn, 2000	BC families (Germany)	36 BRCA1	49 HBC BRCA1 mutation-negative	5.6 yr	—	—	5 yr: 24% vs 6%, 10 yr: 42% vs 6%	0.04

Study	Population	Mutations	Controls	Follow-up	Result		Result	P
Loman et al., 2000	BC families (Lund, Sweden, and Odense, Denmark)	36 BRCA2	214 matched for age and yr of diagnosis; no FH	8.1 yr (cases) 8.9 yr (controls)	—	—	12/54 (22%) vs 22/214 (10%) RR: 2.4 (1.1–5.3)	0.027
Pierce et al., 2000	Stage I–II BC women with BCT (Canada and the USA)	54 BRCA1 17 BRCA2	213 matched for age, yr of diagnosis, and stage	5.3 yr (cases) 4.6 yr (controls)	5 yr: 2% vs 4% HR: 0.85	0.8	5 yr: 20% vs 2% HR: 8.6	<0.0001 <0.0001
Stoppa-Lyonnet et al., 2000	BC families (cohort study) BCT: 74% (Paris, France)	40 BRCA1	143 BRCA1 mutation-negative; FH-positive	7.3 yr (cases) 4.6 yr (controls)	Local recurrence: 5 yr: 17% vs 15%	0.16	Synchronous: 2/40 (5%) vs 7/143 (5%) Metachronous: 14% vs 17%	0.80 NS
Verhoog et al., 2000a	BRCA1-related BC patients (Rotterdam, the Netherlands)	164 BRCA1	—	3.9 yr	—	—	First primary BC <50 yr vs ≥50 yr: 36/124 (29%) vs 3/40 (8%) 5 yr: 30% vs 4% 10 yr: 40% vs 12%	0.005 0.02

[a] Ashkenazi Jewish BRCA1/2 mutations: BRCA1 – 185delAG, 5382insC; BRCA2 – 6174delT.

[b] Synchronous and metachronous.

[c] Combined from two previous studies (Robson et al., 1999; Chappuis et al., 2000b).

AJ, Ashkenazi Jewish; BC, breast cancer; BCT, breast conservative therapy; BOC, breast/ovarian cancer; FH, family history; HBC, hereditary breast cancer; HR, hazard ratio; IBTR, ipsilateral breast tumour recurrence; N0, axillary node negative; NS, not significant (at 5% level); n/s, not stated; OC, ovarian cancer; yr, year(s).

Again, in this study, the median time to IBTR for patients with *BRCA1/2* mutations was nearly 8 years – significantly longer than for patients without *BRCA1/2* mutations (4.7 years; $P = 0.03$). Clinico-histopathological data suggested that late IBTRs were in fact second primary tumours and not true recurrences. All patients carrying *BRCA1/2* mutations underwent successful surgical salvage treatment (mastectomy) at the time of IBTR and were alive without relapse after a median follow-up time of 7.7 years after breast relapse. The design of this later study did not address the question of a higher likelihood of local recurrences associated with *BRCA1/2* mutations, but its findings suggest that there is no increase in early recurrences in patients with *BRCA1/2* mutations.

Under the assumption that new primary cancers should occur at the same frequency in either breast, these data are consistent with the hypothesis that radiotherapy reduces cancer incidence in the treated breast, or significantly delays the appearance of emerging cancers. Prospective studies with long follow-up will be required to confirm the hypothesis of an increased likelihood of late IBTR in *BRCA1/2* mutation carriers after lumpectomy and radiation therapy. A less compelling alternate hypothesis – that radiation scatter may contribute to an increase in contralateral cancers – has also been suggested (Bennett, 1999; Robson et al., 1999). In fact, concern has been expressed that exposure to diagnostic or therapeutic radiation might be hazardous for women who carry *BRCA1* or *BRCA2* mutations (Chakraborty et al., 1998; Bennett, 1999; Formenti et al., 2000). BRCA1 and BRCA2 are involved in the repair of DNA damage of the type that is induced by ionizing radiation, and it is feared that x-rays will be mutagenic and will increase the breast cancer risk. The capability of *BRCA1* heterozygous cells to repair double-strand DNA breaks is impaired, relative to *BRCA1* wild-type cell-lines (Foray et al., 1999). Similarly, mammalian cells lacking functional *BRCA1* or *BRCA2* are hypersensitive to agents that cause oxidative DNA damage or double-strand DNA breaks (Connor et al., 1997; Sharan et al., 1997; Abbott et al., 1998; Chen et al., 1998; Gowen et al., 1998; Morimatsu et al., 1998). Exposing cell-lines that carry *BRCA1* or *BRCA2* mutations to gamma radiation reduces their survival. One interpretation of these data is that the *BRCA1* or *BRCA2* mutation renders the breast cells particularly radiation-sensitive, which results in increased cell death. Therefore, it is possible that those breast cancers that develop in *BRCA1/2* mutation carriers will be particularly sensitive to the effects of radiotherapy. Verhoog et al. reported a rate of contralateral breast cancers of 19% at 5 years in a series of 49 patients with *BRCA1*-related breast cancers (Verhoog et al., 1998) and of 12% among 28 breast cancer patients with *BRCA2* mutations (Verhoog et al., 1999) – a similar rate of contralateral breast cancer seen in the study by Weber and colleagues (Pierce et al., 2000). Two-thirds of the patients in Verhoog et al.'s studies were treated with mastectomy; thus these data do not suggest an increased rate of second cancers in the opposite breast that is attributable to scatter radiation. Moreover, radiotherapy in *BRCA1* and *BRCA2* mutation carriers is not associated with an excess of acute or chronic radiation-induced toxicities (Gaffney et al., 1998; Leong et al., 2000; Pierce et al., 2000).

Regarding the implications of these data for breast cancer screening, Brekelmans et al. reported the first evaluation of a breast cancer surveillance programme among a series of 128 *BRCA1/2* mutation carriers (Brekelmans et al., 2001). Effectiveness of physical examination every 6 months and yearly mammography was evaluated and compared with 449 moderate women and 621 high-risk women. Within a median follow-up of 3 years, the highest cancer detection rates and observed/expected ratio were observed among the *BRCA1/2* mutation carriers ($n = 9$ cases; ratio observed/expected: 23.7), but the cancers were not diagnosed at a particularly early stage (five cases were axillary nodes positive). Even more worrying, five cases were in fact interval cancers, giving the worse sensitivity (56%) of the screening among the *BRCA1/2* mutation carriers. These preliminary data could be interpreted as indicating the need for a more intensive screening scheme or the development of new approaches. For example, the effectiveness of magnetic resonance imaging in the early detection of breast cancer in high-risk women could be of great interest (Kuhl et al., 2000).

Following the publication of the results of the National Surgical Adjuvant Breast and Bowel (NSABP) P1 trial, which showed a significant reduction of invasive ($P<0.0001$) and non-invasive ($P<0.002$) breast cancer among the patients taking tamoxifen as a preventive agent (Fisher et al., 1998b), the question of the efficiency of tamoxifen as a chemopreventive drug in the *BRCA1/2* mutation carrier group became crucial. To date, a single case-control study evaluating the protection against contralateral breast cancer in *BRCA1/2* mutation carriers has been published (Narod et al., 2000). Tamoxifen use was associated with a statistically significant reduction (odds ratio, OR, 0.5; 95% CI 0.3–0.9) in contralateral breast cancer. The protective effect of tamoxifen increased with duration of tamoxifen use by up to 4 years. Interestingly, an even stronger and long-lasting protective effect of oophorectomy (OR 0.4; 95% CI 0.2–0.8) was noted. A similar risk reduction of primary breast cancer after prophylactic oophorectomy among *BRCA1* mutation carriers has been previously published (Rebbeck et al., 1999). Moreover, the effects of tamoxifen and oophorectomy in reducing the risk of contralateral breast cancer were independent (Narod et al., 2000). Despite the absence of studies that have evaluated tamoxifen as a preventive agent of primary breast cancer among *BRCA1/2* mutation carriers, it seems reasonable to speculate that tamoxifen will also reduce the occurrence of primary cancers in *BRCA1* and/or *BRCA2* mutation carriers. Based on the oestrogen receptor status of primary breast cancers in *BRCA1* and *BRCA2* mutation carriers, one would predict that tamoxifen will be effective in preventing BRCA2-, but not BRCA1-, related breast cancer.

In summary, breast conservative surgery associated with radiation is an acceptable option of treatment for patients who harbour BRCA1 or BRCA2 germline mutations. There are currently no definitive data, particularly from prospective studies, that demonstrate a significant increase in IBTR rates among these patients when compared with sporadic breast cancer patients. The best way to explain these data is that therapeutic radiation in BRCA1 or BRCA2 mutation carriers reduces (or delays) the incidence of new cancers in the treated breast. Further observational studies to validate this hypothesis are now underway. Environmental and genetic factors that may modulate the risk of developing a second primary breast cancer (and a fortiori the first one) among BRCA1/2 mutation carriers are also under investigation (Narod et al., 1995a; Gershoni-Baruch et al., 2000b).

Linkage-based studies and survival

In two of the three linkage-based studies (Table 6.3), BRCA1-linked cases were found to have a better prognosis than controls (Porter et al., 1994; Marcus et al., 1996). In the first study, 35 breast cancer patients from eight BRCA1-linked families had an 83% 5-year survival (Porter et al., 1994). The survival for age-matched controls was 61%. Similarly, Lynch and colleagues reported a 5-year survival of 67% in BRCA1-linked cases and 63% in the BRCA2/other gene-linked group, compared with 59% in controls (Marcus et al., 1996). However, after correcting for age and stage, the adjusted crude death HR for BRCA1- and BRCA2/other gene-linked cases was 1.7 ($P=0.12$) and 1.4 ($P=0.18$), respectively. The third linkage-based study examined 42 BRCA2-linked breast cancer patients from five families in Iceland (Sigurdsson et al., 1996). The 10-year overall survival was 45% in cases, compared with 65% in controls ($P<0.05$). No data are yet available regarding the survival rate for the patients linked to the putative breast cancer susceptibility locus identified on 13q21 (Kainu et al., 2000).

The interpretation of linkage-based studies is problematic. There are sources of bias inherent in the study design, and additional confounders exist in each study. In the study by Porter et al. (1994), differences in stage were not taken into account. Secondly, cases and controls were not matched for date of diagnosis, cases being diagnosed from 1942 to 1992, while controls were diagnosed from 1971 to 1973. As such, treatment may have differed. In support of this possibility, the 5-year survival rate in the control group was 59%, which is lower than one would expect now. Also, four families in the study had a probability of linkage of less than 95%. A sporadic early-onset breast cancer case in a family investigated by linkage analysis can result in a negative lod score. In fact, some families with

Table 6.3. Breast cancer and survival: *BRCA1/2* linkage-based studies

Study	Population	BRCA-related BC cases	Controls	Median follow-up	Results (cases vs controls)	P
Porter et al., 1994	*BRCA1*-linked families (Edinburgh, UK)	35 *BRCA1* 8 families	910 age-matched	n/s	5-yr OS: 83% vs 61%	<0.05
Marcus et al., 1996	HBC families (≥3 BC) (Omaha, USA)	72 *BRCA1* 66 *BRCA2*/other	187	3.6 yr (*BRCA1*) (*BRCA2*/other) 8.3 yr (controls)	5-yr OS: (1) *BRCA1*: 67% vs 59% (2) *BRCA2*/other: 63% vs 59%	0.051 0.15
Sigurdsson et al., 1996	HBC families (Reykjavik, Iceland)	42 *BRCA2* 5 families	115 age-matched	n/s	10-yr DFS: 40% vs 55% 10-yr OS: 45% vs 65%	0.009 <0.05

BC, breast cancer; DFS, disease-free survival; HBC, hereditary breast cancer; n/s, not stated; OS, overall survival; yr, years.

negative lod scores at the *BRCA1* locus actually do carry a *BRCA1* germline mutation (Narod et al., 1995b). In the study of Marcus et al. (1996), only 51% of cases were evaluated for survival and they were diagnosed at a younger age than were controls (average age of 42.8 years in cases versus 62.9 years in controls). In addition, there were more stage I and II tumours in the linked groups. It is therefore of interest that, after adjusting for age and stage, there was a non-significant trend towards worse survival in the linked groups ($P = 0.12$ for *BRCA1*-linked cases; $P = 0.18$ for *BRCA2*/other gene-linked cases). In a preliminary report from Icelandic women with breast cancer, *BRCA2*-linked cases had a worse survival than controls (Sigurdsson et al., 1996). Linkage to *BRCA2* was an independent prognostic variable in multivariate analysis. However, this study is based on a small number of individuals from a population with only one common *BRCA2* mutation (999del5), and therefore it may not be possible to generalize from these results. Moreover, a more recent study of this Icelandic *BRCA2* mutation in the same population demonstrated no difference in survival when the control group was matched for age and year of diagnosis (Agnarsson et al., 1998). This probably reflects the impact of the improvement in the management and diagnosis of breast cancer during more recent decades.

Difficulties in linkage-based studies include the fact that they generally contain rather small numbers of living individuals. Families included are those in which several individuals have breast cancer, raising awareness and potentially leading to screening and lead-time bias. Ascertainment bias is probably a more important issue as, inevitably, living cases are preferentially included in the studies. Interestingly, an increased risk for breast cancer associated with recent birth cohort in *BRCA1* mutation carriers has been reported (Narod et al., 1995a). Therefore, results implying improved survival in the linked group must be interpreted with caution.

Mutation-based studies and survival

The mutation-based studies (Table 6.4) can be divided into four categories based on the study population selected. Five papers reported studies from a broad population of women with *BRCA1* mutations (Gaffney et al., 1998; Johannsson et al., 1998; Verhoog et al., 1998) or *BRCA2* mutations (Verhoog et al., 1999; Loman et al., 2000), five studies looked at specific founder *BRCA1/2* mutations in Ashkenazi Jewish women (Foulkes et al., 1997; Robson et al., 1998; Lee et al., 1999; Robson et al., 1999; Chappuis et al., 2000b), five studies reflected the experience of referral cancer clinics (Garcia-Patino et al., 1998; Wagner et al., 1998; Hamann and Sinn, 2000; Pierce et al., 2000; Stoppa-Lyonnet et al., 2000), one study selected *BRCA1* germline mutation carriers with early-onset breast cancer (Ansquer et al.,

1998), and one study reported results from the single *BRCA2* germline mutation identified in Iceland (Agnarsson et al., 1998).

In a previous review of the impact of familial and hereditary factors on breast cancer survival (Chappuis et al., 1999), we noted that 2 out of 10 studies showed a worse survival for women carrying *BRCA1/2* mutations (Foulkes et al., 1997; Ansquer et al., 1998), and no significant difference in survival between cases and controls was shown in the eight other studies (Agnarsson et al., 1998; Gaffney et al., 1998; Garcia-Patino et al., 1998; Johannsson et al., 1998; Robson et al., 1998; Verhoog et al., 1998; Wagner et al., 1998; Lee et al., 1999). Since the publication of this review, seven additional papers have been published. These more recent studies are characterized by a larger number of cases studied with a longer follow-up, and five of those showed a significantly worse survival for *BRCA1* or *BRCA2* mutation carriers (Robson et al., 1999; Chappuis et al., 2000b; Hamann and Sinn, 2000; Loman et al., 2000; Stoppa-Lyonnet et al., 2000). Twenty-eight *BRCA2* mutation carriers had a similar outcome to their age- and year-of-diagnosis-matched study conducted in the Netherlands (Verhoog et al., 1999), and a non-systematic study of stage I or II breast cancer patients with breast-conserving treatment showed no survival difference between *BRCA1/2* mutation carriers and non-carriers after a median follow-up of 5 years (Pierce et al., 2000). Thus, to date, none of the 17 mutation-based studies published has reported a better prognosis for breast cancer related to *BRCA1* or *BRCA2* germline mutations.

BRCA1-related (and to a lesser extent *BRCA2*-related) breast cancers harbour pathological features of tumours that are classically associated with a worse prognosis, such as high histological grade or negativity for oestrogen receptors (Chappuis et al., 2000a; Phillips, 2000). It is particularly interesting to compare the prognostic impact of *BRCA1/2* mutations with well-recognized prognostic factors such as tumour size, axillary node involvement, histological grade or negativity for oestrogen receptors. Using Cox multivariate analyses, Foulkes et al. showed that *BRCA1* mutation status was the only independent prognostic factor for overall survival in a historical cohort of Ashkenazi Jewish women with node-negative breast cancer living in Montreal, Canada (Foulkes et al., 2000b). They subsequently extended their findings in a larger study by including lymph-node-positive and -negative women with breast cancer from the same ethnic group and by lengthening the follow-up (Chappuis et al., 2000b). *BRCA1/2* mutation carrier status, as well as tumour size and p27^{Kip1} low expression, was identified as an independent prognostic factor for distant disease-free survival. Robson et al., using a similar historical cohort approach among Ashkenazi Jewish women from New York, USA, had previously shown in a larger series that *BRCA1/2* mutation status was a prognostic factor for all survival end-points, but only tumour stage and nodal

Table 6.4. Breast cancer and survival: *BRCA1/2* mutation-based studies

Study	Population	BRCA mutation carriers	Controls	Median follow-up	Results (cases vs controls)	P
Foulkes et al., 1997	AJ patients with BC <65 yr (Montreal, Canada)	12 AJ *BRCA1*[a]	100 AJ *BRCA1/2* mutation[a]-negative	3.3 yr	5-yr BCSS: 64% vs 96%	0.0023
Agnarsson et al., 1998	BC families (Reykjavik, Iceland)	40 *BRCA2*	160 matched for age and yr of diagnosis	n/s	10-yr OS: n/s	NS
Ansquer et al., 1998	BC <36 yr (Paris, France)	15 *BRCA1*	108 *BRCA1* mutation[a]-negative	3.6 yr	5-yr DFS: n/s 5-yr OS: 69% vs 83%	NS <0.04
Gaffney et al., 1998	*BRCA1/2* mutation carriers with BC (Utah, USA)	30 *BRCA1* 20 *BRCA2*	17 396 matched for age, yr of diagnosis and tumour	9.8 yr (*BRCA1*) 7.5 yr (*BRCA2*)	5-yr OS: 75% (*BRCA1*), 73% (*BRCA2*), 70% (controls)	NS
Garcia-Patino et al., 1998	Living patients with BC + no FH (Madrid, Spain)	9 *BRCA1*	96 *BRCA1* mutation[a]-negative	n/s	Median survival: 4.3 yr vs 2 yr	NS
Johannsson et al., 1998	BC families (Lund, Sweden)	40 *BRCA1*	112 matched for age, yr of diagnosis and stage	n/s	5-yr OS: 64% vs 80%	NS
Robson et al., 1998	Living AJ patients with BC <42 yr (New York, USA)	30 AJ *BRCA1/2*[a]	61 AJ *BRCA1/2* mutation[a]-negative	5.2 yr	5-yr DFS: 65% vs 69% 5-yr OS: n/s	NS NS
Verhoog et al., 1998	BC families (Rotterdam, the Netherlands)	49 *BRCA1*	196 matched for age, yr of diagnosis and stage	n/s	5-yr DFS: 49% vs 51% 5-yr OS: 63% vs 69%	NS NS
Wagner et al., 1998	BC families or BC <30 yr (Vienna, Austria)	34 *BRCA1*	328 N0	7.5 yr (cases) 6 yr (controls)	DFS: n/s OS: 74% vs 87% (N0 BC)	NS NS
Lee et al., 1999	AJ community-based (Washington DC, USA)	58 BC-affected FDR out of 50 AJ *BRCA1/2* mutation[a] carriers	979 matched for age and yr of diagnosis	n/s	5-yr OS: (1) *BRCA1*: 79% vs 78% (2) *BRCA2*: 65% vs 78% 20-yr OS: *BRCA1/2*: 41% vs 46%	NS NS NS

Reference	Population	Mutation carriers	Comparison group	Follow-up	Outcome	p
Robson et al., 1999	AJ BC patients with BCT (New York, USA)	22 AJ BRCA1[a] 7 AJ BRCA2[a]	277 AJ BRCA1/2 mutation[a]-negative	10.3 yr	5-yr DFS: 74% vs 91% 10-yr DFS: 66% vs 84% 5-yr BCSS: 85% vs 96% 10-yr BCSS: 72% vs 87% 5-yr OS: 82% vs 93% 10-yr OS: 66% vs 81%	0.05 0.02 0.05
Verhoog et al., 1999	BC families (Rotterdam, the Netherlands)	28 BRCA2	112 matched for age and yr of diagnosis	n/s	5-yr DFS: 52% vs 52% 5-yr OS: 74% vs 75%	NS NS
Chappuis et al., 2000b	AJ women with BC <65 yr (Montreal, Canada)	24 AJ BRCA1[a] 8 AJ BRCA2[a]	170 AJ BRCA1/2 mutation[a]-negative	6.4 yr	5-yr DFS: 58% vs 82% 5-yr OS: 61% vs 84%	0.003 0.0007
Foulkes et al., 2000a[b]	AJ BC patients with BCT (Montreal, Canada; New York, USA)	60 AJ BRCA1/2[a]	447 AJ BRCA1/2 mutation[a]-negative	9.3 yr	5-yr BCSS: 76% vs 93% 9.3-yr BCSS: 65% vs 86%	<0.001
Hamann and Sinn, 2000	BC families (Germany)	36 BRCA1	49 BC BRCA1 mutation-negative; FH-positive	5.6 yr	5-yr DFS: 53% vs 87% 5-yr OS: 84% vs 87%	0.02 NS
Loman et al., 2000	BC families (Lund, Sweden; Odense, Denmark)	54 BRCA2	214 matched for age and yr of diagnosis	8.1 yr (cases) 8.9 yr (controls)	5-yr BCSS: 76% vs 89% 10-yr BCSS: 59% vs 79% 5-yr OS: 72% vs 85% 10-yr OS: 58% vs 71%	0.003 0.06
Pierce et al., 2000	Stage I–II BC with BCT (Canada, USA)	54 BRCA1 17 BRCA2	213 matched for age, yr of diagnosis and stage	5.3 yr (cases) 4.6 yr (controls)	5-yr DFS: 78% vs 80% 5-yr OS: 86% vs 91%	NS
Stoppa-Lyonnet et al., 2000	BC families (cohort study) (Paris, France)	40 BRCA1	143 BRCA1 mutation-negative; FH-positive	7.3 yr (cases) 4.7 yr (controls)	5-yr BCSS: 81% vs 91% 5-yr OS: 80% vs 91%	0.015 0.002

[a] Ashkenazi Jewish BRCA1/2 mutations: BRCA1 – 185delAG, 5382insC; BRCA2 – 6174delT.

[b] Combined from two previous studies (Robson et al., 1999; Chappuis et al., 2000b).

AJ, Ashkenazi Jewish; BC, breast cancer; BCSS, breast-cancer-specific survival; BCT, breast-conservative treatment; DFS, disease-free survival; FDR, first-degree relative; FH, family history; N0, axillary node negative; NS, not significant (at 5% level); n/s, not stated; OS, overall survival; T, tumour size; yr, years.

status were predictive of distant disease-free and breast-cancer-specific survival in multivariate analysis (Robson et al., 1999). Interestingly, when the New York and Montreal series were combined, the cohort constituted 507 patients, of whom 60 were identified as *BRCA1/2* mutation carriers, with a median follow-up of 9.3 years (Foulkes et al., 2000a). In association with tumour size and nodal status, *BRCA1/2* mutation status was a strong independent prognostic factor for breast-cancer-specific survival.

Only one prospective study has been so far published. When early-onset breast cancer patients with *BRCA1* mutations were selected to be the cases, a worse 5-year overall survival was seen in the germline mutation carrier group (Ansquer et al., 1998). In a recent study from the same institution, Stoppa-Lyonnet et al. showed, in a series of breast cancer cases from breast/ovarian cancer families, that women identified as *BRCA1* mutation carriers had a significantly worse breast-cancer-specific or overall survival compared with *BRCA1* non-carriers (Stoppa-Lyonnet et al., 2000). In multivariate analyses, *BRCA1* mutation status was identified as an independent prognostic factor for both overall survival (RR: 3.5; 95% CI 1.3–9.7; $P = 0.02$) and metastasis-free survival (RR 2.6; 95% CI 1.0–6.5; $P = 0.05$).

A worse prognosis is not exclusively associated with *BRCA1* germline mutations (Verhoog et al., 2000b). Olsson and colleagues have published the largest series of *BRCA2*-mutation carriers with breast cancer (Loman et al., 2000). These patients had a significantly worse breast-cancer-specific survival when compared with a control group of patients matched for age and year of diagnosis (RR 2.0; 95% CI 1.2–3.4; $P = 0.01$). When stage was corrected for in the multivariate analysis, *BRCA2* mutation status was not an independent prognostic factor. Nevertheless, when the 13 stage-IV breast-cancer cases (six *BRCA2* mutation carriers and seven non-carriers) were excluded from the multivariate Cox model, *BRCA2* status was an independent predictor of a worse breast-cancer-specific survival (N. Loman, personal communication, 2000).

Several sources of bias exist in mutation-based studies. Ascertainment bias is an issue in many, as living affected women are preferentially offered testing (Robson et al., 1998). When Stoppa-Lyonnet et al. restricted the analysis in their series to the patients whose time interval between cancer diagnosis and genetic counselling was less than 3 years, the 5-year overall survival for the *BRCA1* carriers fell from 80% (irrespectively of the time of genetic testing) to 49%, compared with 91% to 85% for the *BRCA1* non-carriers ($P = 0.0001$) (Stoppa-Lyonnet et al., 2000). Verhoog et al. attempted to correct for this by analysing the data with the exclusion of the nine affected probands (Verhoog et al., 1998). This resulted in a non-significant trend towards a higher death and recurrence rate in *BRCA1*-mutation carriers. However, exclusion of the proband does not adequately correct for ascertainment bias. The likelihood of a patient affected with breast cancer to be ascertained also depends on the structure of the pedigree (e.g. small families, predominance of males, deceased relatives) and the knowledge of the family history. Several investigators eliminated survivor bias with their study design, as mutation status was studied from paraffin blocks regardless of whether or not the patient was living. This was the case when only Ashkenazi Jewish women were selected (Foulkes et al., 1997; Robson et al., 1999; Chappuis et al., 2000b; Foulkes et al., 2000b). It may be that different *BRCA1/2* mutations confer a different prognosis, and the results demonstrated in founder populations, as seen in south Sweden (Johannsson et al., 1998), in the Ashkenazim (Foulkes et al., 1997; Robson et al., 1998; Lee et al., 1999; Robson et al., 1999; Chappuis et al., 2000b; Foulkes et al., 2000b) or in the Icelandic population (Agnarsson et al., 1998), may not apply to other populations (Robson, 2000). The absence of prognostic significance of *BRCA1/2* mutations in an Ashkenazi Jewish community-based survey has been reported (Lee et al., 1999). This interesting study evaluated the survival of breast-cancer-affected first-degree relatives of Ashkenazi Jewish mutation carriers compared with breast cancer cases diagnosed in first-degree relatives of non-carriers. Even with an adjustment for age and period of diagnosis, this study has limitations because genetic testing was limited to probands. Mutation status, pathological confirmation, cause of death, and adjustment for stage of the disease in relatives, were not established.

Determining the overall survival of the *BRCA1/2*-affected carriers is not an accurate measure of their survival from breast cancer, as they could die from other *BRCA1/2*-related tumours. In one Swedish study, four of the patients with both breast and ovarian cancer died of ovarian cancer (Johannsson et al., 1998). Non-exclusion of patients with *in situ* breast carcinoma might influence the survival evaluation (Robson et al., 1998).

Another point to be noted in several of the mutation studies is the inclusion of patients with missense mutations (Garcia-Patino et al., 1998; Wagner et al., 1998). Many of these mutations are of unknown biological significance, and including them in the case group may have confounded the results. In addition, in most of the studies the *BRCA1/2* genes were not sequenced in the control group. As such, the presence of mutations in this group cannot be ruled out.

All of the mutation-based studies have a small sample size, making the play of chance more likely to be a problem than in larger studies, and the control group may not be appropriate in all studies, e.g. not adequately stage-matched. One study, designed at the Curie Institute, Paris (Ansquer et al., 1998), is attractive as it was based on a prospective follow-up with the same mutation screening in cases and controls, but for reliable results this kind of approach requires a multicentre recruitment of cases and many years of follow-up. Further large, retrospective, cohort studies using populations with founder mutations, and mutation analysis of archived tissue, may be able to achieve similar results in a shorter time. It is noteworthy that the impact of standard adjuvant chemo- and/or hormonotherapy in *BRCA1/2* mutation carriers has not been properly assessed in the cohort studies so far conducted. This could be particularly important for small, node-negative breast cancers where treatment might not usually be offered (Foulkes et al., 2000b).

Perspectives and conclusion

Based on experimental and clinical data, breast cancer among *BRCA1/2* mutation carriers is at least as radiosensitive as sporadic breast cancer, as demonstrated by similar rates of IBTR in both groups. In the absence of increased risk of early IBTR or proof of contribution of radiotherapy to the significantly increased rates of contralateral breast cancer observed in this subgroup of patients, breast conservative therapy followed by radiation is a valid option of treatment for early-stage breast cancer. Tamoxifen chemoprevention, as well as other options such as prophylactic oophorectomy, should be discussed in the counselling process of breast cancer patients who carry *BRCA1/2* mutations. A better evaluation of the risks for ipsi- and contralateral breast cancer development, efficiency of the preventive procedures and new screening tools should be evaluated in prospective studies.

Some of the discrepancies in the outcome of hereditary breast cancer noted through the literature may be explained by methodological issues. Linkage studies, because of their inherent biases, should be restricted to use as a research tool to confirm or exclude chromosomal regions to be investigated, or interpreted with extreme caution. Because of imperfect molecular assays, small number of patients studied and an insufficient follow-up time, we cannot yet conclude on the precise impact of the breast cancer predisposing genes on the outcome of affected women. Nevertheless, no studies have shown a survival advantage for mutation carriers. This seems to indicate that *BRCA1/2*-related breast cancer is not associated with a survival advantage, and that, in fact, certain *BRCA1/2* germline mutations confer a worse prognosis. However, to adequately answer this question, we need more efficient molecular tools to identify all the genetic changes responsible for breast cancer predisposition, and large prospective studies or well-designed retrospective analyses to evaluate their clinical consequences. These future studies will also provide essential insights into this heterogeneous disease, such as a better understanding of genotype–phenotype correlation, the identification of modifier genes and relevant environmental factors, and a more complete understanding of the tumourigenic process involved in hereditary breast cancer (Narod, 1998).

An accurate appraisal of the survival according to the genetic status is essential for counselling at-risk individuals or breast cancer gene carriers. The prognosis for *BRCA1/2*-mutation-related tumours is important because this knowledge may influence the management of women at risk, by predicting the overall benefit of preventive measures (Hartmann et al., 1999; Schrag et al., 2000). Finally, a thorough understanding of the biological functions of BRCA1 and BRCA2, and their respective influence on the response to radiation or chemotherapy, may also help in the design of the optimal treatment of breast cancer that is developing in *BRCA1/2* mutation carriers.

Acknowledgements

POC is funded by a grant from the University Hospital of Geneva, Switzerland. WDF is a J2 Boursier Chercheur Clinicien of the Fonds de la recherche en Santé du Québec.

REFERENCES

Abbott DW, Freeman ML and Holt JT (1998). Double-strand break repair deficiency and radiation sensitivity in BRCA2 mutant cancer cells. *J Natl Cancer Inst* **90**: 978–85.

Agnarsson BA, Jonasson JG, Bjornsdottir IB, Barkardottir RB, Egilsson V and Sigurdsson H (1998). Inherited BRCA2 mutation associated with high grade breast cancer. *Breast Cancer Res Treat* **47**: 121–7.

Ansquer A, Gautier C, Fourquet A, Asselian B and Stoppa-Lyonnet D (1998). Survival in early-onset BRCA1 breast-cancer patients. *Lancet* **352**: 541.

Arriagada R, Le MG, Rochard F and Contesso G (1996). Conservative treatment versus mastectomy in early breast cancer: patterns of failure with 15 years of follow-up data Institut Gustave-Roussy Breast Cancer Group. *J Clin Oncol* **14**: 1558–64.

Bennett LM (1999). Breast cancer: genetic predisposition and exposure to radiation. *Mol Carcinog* **26**: 143–9.

Bernstein JL, Thompson WD, Risch N and Holford TR (1992). Risk factors predicting the incidence of second primary breast cancer among women diagnosed with a first primary breast cancer. *Am J Epidemiol* **136**: 925–36.

Boice JD, Harvey EB, Blettner M, Stovall M and Flannery JT (1992). Cancer in the contralateral breast after radiotherapy for breast cancer. *N Engl J Med* **326**: 781–5.

Breast Cancer Linkage Consortium (1999). Cancer risks in BRCA2 mutation carriers. *J Natl Cancer Inst* **91**: 1310–6.

Brekelmans CT, Seynaeve C, Bartels CC, et al. (2001). Effectiveness of breast cancer surveillance in BRCA1/2 gene mutation carriers and women with high familial risk. *J Clin Oncol* **19**: 924–30.

Chabner E, Nixon A, Gelman R, et al. (1998). Family history and treatment outcome in young women after breast-conserving surgery and radiation therapy for early-stage breast cancer. *J Clin Oncol* **16**: 2045–51.

Chakraborty R, Little MP and Sankaranarayanan K (1998). Cancer predisposition radiosensitivity and the risk of radiation-induced cancers. IV. Prediction of risks in relatives of cancer-predisposed individuals. *Radiat Res* **149**: 493–507.

Chappuis PO, Rosenblatt J, and Foulkes WD (1999). The influence of familial and hereditary factors on the prognosis of breast cancer. *Ann Oncol* **10**: 1163–70.

Chappuis PO, Nethercot V and Foulkes WD (2000a). Clinico-pathological characteristics of BRCA1- and BRCA2-related breast cancer. *Semin Surg Oncol* **18**: 287–95.

Chappuis PO, Kapusta L, Begin LR, et al. (2000b). Germline BRCA1/2 mutations and p27^{Kip1} protein levels independently predict outcome after breast cancer. *J Clin Oncol* **18**: 4045–52.

Chen PL, Chen CF, Chen Y, Xiao J, Sharp ZD and Lee WH (1998). The BRC repeats in BRCA2 are critical for RAD51 binding and resistance to methyl methanesulfonate treatment. *Proc Natl Acad Sci USA* **95**: 5287–92.

Chen Y, Thompson W, Semenciw R and Mao Y (1999). Epidemiology of contralateral breast cancer. *Cancer Epidemiol Biomarkers Prev* **8**: 855–61.

Connor F, Bertwistle D, Mee PJ, et al. (1997). Tumorigenesis and a DNA repair defect in mice with a truncating Brca2 mutation. *Nat Genet* **17**: 423–30.

Dawson LA, Chow E and Goss PE (1998). Evolving perspectives in contralateral breast cancer. *Eur J Cancer* **34**: 2000–9.

de la Rochefordière A, Asselain B, Campana F, et al. (1993). Age as prognostic factor in premenopausal breast carcinoma. *Lancet* **341**: 1039–43.

Easton DF, Ford D and Bishop DT (1995). Breast and ovarian cancer incidence in BRCA1-mutation carriers Breast Cancer Linkage Consortium. *Am J Hum Genet* **56**: 265–71.

Fisher B, Bauer M, Margolese R, et al. (1985). Five-year results of a randomized clinical trial comparing total mastectomy and segmental mastectomy with or without radiation in the treatment of breast cancer. *N Engl J Med* **312**: 665–73.

Fisher B, Anderson S, Fisher ER, et al. (1991). Significance of ipsilateral breast tumour recurrence after lumpectomy. *Lancet* **338**: 327–31.

Fisher B, Anderson S, Redmond CK, Wolmark N, Wickerham DL and Cronin WM (1995). Reanalysis and results after 12 years of follow-up in a randomized clinical trial comparing total mastectomy with lumpectomy with or without irradiation in the treatment of breast cancer. *N Engl J Med* **333**: 1456–61.

Fisher B, Dignam J, Wolmark N, et al. (1998a). Lumpectomy and radiation therapy for the treatment of intraductal breast cancer: findings from the National Surgical Adjuvant Breast and Bowel Project B-17. *J Clin Oncol* **16**: 441–52.

Fisher B, Costantino JP, Wickerham DL, et al. (1998b). Tamoxifen for prevention of breast cancer: report of the National Surgical Adjuvant Breast and Bowel Project P-1 Study. *J Natl Cancer Inst* **90**: 1371–88.

Foray N, Randrianarison V, Marot D, Perricaudet M, Lenoir G and Feunteun J (1999). Gamma-rays-induced death of human cells carrying mutations of BRCA1 or BRCA2. *Oncogene* **18**: 7334–42.

Ford D, Easton DF, Bishop DT, Narod SA and Goldgar DE (1994). Risks of cancer in BRCA1-mutation carriers Breast Cancer Linkage Consortium. *Lancet* **343**: 692–5.

Ford D, Easton DF, Stratton M, et al (1998). Genetic heterogeneity and penetrance analysis of the BRCA1 and BRCA2 genes in breast cancer families Breast Cancer Linkage Consortium. *Am J Hum Genet* **62**: 676–89.

Formenti SC, Preston-Martin S and Haffty BG (2000). BRCA1/2 germline mutations: a marker for radioresistance or radiosensitivity? *J Clin Oncol* **18**: 1159–60.

Foulkes WD, Wong N, Brunet J-S, et al. (1997). Germ-line BRCA1 mutation is an adverse prognostic factor in Ashkenazi Jewish women with breast cancer. *Clin Cancer Res* **3**: 2465–9.

Foulkes WD, Satagopan JM, Chappuis PO, et al. (2000a). The presence of a germ-line BRCA mutation is an independent poor prognostic marker in breast cancer: a two-center historical cohort study. *Am J Hum Genet* **67** (Suppl 2): 82.

Foulkes WD, Chappuis PO, Wong N, et al. (2000b). Primary node negative breast cancer in BRCA1 mutation carriers has a poor outcome. *Ann Oncol* **11**: 307–13.

Fourquet A, Campana F, Zafrani B, et al. (1989). Prognostic factors of breast recurrence in the conservative management of early breast cancer: a 25-year follow-up. *Int J Radiat Oncol Biol Phys* **17**: 719–25.

Frank TS, Manley SA, Olopade OI, et al. (1998). Sequence analysis of BRCA1 and BRCA2: correlation of mutations with family history and ovarian cancer risk. *J Clin Oncol* **16**: 2417–25.

Futreal PA, Liu Q, Shattuck-Eidens D, et al. (1994). BRCA1 mutations in primary breast and ovarian carcinomas. *Science* **266**: 120–2.

Gaffney DK, Brohet RM, Lewis CM, et al. (1998). Response to radiation therapy and prognosis in breast cancer patients with BRCA1 and BRCA2 mutations. *Radiother Oncol* **47**: 129–36.

Garcia-Patino E, Gomendio B, Provencio M, et al. (1998). Germ-line BRCA1 mutations in women with sporadic breast cancer: clinical correlations. *J Clin Oncol* **16**: 115–20.

Gershoni-Baruch R, Dagan E, Fried G, et al. (2000a). Significantly lower rates of BRCA1/BRCA2 founder mutations in Ashkenazi women with sporadic compared with familial early onset breast cancer. *Eur J Cancer* **36**: 983–6.

Gershoni-Baruch R, Dagan E, Israeli D, Kasinetz L, Kadouri E and Friedman E (2000b). Association of the C677T polymorphism in the MTHFR gene with breast and/or ovarian cancer risk in Jewish women. *Eur J Cancer* **36**: 2313–16.

Gowen LC, Avrutskaya AV, Latour AM, Koller BH and Leadon SA (1998). BRCA1 required for transcription-coupled repair of oxidative DNA damage. *Science* **281**: 1009–12.

Haffty BG, Fischer D, Beinfield M and Mckhann C (1991a). Prognosis following local recurrence in the conservatively treated breast cancer patient. *Int J Radiat Oncol Biol Phys* **21**: 293–8.

Haffty BG, Fischer D, Rose M, Beinfield M and Mckhann C (1991b). Prognostic factors for local recurrence in the conservatively treated breast cancer patient: a cautious interpretation of the data. *J Clin Oncol* **9**: 997–1003.

Haffty BG, Ward BA, Matloff E, et al. (2000). Patients with germline BRCA1/2 mutations treated by lumpectomy and radiation therapy (L + RT) have similar risks of ipsilateral and contralateral second primary tumors. *Proc ASCO* **19**: 77a.

Hamann U and Sinn HP (2000). Survival and tumor characteristics of German hereditary breast cancer patients. *Breast Cancer Res Treat* **59**: 185–92.

Hankey BF, Curtis RE, Naughton MD, Boice JD and Flannery JT (1983). A retrospective cohort analysis of second breast cancer risk for primary breast cancer patients with an assessment of the effect of radiation therapy. *J Natl Cancer Inst* **70**: 797–804.

Harrold EV, Turner BC, Matloff ET, et al. (1998). Local recurrence in the conservatively treated breast cancer patient: a correlation with age and family history. *Cancer J Sci Am* **4**: 302–7.

Hartmann LC, Schaid DJ, Woods JE, et al. (1999). Efficacy of bilateral prophylactic mastectomy in women with a family history of breast cancer. *N Engl J Med* **340**: 77–84.

Hedenfalk I, Duggan D, Chen Y, et al. (2001). Gene-expression profiles in hereditary breast cancer. *N Engl J Med* **344**: 539–48.

Jacobson JA, Danforth DN, Cowan KH, et al. (1995). Ten-year results of a comparison of conservation with mastectomy in the treatment of stage I and II breast cancer. *N Engl J Med* **332**: 907–11.

Johannsson OT, Ranstam J, Borg A and Olsson H (1998). Survival of BRCA1 breast and ovarian cancer patients: a population-based study from Southern Sweden. *J Clin Oncol* **16**: 397–404.

Kainu T, Juo SH, Desper R, et al. (2000). Somatic deletions in hereditary breast cancers implicate 13q21 as a putative novel breast cancer susceptibility locus. *Proc Natl Acad Sci USA* **97**: 9603–8.

Kuhl CK, Schmutzler RK, Leutner CC, et al. (2000). Breast MR imaging screening in 192 women proved or suspected to be carriers of a breast cancer susceptibility gene: preliminary results. *Radiology* **215**: 267–79.

Kurtz JM, Amalric R, Brandone H, et al. (1989). Local recurrence after breast-conserving surgery and radiotherapy. Frequency time course and prognosis. *Cancer* **63**: 1912–17.

Lakhani SR, Easton DF, Stratton MR, et al. (1997). Pathology of familial breast cancer: differences between breast cancers in carriers of BRCA1 or BRCA2 mutations and sporadic cases. *Lancet* **349**: 1505–10.

Lakhani SR, Jacquemier J, Sloane JP, et al. (1998). Multifactorial analysis of differences between sporadic breast cancers and cancers involving BRCA1 and BRCA2 mutations. *J Natl Cancer Inst* **90**: 1138–45.

Lee JS, Wacholder S, Struewing JP, et al. (1999). Survival after breast cancer in Ashkenazi Jewish BRCA1 and BRCA2 mutation carriers. *J Natl Cancer Inst* **91**: 259–63.

Leong T, Whitty J, Keilar M, et al. (2000). Mutation analysis of BRCA1 and BRCA2 cancer predisposition genes in radiation hypersensitive cancer patients. *Int J Radiat Oncol Biol Phys* **48**: 959–65.

Loman N, Johannsson O, Bendahl PO, et al. (2000). Prognosis and clinical presentation of BRCA2-associated breast cancer. *Eur J Cancer* **36**: 1365–73.

Marcus JN, Watson P, Page DL, et al. (1996). Hereditary breast cancer: pathobiology prognosis and BRCA1 and BRCA2 gene linkage. *Cancer* **77**: 697–709.

Morimatsu M, Donoho G and Hasty P (1998). Cells deleted for Brca2 COOH terminus exhibit hypersensitivity to gamma-radiation and premature senescence. *Cancer Res* **58**: 3441–7.

Narod SA (1998). Host susceptibility to cancer progression. *Am J Hum Genet* **63**: 1–5.

Narod SA, Goldgar D, Cannon-Albright L, et al. (1995a). Risk modifiers in carriers of BRCA1 mutations. *Int J Cancer* **64**: 394–8.

Narod SA, Ford D, Devilee P, et al. (1995b). Genetic heterogeneity of breast–ovarian cancer revisited Breast Cancer Linkage Consortium. *Am J Hum Genet* **57**: 957–8.

Narod SA, Brunet J-S, Ghadirian P, et al. (2000). Tamoxifen and risk of contralateral breast cancer in BRCA1 and BRCA2 mutation carriers: a case-control study. *Lancet* **356**: 1876–81.

Neugut AI, Weinberg MD, Ahsan H and Rescigno J (1999). Carcinogenic effects of radiotherapy for breast cancer. *Oncology (Huntingt)* **13**: 1245–56.

Noguchi S, Kasugai T, Miki Y, Fukutomi T, Emi M and Nomizu T (1999). Clinicopathologic analysis of BRCA1- or BRCA2-associated hereditary breast carcinoma in Japanese women. *Cancer* **85**: 2200–5.

Phillips KA (2000). Immunophenotypic and pathologic differences between BRCA1 and BRCA2 hereditary breast cancers. *J Clin Oncol* **18** (Suppl) S107–12.

Pierce LJ, Strawderman M, Narod SA, et al. (2000). Effect of radiotherapy after breast-conserving treatment in women with breast cancer and germline BRCA1/2 mutations. *J Clin Oncol* **18**: 3360–9.

Porter DE, Cohen BB, Wallace MR, et al. (1994). Breast cancer incidence penetrance and survival in probable carriers of BRCA1 gene mutation in families linked to BRCA1 on chromosome 17q12–21. *Br J Surg* **81**: 1512–15.

Rahman N and Stratton MR (1998). The genetics of breast cancer susceptibility. *Annu Rev Genet* **32**: 95–121.

Rebbeck TR, Levin AM, Eisen A, et al. (1999). Breast cancer risk after bilateral prophylactic oophorectomy in BRCA1 mutation carriers. *J Natl Cancer Inst* **91**: 1475–9.

Recht A, Silen W, Schnitt SJ, et al. (1988). Time-course of local recurrence following conservative surgery and radiotherapy for early stage breast cancer. *Int J Radiat Oncol Biol Phys* **15**: 255–61.

Robson M (2000). Are BRCA1- and BRCA2-associated breast cancers different? Prognosis of BRCA1-associated breast cancer. *J Clin Oncol* **18** (Suppl.) S113–18.

Robson M, Gilewski T, Haas B, et al. (1998). BRCA-associated breast cancer in young women. *J Clin Oncol* **16**: 1642–9.

Robson M, Levin D, Federici M, et al. (1999). Breast conservation therapy for invasive breast cancer in Ashkenazi women with BRCA gene founder mutations. *J Natl Cancer Inst* **91**: 2112–17.

Sankila R, Aaltonen L, Jarvinen HJ and Mecklin JP (1996). Better survival rates in patients with

MLH1-associated hereditary colorectal cancer. *Gastroenterology* **110**: 682–7.

Schnitt SJ, Connolly JL, Harris JR, Hellman S and Cohen RB (1984). Pathologic predictors of early local recurrence in Stage I and II breast cancer treated by primary radiation therapy. *Cancer* **53**: 1049–57.

Schrag D, Kuntz KM, Garber JE and Weeks JC (2000). Life expectancy gains from cancer prevention strategies for women with breast cancer and BRCA1 or BRCA2 mutations. *JAMA* **283**: 617–24.

Sharan SK, Morimatsu M, Albrecht U, et al. (1997). Embryonic lethality and radiation hypersensitivity mediated by Rad51 in mice lacking Brca2. *Nature* **386**: 804–10.

Sigurdsson H, Agnarsson BA, Jonasson JG, et al. (1996). Worse survival among breast cancer patients in families carrying the BRCA2 susceptibility gene. *Breast Cancer Res Treat* **37** (Suppl): 33.

Smith TE, Lee D, Turner BC, Carter D and Haffty BG (2000). True recurrence vs new primary ipsilateral breast tumor relapse: an analysis of clinical and pathologic differences and their implications in natural history, prognoses and therapeutic management. *Int J Radiat Oncol Biol Phys* **48**: 1281–9.

Stoppa-Lyonnet D, Ansquer Y Dreyfus H. et al. (2000). Familial invasive breast cancer: worse outcome related to BRCA1 mutations. *J Clin Oncol* **18**: 4053–9.

Storm HH, Andersson M, Boice JDJ, et al. (1992). Adjuvant radiotherapy and risk of contralateral breast cancer. *J Natl Cancer Inst* **84**: 1245–50.

Tirkkonen M, Johannsson O, Agnarsson BA, et al. (1997). Distinct somatic genetic changes associated with tumor progression in carriers of BRCA1 and BRCA2 germ-line mutations. *Cancer Res* **57**: 1222–7.

Turner BC, Harrold E, Matloff E, et al. (1999). BRCA1/BRCA2 germline mutations in locally recurrent breast cancer patients after lumpectomy and radiation therapy: implications for breast-conserving management in patients with BRCA1/BRCA2 mutations. *J Clin Oncol* **17**: 3017–24.

Verhoog LC, Brekelmans CT, Seynaeve C, et al. (1998). Survival and tumor characteristics of breast-cancer patients with germline mutations of BRCA1. *Lancet* **351**: 316–21.

Verhoog LC, Brekelmans CT, Seynaeve C, et al. (1999). Survival in hereditary breast cancer associated with germline mutations of BRCA2. *J Clin Oncol* **17**: 3396–402.

Verhoog LC, Brekelmans CT, Seynaeve C, Meijers-Heijboer EJ and Klijn JG (2000a). Contralateral breast cancer risk is influenced by the age at onset in BRCA1-associated breast cancer. *Br J Cancer* **83**: 384–6.

Verhoog LC, Berns EM, Brekelmans CT, Seynaeve C, Meijers-Heijboer EJ and Klijn JG (2000b). Prognostic significance of germline BRCA2 mutations in hereditary breast cancer patients. *J Clin Oncol* **18** (Suppl.): S119–S124.

Veronesi U, Luini A, Galimberti V and Zurrida S (1994). Conservation approaches for the management of stage I/II carcinoma of the breast: Milan Cancer Institute trials. *World J Surg* **18**: 70–5.

Veronesi U, Marubini E, Del Vecchio M, et al. (1995). Local recurrences and distant metastases after conservative breast cancer treatments: partly independent events. *J Natl Cancer Inst* **87**: 19–27.

Wagner TM, Moslinger RA, Muhr D, et al. (1998). BRCA1-related breast cancer in Austrian breast and ovarian cancer families: specific BRCA1 mutations and pathological characteristics. *Int J Cancer* **77**: 354–60.

Watson P, Lin KM, Rodriguez-Bigas MA, et al. (1998). Colorectal carcinoma survival among hereditary nonpolyposis colorectal carcinoma family members. *Cancer* **83**: 259–66.

Wilson CA, Ramos L, Villasenor MR, et al. (1999). Localization of human BRCA1 and its loss in high-grade non-inherited breast carcinomas. *Nat Genet* **21**: 236–40.

Winchester DJ, Menck HR and Winchester DP (1997). The National Cancer Data Base report on the results of a large nonrandomized comparison of breast preservation and modified radical mastectomy. *Cancer* **80**: 162–7.

7

Pathology of the breast and ovary in mutation carriers

Sunil R. Lakhani[1] and Adrienne M. Flanagan[2]

[1]Institute of Cancer Research, London, UK
[2]Royal Free and University College Medical School, London, UK

Introduction

Breast cancer is a leading cause of cancer death in women. It is estimated that 1 in 12 women will develop breast cancer in their lifetime. Risk factors for breast cancer include: age, early menarche, late menopause, obesity (particularly in post-menopausal women), oestrogen replacement therapy and a positive family history.

The majority of breast cancer (95%) is sporadic in nature and only a small proportion, in particular those diagnosed in young women, is due to a hereditary predisposition. This predisposition is transmitted as a highly penetrant autosomal dominant trait. Over the last 5–10 years, there has been considerable progress in the identification and localization of the genes responsible for hereditary breast cancer. In particular, two have attracted the most attention – *BRCA1* and *BRCA2* (Miki et al., 1994; Wooster et al., 1995).

The *BRCA1* gene is located on chromosome 17q21 and encodes for a protein of 1863 amino acids (Miki et al., 1994). The protein includes a zinc finger motif, which suggests a possible role in transcription. Evidence is also accumulating for a role in DNA repair. Mutations in the *BRCA1* gene are associated with a risk of breast cancer of approximately 80% and a risk of ovarian cancer of approximately 40% by the age of 70 years (Ford et al., 1994; Easton et al., 1995). The *BRCA1* gene accounts for approximately 45% of all hereditary breast-cancer-prone families. Patients with mutations in the *BRCA1* gene also have a slightly increased risk of colon and prostate cancer (Ford et al., 1994).

The *BRCA2* gene is located on chromosome 13q12–13 and encodes for a protein of 3418 amino acids. (Wooster et al., 1994, 1995; Tavtigian et al., 1996). It has been estimated that mutations in the *BRCA2* gene are associated with a risk of breast cancer that is similar or higher than that for *BRCA1*, but a lower risk of ovarian cancer. *BRCA2* gene mutations, however, confer a higher risk of male breast cancer.

Other cancers occurring in patients with *BRCA2* gene mutations include carcinoma of the pancreas, head and neck, and cutaneous malignant melanoma. Mutations in *BRCA1* and *BRCA2* genes together account for approximately 80% of families with four or more cases of breast cancer diagnosed under the age of 60 years. Other genes that are known to increase the risk of breast cancer include the *TP53* gene (Malkin et al., 1990), the gene on chromosome 10q22–23 responsible for Cowden disease (Nelen et al., 1996) and, in man, the androgen receptor gene (Wooster et al., 1992). Mutations in these genes are rare compared with mutations in *BRCA1* and *BRCA2*. In addition, certain alleles of the H-*ras*-1 gene (Krontiris et al., 1993), which are common compared with disease-associated variants of *BRCA1* and *BRCA2*, may slightly increase the risk of breast and other types of cancers.

For more than half a century, the association of cancer type with a history of familial predisposition has fascinated breast cancer researchers. Certain morphological types, including medullary carcinoma, tubular carcinoma, lobular carcinoma *in situ*, and invasive lobular carcinoma, have all been reported to be more commonly associated with a positive family history of breast cancer than other subtypes (Erdreich et al., 1980; Lagios et al., 1980; LiVolsi et al., 1982; Rosen et al., 1982; Lynch et al., 1984). It has been difficult to interpret the data in some studies owing to the small number of samples, the differing criteria of a 'positive family history' and the changing criteria and classification for the diagnosis of breast cancer. The morphological classification of breast disease is subjective and, despite an attempt to provide clear guidelines, the inter-observer variability is known to be high (Sloane et al., 1994). Because of this inter-observer variability and the factors outlined above, no clear agreement has emerged, until recently, that any particular phenotype is more commonly associated with a positive family history than any other. Nonetheless, in a histological review of the population-based series of 4071 breast cancers diagnosed between the ages of 20 and 54 years in the Cancer and Steroids Hormone Study, lobular carcinoma *in situ* showed a strong association with familial risk (Claus et al., 1993). In the Utah population database, invasive lobular carcinoma has been shown to have an association with familiality (Cannon-Albright et al., 1994).

Pathology of breast cancers in mutation carriers

BRCA1-associated tumours

There are a number of published studies indicating that breast cancers arising in mutation carriers are of higher grade than sporadic cancers (Bignon et al., 1995;

Jacquemier et al., 1995; Eisinger et al., 1996; Marcus et al., 1996). Eisenger et al. studied 27 *BRCA1*-associated breast cancers from 14 families and compared these to sporadic breast cancers, matching for grade. They found an excess of grade III carcinomas in the *BRCA1*-associated group. Marcus et al. reported the first large series of the pathology of *BRCA1*-related tumours. They had 90 *BRCA1*-related breast cancers assigned to the group on the basis of linkage to chromosomes 17q and/or the presence of ovarian cancer and male breast cancer. The control set comprised 187 predominantly non-familial cases. They reported that *BRCA1*-associated tumours were more likely to be of medullary or atypical medullary type, to be of higher grade, to be aneuploid, and to have a higher tumour cell proliferation rate. When adjusted for age, the association with medullary carcinoma lost formal significance.

A large collaborative study organized through the Breast Cancer Linkage Consortium (BCLC) compared the pathology of familial cancers with those of controls unselected for a family history of the disease (BCLC, 1997; Lakhani et al., 1998). There were 118 (27%) cases in the *BRCA1* group, selected on the basis of linkage or mutational data. The control group comprised 548 breast cancers without a known family history.

The BCLC review produced some intriguing data. The proportion of invasive ductal carcinoma of no special type (IDC-NST) was similar between *BRCA1* and control breast cancers. In keeping with the study by Marcus et al. (1996), more carcinomas were reported as medullary or atypical medullary in a *BRCA1* group (14%) compared with controls (2%) ($P<0.0001$).

The overall grade of *BRCA1* breast cancers was significantly higher than that of the control population. The grading of breast cancers is achieved by giving a score of 1–3 for each of three parameters: (i) tubule formation, (ii) pleomorphism and (iii) mitotic count. If more than 75% of the tumour has good tubules, the score is 1; if less than 10% of the tumour has good tubules, the score is 3. For pleomorphism, the greater the degree of pleomorphism, the worse the score, and similarly, the higher the mitotic count per 10 high-powered fields, the higher the score. A total score of 3–5 = grade 1, score 6–7 = grade 2 and score 8–9 = grade 3 (NHSBSP Publication, 1995). Interestingly, the higher grade of the *BRCA1* tumours was a result of a higher score in all three parameters of grade. This was different from *BRCA2* tumours (see below).

The presence of *in situ* disease was also recorded from the analysis. Although there are inherent difficulties with these data due to the limited examination of each case, ductal carcinoma *in situ* was seen less frequently in *BRCA1* cases (41%) than in controls (56%) ($P=0.01$). Lobular carcinoma *in situ* was also seen less frequently compared with controls; however, the results were not statistically significant.

Medullary carcinoma is a controversial entity. It is defined as a tumour that grows in solid sheets with an indistinct cell border (syncytial growth pattern), has large vesicular nuclei and prominent nucleoli, and has a broad pushing margin and a prominent lymphocytic infiltrate both at the periphery and within the tumour. These features must be present in the entire tumour for it to be regarded as a classic medullary carcinoma. If the tumours have less lymphocytic infiltrate or an infiltrating margin in part of the tumour, it is regarded as an atypical medullary carcinoma. The presence of a classic IDC-NST that forms less than 25% of the tumour also pushes it into an atypical medullary carcinoma category. Although these features appear to be fairly specific, pathologists have a great deal of difficulty in making a diagnosis of medullary carcinoma and atypical medullary carcinoma, and, in the BCLC study, the agreement amongst the pathologists was low. Because of the strong associations of the medullary and atypical medullary carcinoma with the *BRCA1* phenotype, a further review to identify the features that were predictive for *BRCA1* phenotype was carried out. Hence, in the second review (Lakhani et al., 1998) the pathologists were asked to evaluate specific features of the tumour (e.g. the presence of continuous pushing margins, confluent necrosis and a lymphocytic infiltrate) rather than assigning a specific type to the tumour. In a multifactorial analysis using the data from both reviews, the only factors found to be significant were total mitotic count, continuous pushing margins and lymphocytic infiltrate. All other features, including the diagnosis of medullary and atypical medullary carcinoma, were no longer significant in the analysis (Lakhani et al., 1998).

Two out of the three features that are independently associated with cancers from the *BRCA1* patient (continuous pushing margins and lymphocytic infiltrate) are part of the subset of the characteristics that define medullary carcinoma. High mitotic count, which is the third feature associated with these tumours, is also often seen in medullary carcinomas since these tend to be of higher grade, but it is not regarded as a defining feature. It appears that although an increase in the frequency of classic and atypical medullary carcinoma may contribute to the observed *BRCA1* phenotype, these cancers are likely to account for only a small proportion of the differences observed between *BRCA1* mutation carriers and control groups.

BRCA2-associated tumours

Unlike *BRCA1*, data on the pathology of tumours associated with *BRCA2* are limited. The study by Marcus et al. (1996) attempted to delineate the pathology of *BRCA2* tumours. Their study groups comprised *BRCA1*-associated tumours and 'others', which would include the *BRCA2* cases. Although this group had 85 cases, only nine were linked to *BRCA2* and three were of male breast cancer. They suggested that tumours arising in patients with *BRCA2* mutations were different from those arising in patients with *BRCA1* mutations. These tumours were of lower grade than those of *BRCA1*, were less aneuploid and did not have the high proliferation seen in tumours from *BRCA1* patients. They found an association of *BRCA2* tumours with invasive lobular carcinoma, tubular–lobular carcinoma, tubular carcinoma and cribriform carcinoma, which they designated as a 'tubular–lobular group' (TLG). This is in contrast to the findings of Agnarsson et al. (1998), who found that *BRCA2* tumours in the Icelandic population were of higher grade than tumours of sporadic controls. Their data are, however, based on one particular *BRCA2* mutation – 999del5 – and hence it is possible that this phenotype represents a peculiarity of the particular mutation. The studies carried out by the BCLC (1997) analysed 78 (18%) patients assigned to the *BRCA2* group on the basis of linkage analysis or mutation testing. This represents the largest dataset on *BRCA2* tumours to date. Unlike the study by Marcus et al., no difference in the frequency of invasive lobular carcinoma or tubular carcinoma between the control group and the *BRCA2* mutation group was identified. There was also no evidence of an excess of medullary or atypical medullary carcinoma in the *BRCA2* group. Hence, no particular type of breast cancer was over-represented in patients with *BRCA2* mutations.

BRCA2 breast cancers were, overall, of higher grade than those from the control population. Interestingly, in contrast to *BRCA1*, the higher grade of *BRCA2* tumour was only due to the higher score for tubule formation. No differences were identified in pleomorphism or mitotic count between *BRCA2* tumours and sporadic cancers.

There was no difference in the incidence of ductal carcinoma *in situ* between the *BRCA2* group and the control group. Lobular carcinoma *in situ* was seen less frequently in *BRCA2* mutation carriers compared with controls; however, the results were not statistically significant.

Multifactorial analysis from the two *BRCA2* mutation carrier reviews showed that the only significant features were tubule score and continuous pushing margins (Lakhani et al., 1998).

Molecular pathology of *BRCA1/2*-associated breast cancers

Steroid hormone receptors

Since its discovery in 1960, oestrogen receptor (ER) has become an important prognostic and predictive marker for breast cancer (Osborne, 1998). ER expression is inversely correlated with tumour grade (Henderson and Patek, 1998); hence, *BRCA*-associated tumours, which are more often of a higher grade than those of sporadic breast cancer, would be predicted to be more often ER-negative.

Many studies have shown low levels of ER expression in familial breast cancers (Johannsson et al., 1997; Osin et al., 1998a,b; Robson et al., 1998; Armes et al., 1999). This is also true when ER expression in *BRCA*-associated tumours is compared with a grade-matched control group (Osin et al., 1998a). In contrast, the expression of ER in *BRCA2* tumours appears to be similar to that in sporadic breast cancer tumours (Osin et al., 1998a,b). The detection of ERs immunohistochemically does not necessarily reflect their functional competence, and a percentage of cancers expressing ER are known to be resistant to anti-oestrogen therapy. The function of ER is dependent on the ability to transactivate ER-dependent genes. Expression of progesterone receptor (PgR) and PS2 protein is indirect evidence of retained transcriptional activation activity of ER and it has been shown that PgR and PS2 expression has a stronger correlation with prognosis in breast cancer than ER expression alone (Ioakim-Liossi et al., 1997). The finding of PgR negativity in familial cases of breast cancer that are ER-positive suggests that their functional ability may be compromised. It has been demonstrated that both the invasive and the *in situ* components in *BRCA* tumours have a similar status of steroid hormone receptor expression, suggesting that loss of hormonal response is a relatively early event in the progression of these tumours (Osin et al., 1998a,b).

c-erb-b2

HER2/neu product is a tyrosine kinase receptor belonging to the same family as epidermal growth factor receptor. It is over-expressed in approximately 20–30% of high-grade invasive breast cancers and is a poor prognostic indicator. HER2/neu status also predicts response to anti-oestrogen and cytotoxic chemotherapy. Antibodies directed against the HER2/neu protein have attracted attention recently owing to the availability of the monoclonal antibody Herceptin for the treatment of breast cancer (Ross and Fletcher, 1999). Clearly, the role of HER2/neu in familial breast cancer would therefore be of interest. Data on HER2/neu are limited and conflicting. Robson et al. (1998) and Armes et al. (1999) have not shown a difference in HER2/neu expression between sporadic and familial cancers. However, the study by Johannsson et al. (1997) demonstrated that c-erb-b2 expression in *BRCA1*-associated cancers is lower than would be predicted on the basis of their histological grade. Data from a large BCLC study are similar to those of Johannsson et al. (Lakhani and Easton, unpublished observations).

TP53

Mutations in the *TP53* gene are the most common genetic alterations in human cancers and are encountered in 20–40% of sporadic breast cancers. The frequency of these mutations correlates with tumour grade. Detection of p53 protein by immunohistochemistry correlates with higher histopathological grade, increased mitotic activity, aggressive behaviour and, therefore, a worse prognosis (Elledge and Allred, 1998; Rudolph et al., 1999). Using immunohistochemistry, Crook et al. (1997, 1998) reported that *BRCA*-associated tumours were more often p53-positive compared with grade-matched sporadic breast cancers (77% *BRCA1*, 45% *BRCA2*, 35% sporadics). Mutations in p53 have also been identified and these were often multiple and their locations unusual, which is in marked contrast to sporadic cancer. Studies of p53 gene function in *BRCA* tumours have been performed using *in vitro* models. These show that the identified mutants are unique not only in their number and location but also in their function. In sporadic breast cancer, an inverse correlation between loss of p53 expression and high proliferation index on one side, and low expression of anti-apoptotic gene *BCL2* on the other, has been demonstrated. Surprisingly, two studies show that *BRCA1/2* tumours have the same level of *BCL2* expression as the control group, despite being highly proliferative and with frequent p53 mutations (Robson et al., 1998; Armes et al., 1999). Clearly the regulation of both cell cycle and apoptosis is multifactorial, and a relatively high expression of anti-apoptotic *BCL2* is probably one of the mechanisms of tumour survival in conditions where apoptosis-inducing genes are still transactivated by mutant p53.

Cell cycle proteins

Cyclin-dependent kinase inhibitor p21 blocks transition from G1 to S phase and suppresses cell proliferation. The p21 is thought to be a major downstream effector of the wild-type, p53-mediated, growth arrest pathway that is induced by DNA damage. In sporadic breast tumours the expression of p21 is inversely correlated with p53 expression and high tumour grade (Elledge and Allred, 1998; McClelland et al., 1999). Immunohistochemical studies have failed to demonstrate a relationship between p21 and p53 in *BRCA1/2* tumours, suggesting that p21 transactivation in this group could be mediated by a p53-independent mechanism (Crook et al., 1998). Another cyclin-dependent kinase complex inhibitor that plays an important role in breast cancer pathogenesis is p27. There are reports that patients whose tumours over-express p27 have significantly higher survival rates. In small breast cancers (stages T1a and b), p27 expression was reported as the only independent prognostic factor (Tan et al., 1997). Data regarding p27 expression in familial *BRCA*-associated breast cancer are scarce and contradictory. Robson et al. (1998) reported that p27 expression does not differ between sporadic and *BRCA*-associated cancers; however, this is contrary to data from other groups (86% in familial tumours vs 65% in sporadics: P.P. Osin, unpublished observations). Cyclin D1 is a regulator of progression from G1 to S phase in the cell cycle. It represents an important part of hormonal regulation of mammary epithelium growth: Cyclin D1 is known to be unregulated by oestrogen and progestins and down-regulated by anti-oestrogens (Gillett et al., 1998). Cyclin D1 also modulates the transcription of ER-regulated genes (Neuman et al., 1997; McMahon et al., 1999). Cyclin D1 over-expression is a common event in breast cancer and is especially frequent in early-onset breast cancer, probably because of the high level of oestrogens in this age group (Barnes and Gillett, 1998). However, *BRCA1/2*-associated tumours show very low expression of Cyclin D1 in both the invasive and *in situ* components (14% in both invasive and ductal carcinoma *in situ* (DCIS) in *BRCA1/2* tumours vs 35–36% in invasive and DCIS in sporadics) (Osin et al., 1998a). Taken together with the absence of ER and PgR in *BRCA1/2* cancers, the absence of Cyclin D1 in these tumours could be additional evidence of hormone independence of *BRCA*-associated familial breast cancers.

Familial ovarian cancer

Ovarian cancer is the fifth most common cancer in women (excluding skin) in the USA and UK. Since the prognosis of this neoplasm is largely determined by the stage of the disease at presentation, and approximately 80% of cases have spread beyond the ovary when first diagnosed, ovarian cancer accounts for a disproportionate number of deaths compared with other cancers of the female genital tract. A family history of ovarian cancer confers the highest known risk factor for developing the disease. Other risk factors include gonadal dysgenesis (Szamborski et al., 1981), early menarche and late menopause, whereas reducing the number of ovulation events either by use of an oral contraceptive or through pregnancy reduces the risk of ovarian cancer. The oral contraceptive pill appears to offer protection against the risk of developing both sporadic and familial cancer and continues to provide protection for some years after the contraceptive has been terminated (Anonymous, 1987).

Families with a history of ovarian cancer are classified into three main groups: (1) families with a history of ovarian cancer only (site specific), (2) families that develop either ovarian and/or breast carcinoma, and (3) families with a history of non-polyposis colorectal neoplasms and endometrial, prostate and lung cancers (Lynch II syndrome) (Lynch et al., 1997). It is estimated that 5–10% of ovarian cancers result from a hereditary predisposition and that these are caused, in the vast majority of cases (90%), by germline mutations in tumour suppressor genes, *BRCA1* and *BRCA2* (Miki et al., 1994; Wooster et al., 1995). The remaining 10% of familial cases are likely to be accounted for by the Lynch II syndrome.

Classification of ovarian neoplasms

Ovarian neoplasms are typed according to the World Health Organization and International Federation of Gynaecology and Obstetrics classifications. There are three major categories, these being determined by the cell of origin from which the neoplasm is considered to arise. These include: (a) epithelial neoplasms (which are thought to originate from the surface ovarian epithelium or epithelial inclusion cysts – a smaller proportion arise from ovarian endometrial foci), (b) germ cells, and (c) stromal lesions. Epithelial neoplasms are the most common in the ovary, constituting approximately two-thirds of the total, 90% of which are malignant. Epithelial ovarian neoplasms include five subtypes: serous, mucinous, endometrioid, clear cell and transitional cell (otherwise known as 'Brenner tumour'). These are classified as 'benign', 'borderline' and 'malignant'.

Pathology of ovarian cancers in mutation carriers

BRCA1-associated tumours

All studies performed to date indicate that carcinoma is the most common histological diagnosis observed in *BRCA1*- and *BRCA2*-associated ovarian cancer. Most of the information available on familial ovarian cancer is based on *BRCA1*-linked disease because, unlike familial breast cancer patients, *BRCA1* germline mutations are approximately four times more common than *BRCA2* mutations in ovarian cancer patients (Gayther et al., 1999; Boyd et al., 2000). All five subtypes of malignant epithelial ovarian neoplasms have occurred in *BRCA1* mutation carriers. Even a case of a malignant transitional cell carcinoma – a very rare entity – has been found to occur in an individual carrying a *BRCA1* mutation (Werness et al., 2000a). It is generally agreed that the frequency of endometrioid and clear-cell carcinoma occurring in *BRCA1* mutation carriers is similar to that of sporadic cases (Rubin et al., 1996; Stratton et al., 1997; Aida et al., 1998; Berchuck et al., 1998; Johannsson et al., 1998; Zweemer et al., 1998; Pharoah et al., 1999; Werness et al., 2000a). In no studies was a particular mutation found to be associated with a specific histological subtype.

It is agreed that significant inter-observer variation commonly occurs in typing of ovarian carcinoma, particularly when a lesion is high grade (Sakamoto et al., 1994). Furthermore, consensus criteria for grading ovarian carcinomas have not been agreed and consequently differ between individuals (Cramer et al., 1987; Lund et al., 1991). The difficulty in subtyping ovarian carcinomas is clearly shown in the publication by Pharoah et al. (1999), in which 59% (61/133 cases) of the *BRCA1*-associated neoplasms and 36% (8/26 cases) of the *BRCA2*-associated cancers were classified as carcinomas, unspecified. The subjectivity of typing and grading is likely to account, at least in part, for the different results generated from studies undertaken to date. Systematic reviewing of the slides included in familial cancer studies by a group of histopathologists with a specialist interest in gynaeco-logical pathology has the benefit of reducing the inter-observer diagnostic vari-ation, but this was only performed in studies by Zweemer et al. (1998), Shaw et al. (1999) and Werness et al. (2000a). All studies have found that papillary serous adenocarcinoma is the predominant ovarian cancer in familial ovarian cancer syndromes. Some, but not all, researchers have found that this subtype occurs more commonly in *BRCA* germline mutation carriers than in sporadic cases. Rubin et al. (1996) reported that 43 out of 53 women with ovarian neoplasms who carried *BRCA1* germline mutations were diagnosed as having papillary serous adenocarcinoma. Stratton et al. (1997) and Berchuck et al. (1998) obtained similar results in studies of 12 out of 13, and 15 out of 15, individuals studied respectively. These data are further supported by data in brief reports provided by Shaw et al. (1999) and Risch et al. (1999). The obvious weakness of these studies is the small number of cases examined. In contrast, three larger investigations reported that papillary serous carcinomas occurred with similar frequency in *BRCA* mutation carriers as in the control groups obtained from sporadic cases (Pharoah et al., 1999; Boyd et al. 2000; Werness et al., 2000a). Currently, a systematic, blinded, detailed review of approximately 220 *BRCA*-associated ovarian cancers, and a similar number of non-familial cases, is being studied by a group of gynaepatholo-gists organized by the UK Coordinating Committee on Cancer Research (UKCCCR) Familial Ovarian Cancer Study Group. A study of this size may help to determine which, if any, tumour type or particular histological features correlate with *BRCA*-associated ovarian cancers.

The large majority of familial ovarian cancer studies performed have shown malignant mucinous carcinoma to be under-represented in *BRCA1* mutation carriers (Narod et al., 1994; Rubin et al., 1996; Stratton et al., 1997; Aida et al., 1998; Berchuck et al., 1998; Pharoah et al., 1999; Werness et al., 2000a), suggesting that aberrations in this gene do not generally play a role in the development of this subtype of epithelial neoplasm. Interestingly, this observation was originally made prior to the cloning of the ovarian cancer-associated genes (Bewtra et al., 1992). However, occasional invasive (Rubin et al., 1996; Zweemer et al., 1998) and borderline (Stratton et al., 1997) mucinous neoplasms have occurred in *BRCA1* mutation carriers.

BRCA2-associated tumours

Compared with the information on the pathology of *BRCA1*-associated ovarian cancers, little is reported on *BRCA2* mutation-related ovarian tumours. The paucity of information is accounted for by the low incidence of this disease compared with that of *BRCA1*-linked cases (Gayther et al., 1999; Boyd et al., 2000). Recently, studies, although small, indicate that the histological phenotype of these ovarian neoplasms is similar to that of *BRCA1*-associated carcinomas and is predominantly of papillary serous type (Zweemer et al., 1998; Pharoah et al., 1999; Risch et al., 1999; Shaw et al., 1999; Boyd et al., 2000). Finally, a single case of an ovarian carcinosarcoma – otherwise referred to as a 'malignant mixed müllerian tumour' – has been reported as occurring in a *BRCA2* mutation carrier (Sonada et al., 2000).

Grading and staging of familial ovarian cancers

The first report on *BRCA1*-associated ovarian carcinoma found that, overall, the tumours were of higher grade and higher stage than their historic age-matched controls (Rubin et al., 1996). However, grade I/stage I tumours have been observed, suggesting that loss of differentiation occurs in parallel with spread of disease. These findings have been largely reproduced by a number of other groups (Aida et al., 1998). Werness et al. (2000a) and Boyd et al. (2000) also found fewer low-grade carcinomas in the mutation carriers. Zweemer et al. (1998) and Pharoah et al. (1999) found that a greater number of high-stage (III/IV) cancers and fewer low-stage (I) cancers occurred in individuals with *BRCA1* and *BRCA2* germline mutations. Shaw et al. (1999) also studied a familial ovarian cancer group comprising *BRCA1* and *BRCA2* carriers and reported that they had a higher grade of cancer than their sporadic counterparts. However, Berchuck et al. (1998) found that, although the *BRCA1* cases in their study were all of advanced stage (III/IV), they were half as likely to be as poorly differentiated compared with cases without mutations, and Johannsson et al. (1998) did not identify a difference in grade between the ovarian cancers in their *BRCA* mutation carriers and the population-based, cancer registry control group.

Malignant germ-cell and stromal-cell neoplasms in *BRCA1* and *BRCA2* mutation carriers

Occasional reports exist of siblings and first-degree relatives with malignant, germ-cell, ovarian neoplasms, which comprise 1–3% of all malignant ovarian cancers (Jackson, 1967; Talerman et al., 1973; Mandel et al., 1994; Stettner et al., 1999), but a hereditary predisposition for such neoplasms has never been substantiated. However, a single report of a dysgerminoma arising in an individual with a *BRCA1* germline mutation has been published recently (Werness et al., 2000b). Another group of malignant ovarian neoplasms, which comprises approximately 5% of all ovarian cancers, are stromal-cell cancers and include malignant granulosa cell neoplasms, fibrosarcomas and other rare entities. To date, none of these lesions has been found to be associated with *BRCA* germline mutations, suggesting that such mutations do not predispose individuals to the development of this subtype of ovarian cancer.

Borderline ovarian neoplasms and *in situ* lesions in women with and without *BRCA* germline mutations

Approximately 20% of all ovarian neoplasms are categorized as borderline ovarian neoplasms, otherwise known as 'tumours of low-grade malignancy', and a large proportion of these are serous lesions. Hence, they constitute an important clinical problem. The current data suggest that germline mutations in *BRCA* genes do not predispose individuals to the development of borderline neoplasms. This is demonstrated most convincingly in two manuscripts. Firstly, Gotlieb et al. (1998) found that only one out of 46 Ashkenazi Jewish patients with frequently occurring *BRCA* mutations in this population had a borderline neoplasm. This contrasted the finding of 17 carriers of the 18delTAG-*BRCA1/2* carriers of the 6174delT-*BRCA2* mutations in a group of 59 patients with invasive carcinoma. Furthermore, in this study one patient with a borderline tumour, who had a family history of ovarian and breast cancer, which co-segregated with a 185delAG-*BRCA1* mutation, was not a carrier for this mutation. Secondly, Lu et al. (1999) reported that 14 out of 32 Jewish patients (44%) with ovarian cancer were carriers for either a 185delAG-*BRCA1* mutation ($n = 8$) or a 6174delT-*BRCA2* mutation ($n = 6$), whereas neither of these mutations were found in 16 borderline tumours from Jewish women or in 33 controls. These data support the view that borderline ovarian neoplasms do not progress to frankly invasive adenocarcinoma (for review, see Seidman and Kurman, 2000).

Studies have been performed with the aim of identifying pre-neoplastic histological features in ovaries removed prophylactically from *BRCA* mutation carriers. However, *in situ* neoplastic change was rarely observed in ovarian neoplasms, irrespective of whether they develop in familial or sporadic cases (Stratton et al., 1999; Werness et al., 1999; Casey et al., 2000). However, the importance of such studies being performed without prior knowledge of the mutation status cannot be over-emphasized. Barakat et al. (2000) also found no histological difference and no difference in the expression of *erb*-b2, p53, *BRCA1* and Ki67 between the 18 ovaries removed prophylactically from *BRCA1* mutation carriers and control ovaries.

REFERENCES

Agnarsson BA, Jonasson JG, Bjornsdottir IB, Barkardottir RB, Egilsson V and Sigurdsson H (1998). Inherited *BRCA2* mutation associated with high grade breast cancer. *Breast Cancer Res Treat* **47**: 121–7.

Aida H, Takakuwa K, Nagata H, et al. (1998). Clinical features of ovarian cancer in Japanese women with germ-line mutations of *BRCA1*. *Clin Cancer Res* **4**: 235–40.

Anonymous (1987). The reduction in risk of ovarian cancer associated with oral-contraceptive use: the cancer and steroid hormone study of the Centers of Disease Control and the National Institute of Child Health and Human Development. *New Engl J Med* **316**: 650–5.

Armes JE, Trute L, White D, et al. (1999). Distinct molecular pathogeneses of early-onset breast cancers in *BRCA1* and *BRCA2* mutation carriers: a population-based study. *Cancer Res* **59**: 2011–17.

Barakat RR, Federici MG, Robson ME, Offit K and Boyd J (2000). Absence of premalignant histologic, molecular, or cell biological alterations in prophylactic oophorectomy specimens from *BRCA1* heterozygotes. *Cancer* **89**: 383–90.

Barnes DM and Gillett CE (1998). Cyclin D1 in breast cancer. *Breast Cancer Res Treat* **52**: 1–15.

Berchuck A, Heron K-A, Carney ME, et al. (1998). Frequency of germline and somatic *BRCA1* mutations in ovarian cancer. *Clin Cancer Res* **4**: 2433–7.

Bewtra C, Watson P, Conway T, Read-Hippee C and Lynch HT (1992). Hereditary ovarian cancer: a clinicopathological study. *Int J Pathol* **11**: 180–7.

Bignon YJ, Fonck Y and Chassagne MC (1995). Histoprognostic grade in tumours from families with hereditary predisposition to breast cancer. *Lancet* **346**: 258.

Boyd J, Sonada Y, Federici MG, et al. (2000). Clinicopathological features of *BRCA*-linked and sporadic ovarian cancer. *JAMA* **283**: 2260–5.

Breast Cancer Linkage Consortium (1997). Pathology of familial breast cancer: differences between breast cancers in carriers of *BRCA1* or *BRCA2* mutations and sporadic cases. Breast Cancer Linkage Consortium. *Lancet* **349**: 1505–10.

Cannon-Albright LA, Thomas A, Goldgar DE, et al. (1994). Familiality of cancer in Utah. *Cancer Res* **54**: 2378–85.

Casey MJ, Bewtra C, Hoehne LL, Tatpti AD, Lynch HT and Watson PW (2000). Histology of prophylactically removed ovaries from *BRCA1* and *BRCA2* mutation carriers compared with non-carriers in hereditary breast ovarian cancer syndrome kindreds. *Gynecol Oncol* **78**: 278–87.

Claus EB, Risch N, Thompson WD and Carter D (1993). Relationship between breast histopathology and family history of breast cancer. *Cancer* **71**: 147–53.

Cramer SF, Roth LM and Ulbright TM (1987). Evaluation of the reproducibility of the World Health Organization of common ovarian cancers: with emphasis on methodology. *Arch Pathol Lab Med* **111**: 819–29.

Crook T, Crossland S, Crompton MR, Osin P and Gusterson BA (1997). p53 mutations in

BRCA1-associated familial breast cancer. *Lancet* **350**(9078): 638–9.

Crook T, Brooks LA, Crossland S, et al. (1998). p53 mutation with frequent novel codons but not a mutator phenotype in *BRCA1*- and *BRCA2*-associated breast tumours. *Oncogene* **17**: 1681–9.

Easton DF, Ford D and Bishop DT (1995). Breast and ovarian cancer incidence in *BRCA1*-mutation carriers. Breast Cancer Linkage Consortium. *Am J Hum Genet* **56**: 265–71.

Eisinger F, Stoppa-Lyonnet D, Longy M, et al. (1996). Germline mutation at *BRCA1* affects the histoprognostic grade in hereditary breast cancer. *Cancer Res* **56**(3): 471–4.

Elledge RM and Allred DC (1998). Prognostic and predictive value of p53 and p21 in breast cancer. *Breast Cancer Res Treat* **52**: 79–98.

Erdreich LS, Asal NR and Hoge AF (1980). Morphologic types of breast cancer: age, bilaterality, and family history. *South Med J* **73**: 28–32.

Ford D, Easton DF, Bishop DT, Narod SA and Goldgar DE (1994). Risks of cancer in *BRCA1*-mutation carriers. Breast Cancer Linkage Consortium. *Lancet* **343**: 692–5.

Gayther SA, Russell P, Harrington P, Antoniou AC, Easton DF and Ponder BAJ (1999). The contribution of germline *BRCA1* and *BRCA2* mutations to familial ovarian cancer: no evidence for other ovarian cancer-susceptibility genes. *Am J Hum Genet* **65**: 1021–9.

Gillett CE, Lee AH, Millis RR and Barnes DM (1998). Cyclin D1 and associated proteins in mammary ductal carcinoma in situ and atypical ductal hyperplasia. *J Pathol* **184**: 396–400.

Gotlieb WH, Friedman E, Bar-Sade BR, et al. (1998). Rates of Jewish ancestral mutations in *BRCA1* and *BRCA2* in borderline ovarian tumours. *J Natl Cancer Inst* **90**: 995–1000.

Henderson IC and Patek AJ (1998). The relationship between prognostic and predictive factors in the management of breast cancer. *Breast Cancer Res Treat* **52**: 261–88.

Ioakim-Liossi A, Karakitsos P, Markopoulos C, et al. (1997). Expression of pS2 protein and estrogen and progesterone receptor status in breast cancer. *Acta Cytol* **41**: 713–16.

Jackson SM (1967). Ovarian dysgerminoma. *Br J Radiol* **40**: 459–62.

Jacquemier J, Eisinger F, Birnbaum D and Sobol H (1995). Histoprognostic grade in *BRCA1*-associated breast cancer. *Lancet* **345**: 1503.

Johannsson OT, Idvall I, Anderson C, et al. (1997). Tumour biological features of *BRCA1*-induced breast and ovarian cancer. *Eur J Cancer* **33**: 362–71.

Johannsson OT, Ranstam J, Borg A and Olsson H (1998). Survival of *BRCA1* breast and ovarian cancer patients: a population-based study from Southern Sweden. *J Clin Oncol* **16**: 397–404.

Krontiris TG, Devlin B, Karp DD, Robert NJ and Risch N (1993). An association between the risk of cancer and mutations in the HRAS1 minisatellite locus. *N Engl J Med* **329**: 517–23.

Lagios MD, Rose MR and Margolin FR (1980). Tubular carcinoma of the breast: association with multicentricity, bilaterality, and family history of mammary carcinoma. *Am J Clin Pathol* **73**: 25–30.

Lakhani SR, Jacquemier J, Sloane JP, et al. (1998). Multifactorial analysis of differences between sporadic breast cancers and cancers involving *BRCA1* and *BRCA2* mutations. *J Natl Cancer Inst* **90**: 1138–45.

LiVolsi VA, Kelsey JL, Fischer DB, Holford TR, Mostow ED and Goldenberg IS (1982). Effect of age at first childbirth on risk of developing specific histologic subtype of breast cancer. *Cancer* **49**: 1937–40.

Lu KH, Cramer DW, Muto MG, Li EY, Niloff J and Mok SC (1999). A population-based study of *BRCA1* and *BRCA2* mutations in Jewish women with epithelial ovarian cancer. *Obstet Gynecol* **93**: 34–7.

Lund B, Thomsen H and Olsen J (1991). Reproducibility of histopathological evaluation in epithelial ovarian carcinoma. Clinical implications. *APMIS* **99**: 353–8.

Lynch HT, Albano WA, Heieck JJ, et al. (1984). Genetics, biomarkers, and control of breast cancer: a review. *Cancer Genet Cytogenet* **13**: 43–92.

Lynch HT, Smyrk T, Lynch J (1997). An update of HNPCC (Lynch syndrome). *Cancer Genet Cytogenet* **93**: 84–99.

Malkin D, Li FP, Strong LC, et al. (1990). Germ line p53 mutations in a familial syndrome of breast cancer, sarcomas, and other neoplasms. *Science* **250**: 1233–8.

Mandel M, Toren A, Kende G, Neuman Y, Kenet G and Rechavi G (1994). Familial clustering of malignant germ cell tumours and Langerhans' histiocytosis. *Cancer* **73**: 1980–3.

Marcus JN, Watson P, Page DL, et al. (1996). Hereditary breast cancer: pathobiology, prognosis, and *BRCA1* and *BRCA2* gene linkage. *Cancer* **77**: 697–709.

McClelland RA, Gee JM, O'Sullivan L, et al. (1999). p21(WAF1) expression and endocrine response in breast cancer. *J Pathol* **188**: 126–32.

McMahon C, Suthiphongchai T, DiRenzo JE and Ewen ME (1999). P/CAF associates with cyclin D1 and potentiates its activation of the estrogen receptor. *Proc Natl Acad Sci USA* **96**: 5382–7.

Miki Y, Swensen J, Shattuck ED, et al. (1994). A strong candidate for the breast and ovarian cancer susceptibility gene *BRCA1*. *Science* **266**: 66–71.

Narod S, Tonin P, Lynch H, Watson P, Feunteun J and Lenoir G (1994). Histology of *BRCA1*-associated ovarian tumours. *Lancet* **343**: 236.

Nelen MR, Padberg GW, Peeters EA, et al. (1996). Localization of the gene for Cowden disease to chromosome 10q22–23. *Nat Genet* **13**: 114–16.

Neuman E, Ladha MH, Lin N, et al. (1997). Cyclin D1 stimulation of estrogen receptor transcriptional activity independent of cdk4. *Mol Cell Biol* **17**: 5338–47.

NHSBSP Publication (1995). *Pathology Reporting in Breast Cancer Screening*, 2nd edn. Sheffield: NHSBSP Publications, National Breast Screening Programme.

Osborne CK (1998). Steroid hormone receptors in breast cancer management. *Breast Cancer Res Treat* **51**(3): 227–38.

Osin P, Gusterson BA, Philip E, et al. (1998a). Predicted anti-oestrogen resistance in *BRCA*-associated familial breast cancers. *Eur J Cancer* **34**: 1683–6.

Osin P, Crook T, Powles T, Peto J and Gusterson B (1998b). Hormone status of in-situ cancer in *BRCA1* and *BRCA2* mutation carriers. *Lancet* **351**: 1487.

Pharoah PDP, Easton DF, Stockton DL, Gayther S, Ponder BAJ and the UK Coordinating

Committee for Cancer Research (1999). Survival in familial, *BRCA1*-associated, and *BRCA2*-associated epithelial cancer. *Cancer Res* **59**: 868–71.

Risch H, Vesprini D, McLaughlin J, et al. (1999). Factors predicting carrier status in a population-based study of germline *BRCA1/2* mutations in ovarian cancer (OC) patients. *Gynecol Oncol* **72**: 450.

Robson M, Rajan P, Rosen PP, et al. (1998). *BRCA*-associated breast cancer: absence of a characteristic immunophenotype. *Cancer Res* **58**: 1839–42.

Rosen PP, Lesser ML, Senie RT and Kinne DW (1982). Epidemiology of breast carcinoma III: relationship of family history to tumour type. *Cancer* **50**: 171–9.

Ross JS and Fletcher JA (1999). HER-2/neu (c-erb-B2) gene and protein in breast cancer. *Am J Clin Pathol* **112**(1 Suppl): S53–67.

Rubin SC, Benjamin I, Behbakht K, et al. (1996). Clinical and pathological features of ovarian cancer in women with germ-line mutations of *BRCA1*. *New Engl J Med* **335**: 1413–16.

Rudolph P, Olsson H, Bonatz G, et al. (1999). Correlation between p53, c-erbB-2, and topoisomerase II alpha expression, DNA ploidy, hormonal receptor status and proliferation in 356 node-negative breast carcinomas: prognostic implications. *J Pathol* **187**: 207–16.

Sakamoto A, Sasaki H, Furusato M, et al. (1994). Observer disagreement in histological classification of ovarian tumours in Japan. *Gynecol Oncol* **54**: 54–8.

Seidman JD and Kurman RJ (2000). Ovarian serous borderline tumors: a critical review of the literature with emphasis on prognostic indicators. *Hum Pathol* **31**: 539–57.

Shaw PA, Zweemer RP, McLaughlin JR, Narod SA, Risch H and Jacobs IJ (1999). Characteristics of genetically determined ovarian cancer. *Gynecol Oncol* **72**: 49.

Sloane JP, Ellman R, Anderson TJ, et al. (1994). Consistency of histopathological reporting of breast lesions detected by screening: findings of the U.K. National External Quality Assessment (EQA) Scheme. *Eur J Cancer* **30A**: 1414–19.

Sonada Y, Saigo PE, Federici MG and Boyd J (2000). Carcinosarcoma of the ovary in a patient with a germline *BRCA2* mutation: evidence for monoclonal origin. *Gynecol Oncol* **76**: 226–9.

Stettner A, Hartenbach E and Schink J (1999). Familial ovarian germ cell cancer: report and review. *Am J Med Genet* **84**: 43–6.

Stratton JF, Gayther SA, Russell P, et al. (1997). Contribution of *BRCA1* mutations to ovarian cancer. *New Engl J Med* **336**: 1125–30.

Stratton JF, Buckley CH, Lowe D, Ponder BAJ and the UK Coordinating Committee on Cancer Research (UKCCCR) Familial Ovarian Cancer Study Group (1999). Comparison of prophylactic oophorectomy specimens from carriers and non-carriers of a *BRCA1* or *BRCA2* gene mutation. *J Natl Cancer Inst* **91**: 626–8.

Szamborski J, Obreski T and Starzynska J (1981). Germ cell tumors in monozygous twins with gonadal dysgenesis. *Obstet Gynecol* **58**: 120–2.

Talerman A, Huyzinga WT and Kuipers T (1973). Dysgerminoma. Clinicopathological study of 22 cases. *Obstet Gynecol* **41**: 137–47.

Tan P, Cady B, Wanner M, et al. (1997). The cell cycle inhibitor p27 is an independent prognostic marker in small (T1a,b) invasive breast carcinomas. *Cancer Res* **57**: 1259–63.

Tavtigian SV, Simard J, Rommens J, et al. (1996). The complete *BRCA2* gene and mutations in chromosome 13q-linked kindreds. *Nat Genet* **12**: 333–7.

Werness BA, Afify AM, Bielat KL, Eltabbakh GH, Piver MS and Patterson JM (1999). Altered surface epithelium and cyst epithelium of ovaries removed prophylactically from women with a family history of ovarian cancer. *Hum Pathol* **30**: 151–7.

Werness BA, Ramus SJ, Whittemore AS, et al. (2000a). Histopathology of familial ovarian tumors in women from families with and without germline *BRCA1* mutations. *Hum Pathol* **31**: 1420–4.

Werness BA, Ramus SJ, Whittemore AS, et al. (2000b). Primary ovarian dysgerminoma in a patient with a germline *BRCA1* mutation. *Int J Gynecol Pathol* **19**: 390–4.

Wooster R, Mangion J, Eeles R, et al. (1992). A germline mutation in the androgen receptor gene in two brothers with breast cancer and Reifenstein syndrome. *Nat Genet* **2**: 132–4.

Wooster R, Neuhausen SL, Mangion J, et al. (1994). Localization of a breast cancer susceptibility gene, *BRCA2*, to chromosome 13q12–13. *Science* **265**: 2088–90.

Wooster R, Bignell G, Lancaster J, et al. (1995). Identification of the breast cancer susceptibility gene *BRCA2*. *Nature* **378**: 789–92.

Zweemer RP, Verheijen RHM, Gille JJP, van Diest PJ, Pals G and Menko FH (1998). Clinical and genetic evaluation of thirty ovarian cancer families. *Am J Obstet Gynecol* **178**: 85–90.

8

Risk estimation for familial breast and ovarian cancer

Jenny Chang-Claude and Heiko Becher

Deutsches Krebsforschungszentrum, University of Heidelberg, Germany

Introduction

The awareness of genetic predisposition to breast cancer has increased tremendously since the identification of the two highly penetrant breast and ovarian cancer genes – *BRCA1* and *BRCA2* (Miki et al., 1994; Wooster et al., 1995). Women with a family history of breast cancer are particularly concerned about their own risk, thus creating a greater demand for risk assessment and genetic counselling as well as for genetic testing. Mutations in *BRCA1* or *BRCA2* account for the majority of high-risk families in which the segregation of a dominant high-penetrance susceptibility gene has quite clearly manifested itself in multiple cases of breast cancer over several generations of close relatives (Ford et al., 1998). Only a small proportion of families with a less striking family history and isolated early-onset breast cancer can also be attributed to mutations in these genes (Frank et al., 1998; Malone et al., 1998; Newman et al., 1998) except in founder populations with recurrent mutations (Andersen et al., 1996; Johannesdottir et al., 1996; Fodor et al., 1998; Thorlacius et al., 1998). Screening for mutations is, however, still a technically demanding and labour-intensive task, and gene testing is usually only offered to persons with a greater than three-fold increase in risk compared with the general population (Gayther and Ponder, 1997). Generally, for genetic counselling on familial breast cancer, an accurate evaluation is needed of the probability that a woman carries a mutation before any decisions are made regarding genetic testing. Furthermore, knowledge of a women's underlying risk of breast cancer may affect important medical decisions to be made with respect to primary and/or secondary prevention. These decisions include: at what age to begin mammographic screening, whether to use tamoxifen to prevent breast cancer, and whether to perform prophylactic mastectomy to prevent breast cancer.

Different basis for risk prediction

Without consideration of family history or other risk factors, lifetime risk for breast cancer for an individual can be estimated by using the cumulative risk of breast cancer in the general population, which varies considerably between countries. It is 10% in the UK female population or approximately 1 in 10. The longer a woman lives without cancer, the lower is her risk of developing breast cancer in the remainder of her lifetime.

Menstrual and reproductive history, such as early age at menarche, late age at menopause, nulliparity or late age at first birth, as well as family history of breast cancer and history of benign breast disease, have been shown in epidemiological studies to increase the risk of breast cancer in women relative to those without these characteristics. Risk prediction models accounting for some of these factors have been developed. The Gail model was based on data from the Breast Cancer Detection and Demonstration Project – a large mammographic screening programme conducted in the 1970s (Gail et al., 1989). Risk factors accounted for included: age at menarche (≥ 14, 12–13, <12 years), number of breast biopsies and woman's age (0, 1, ≥ 2 biopsies at <50 or ≥ 50 years), number of first-degree relatives with breast cancer (0, 1 or ≥ 2) and woman's age at first live birth (<20, 20–24, 25–29, ≥ 30 years, or nulliparous). The calculation of breast cancer risk with the Gail model requires translating a woman's risk factors into a risk score and then multiplying by an adjusted population breast cancer risk. It is most easily performed using a software program, which is available from the National Cancer Institute at http://cancernet.nci.nih.gov/h_detect.html. In validation studies, it has been shown that this risk prediction model is more accurate for women undergoing regular mammographic screening (Bondy et al., 1994).

Pedigree analysis

For genetic counselling of women with a family history of breast cancer, the commonly employed model for estimating breast cancer risk is based on the Cancer and Steroid Hormone (CASH) study – a large population-based, case-control study of breast cancer comprising 4730 patients diagnosed at 20–54 years and 4688 control subjects. The Claus model is based on a genetic model of rare highly penetrant genes for susceptibility to breast cancer and therefore includes more information about family history but excludes other risk factors (Claus et al., 1991). Since the effect of family history on breast cancer risk is much stronger than other risk factors, the Claus model is more appropriate than the Gail model for assessing risk in women with a family history of breast cancer.

Claus et al. (1994) have used the model to construct detailed tables that predict the cumulative risk of breast cancer according to decades from 29 to 79 years of age, based on age at diagnosis of one or two first- and/or second-degree relatives with breast cancer. Predictions using the Claus model for women with one first-degree relative with breast cancer, one second-degree relative with breast cancer, and two first-degree relatives with breast cancer are shown in Table 8.1. Cumulative risk based on other combinations of relatives with breast cancer (mother and maternal aunt, mother and paternal aunt, and two second-degree relatives) are available in the publication by Claus et al. (1994). As an example, the risk of breast cancer by 79 years for a woman who is 35 years old at counselling and has an affected mother and an affected maternal aunt would be 0.37 and 0.18 according to whether the breast cancers occurred before or after menopause (Table 8.2). The risk of the same woman would be 0.22 even if the breast cancers occurred before menopause in two maternal aunts but not in the mother. The method of Claus et al. (1994) has been generalized by Becher and Chang-Claude (1996) to be applicable to different populations, taking into account the different baseline breast cancer risk of specific populations.

However, the Claus tables were not generated to consider the complete pedigree structure, i.e. the number and ages of unaffected relatives and the exact genealogical relationship between the proband and her affected relatives. A more sophisticated method of risk prediction allows the estimation of the proband's genetic risk under a particular genetic model, given her family history, and can be performed using the software package LINKAGE (Lathrop et al., 1984). This calculation takes into account the entire pedigree information, including family size, relationships, ages and disease phenotypes of all members. The method can be used to estimate the probability that the proband is a carrier of a highly penetrant breast cancer susceptibility gene, as characterized by the Claus model (Claus et al., 1991). This measure of genetic risk can then be used to estimate the risk of developing breast cancer risk at a certain age and has been shown to provide more accurate risk estimation, particularly in families with smaller numbers of affected members (Schmidt et al., 1998). This can be illustrated by comparing, for three different family sizes, the risk of breast cancer by 79 years for a woman who is 35 years old at counselling and whose mother and a sister are affected with breast cancer (Figure 8.1).

The calculation of breast cancer risk with the Claus model can be easily performed using the software package MLINK/LINKAGE (Lathrop et al., 1984), which is publicly available from the web resources of Rockefeller University at http://linkage.rockefeller.edu/. The genetic model and the parameters (gene frequency and age-specific penetrances for gene carriers and non-gene carriers) need to be specified. It should be mentioned that the magnitude of the estimated genetic risk depends upon the genetic model assumed and may vary with different

Table 8.1. Cumulative risk of breast cancer according to the Claus model

Number of relatives with breast cancer and their age (years) at diagnosis	Cumulative risk of breast cancer (%)				
	Age (years)				
	39	49	59	69	79
One first-degree relative					
20–29	2.5	6.2	11.6	17.1	21.1
30–39	1.7	4.4	8.6	13.0	16.5
40–49	1.2	3.2	6.4	10.1	13.2
50–59	0.8	2.3	4.9	8.2	11.0
60–69	0.6	1.8	4.0	7.0	9.6
70–79	0.5	1.5	3.5	6.2	8.8
One second-degree relative					
20–29	1.4	3.5	7.0	11.0	14.2
30–39	1.0	2.7	5.6	9.0	12.0
40–49	0.7	2.1	4.5	7.6	10.4
50–59	0.6	1.7	3.8	6.7	9.4
60–69	0.5	1.7	3.8	6.7	9.4
70–79	0.4	1.3	3.2	5.8	8.3
Two first-degree relatives					
Age at diagnosis of younger relative: 20–29					
Age at diagnosis of older relative:					
20–29	6.9	16.6	29.5	41.2	48.4
30–39	6.6	15.7	27.9	39.1	46.0
40–49	6.1	14.6	26.1	36.6	43.4
50–59	5.5	13.3	23.8	33.5	39.7
60–69	4.8	11.7	21.0	29.7	35.4
70–79	4.1	9.9	17.9	25.6	30.8
Age at diagnosis of younger relative: 30–39					
Age at diagnosis of older relative:					
30–39	6.2	14.8	26.5	37.1	43.7
40–49	5.6	13.4	23.9	33.7	39.9
50–59	4.8	11.6	20.9	29.6	35.3
60–69	4.0	9.6	17.5	25.1	30.2
70–79	3.2	7.7	14.3	20.7	25.2
Age at diagnosis of younger relative: 40–49					
Age at diagnosis of older relative:					
40–49	4.8	11.7	21.0	29.8	35.4
50–59	3.9	9.6	17.4	24.9	30.0
60–69	3.0	7.5	13.9	20.2	24.6
70–79	2.3	5.8	10.8	16.1	20.0

Table 8.1. (*cont.*)

Number of relatives with breast cancer and their age (years) at diagnosis	Cumulative risk of breast cancer (%)				
	Age (years)				
	39	49	59	69	79
Age at diagnosis of younger relative: 50–59					
Age at diagnosis of older relative:					
50–59	3.0	7.5	13.8	20.0	24.5
60–69	2.2	5.6	10.5	15.7	19.5
70–79	1.6	4.2	8.1	12.4	15.8
Age at diagnosis of younger relative: 60–69					
Age at diagnosis of older relative:					
60–69	1.6	4.1	8.0	12.2	15.6
70–79	1.2	3.0	6.1	9.8	12.8
Age at diagnosis of younger relative: 70–79					
Age at diagnosis of older relative:					
70–79	0.8	2.3	4.9	8.1	10.9

Table 8.2. Risk of breast cancer (by 79 years) for a 35-year-old woman with two first- or second-degree relatives with breast cancer

Relatives with breast cancer	Age at diagnosis (years)	Risk for 35-year-old woman
Mother and maternal aunt	37, 40	0.37
Mother and maternal aunt	64, 58	0.18
Two maternal aunts	37, 40	0.22

From Claus et al. (1994).

gene frequency and penetrance estimates. Risk prediction based on a genetic model can also be performed with the software program MENDEL (Lange and Weeks, 1988), which can be obtained at http://www.biomath.medsch.ucla.edu/faculty/klange/software.html (from Ken Lange) but which is less user friendly. The commercial software package Cyrillic has implemented risk estimation for breast cancer based on the Claus model, with parameter specification based on data from the UK, whereby version 2.1 uses LINKAGE and version 3.0 employs MENDEL. However, the genetic model employed is not clearly documented in Cyrillic version 2.1 and options for changing model parameters do not appear to be well tested in version 3.0. Therefore, some experience with, and understanding of,

Table 8.3. Estimated proportion of *BRCA1* and *BRCA2*[a] in families with breast/ovarian cancer

Type of family	Estimated proportion (95% CI)	
	BRCA1	*BRCA2*
Families with 4 or more breast cancers in cases		
≤ 60 years		
All families	0.52 (0.42–0.62)	0.35 (0.24–0.46)
Female breast cancer only	0.28 (0.13–0.45)	0.37 (0.20–0.56)
≥ 1 ovarian cancer (without male breast cancer)	0.80 (0.66–0.92)	0.15 (0.05–0.28)
≥ 1 male breast cancer	0.19 (0.01–0.47)	0.77 (0.43–0.97)

[a]From Ford et al. (1998).

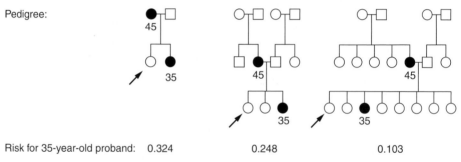

Pedigree:

Risk for 35-year-old proband: 0.324   0.248   0.103

Figure 8.1   Three pedigrees of different size and the predicted cumulative risk of breast cancer for a 35-year-old woman with two first-degree relatives affected with breast cancer at 45 and 35 years, as calculated under the genetic model with parameters according to Claus et al. (1991).

genetic risk calculation will be required for the application of Cyrillic for risk estimation.

Pedigree analysis generally precedes genetic analysis and is employed for women who want to know the magnitude of their familial breast cancer risk before making decisions about mutation testing of known highly penetrant genes, such as *BRCA1* or *BRCA2*. Some estimates have been reported regarding the proportions of *BRCA1* and *BRCA2* mutations in families with breast/ovarian cancer defined by number and age at diagnosis of the cancer, based on data from the Breast Cancer Linkage Consortium, and these have recently been updated (Ford et al., 1998) (Table 8.3). However, they do not account for families that may actually be harbouring mutations in a highly penetrant susceptibility gene, but who are presenting a less extensive family history that does not provide conclusive evidence for the involvement of such a gene. Therefore, risk estimation based on pedigree information can provide more accurate assessment of familial risk. These methods of risk estimation will be employed where genetic testing is not available or only for certain gene mutations. Furthermore, since not all predisposing genes are known, risk estimation will have to rely on pedigree information when the genetic test result is negative.

Genetic analysis (mutation screening)

Screening for mutation in the two highly penetrant breast cancer susceptibility genes, *BRCA1* and *BRCA2*, in affected family members is the preferred method for obtaining a more accurate risk estimate for unaffected women in high-risk families. The identification of a functionally relevant mutation in an affected woman will permit differentiation between gene carrier and non-gene carrier status in family members tested for the identified mutation and thus more accurate quantification of risk for the unaffected family members. Women with an inherited mutation in either *BRCA1* or *BRCA2* have an equally high lifetime risk of developing breast cancer. The estimates of risk range between 40% and 85%, depending upon the population and the type of families studied (Easton et al., 1995; Struewing et al., 1997; Ford et al., 1998; Thorlacius et al., 1998; Hopper et al., 1999). Generally, risk estimates obtained from analysis of breast cancer patients unselected for family history were lower than those from analysis of families with multiple cases of breast cancer (Table 8.4). *BRCA1* confers a higher risk of ovarian cancer than *BRCA2* (63% vs 27%) and *BRCA2* confers, in addition, an elevated risk of male breast cancer (Stratton, 1996; Easton et al., 1997; Ford et al., 1998). Those who are non-carriers in a family with an inherited mutation will have the population risk of developing breast cancer, which is 8–12% in western European countries.

However, women from families who test negative for *BRCA1/2* mutations will remain at elevated risk owing to their family history: (1) because the involvement of unknown predisposing genes cannot be excluded, and (2) the sensitivity of the mutation analysis is less than 100%. Their risk reduces by an amount related to the a priori probability of carrying a high-penetrance breast cancer susceptibility gene, which is estimated from pedigree information as described in the previous section. The a posteriori risk can be estimated from the a posteriori carrier probability, which can be calculated using a Bayesian approach (accounting for sensitivity of genetic testing, s, and assuming a specificity of 1 by:

$$\frac{\text{a priori carrier prob} \times (1-s)}{\text{a priori carrier prob} \times (1-s) + (1 - \text{a priori carrier prob})}$$

Table 8.4. Cumulative risk of breast cancer (95% CI) in carriers of *BRCA* mutations

	Cumulative risk of breast cancer (95% CI)			
	BCLC families[1]	Ashkenazi Jewish[2]	Icelandic[3]	Australian[4]
BRCA1				
By 60 years	0.49 (0.28–0.64)	0.33 (0.23–0.44)	—	0.10 (0–0.24)
By 70 years	0.71 (0.53–0.82)	0.56 (0.40–0.73)	—	0.40 (0.16–0.64)
BRCA2				
By 60 years	0.28 (0.09–0.44)	0.33 (0.23–0.44)	0.18 (0.09–0.26)	0.10 (0–0.24)
By 70 years	0.84 (0.43–0.95)	0.56 (0.40–0.73)	0.37 (0.22–0.54)	0.40 (0.16–0.64)

[1] Ford et al. (1998): 237 families with ≥ 4 cases of breast cancer (females < 60 years, males any age).

[2] Struewing et al. (1997): 5318 Ashkenazi Jewish subjects (120 *BRCA1/2* carriers: 185delAG, 5382insC, 6174delT); risk in first-degree relatives of carriers.

[3] Thorlacius et al. (1998): 573 breast cancer patients (841 women, 34 men), 69 carriers of 999del5 mutation (56 women, 13 men).

[4] Hopper et al. (1999): 388 breast cancer patients diagnosed before age 40 years, 18 mutation carriers (9 *BRCA1*, 9 *BRCA2*).

Here, the prior probability refers to being the carrier of any breast cancer susceptibility gene and not only *BRCA1* and *BRCA2*. Therefore, the term 'sensitivity' as used here refers to a genetic test for any breast cancer susceptibility gene and comprises both the sensitivity of mutation analysis of the *BRCA1/2* genes and the prior probability of the involvement of the *BRCA1/2* genes. This sensitivity can be estimated from empirical data (see next section). Therefore, given a family who tested negative for *BRCA* mutations, the risk of breast cancer for a 35-year-old woman with a 36% a priori probability of carrying a breast cancer susceptibility gene will be 19%, assuming that the sensitivity of genetic testing is 60% (Figure 8.2).

Generally, the molecular genetic techniques used for mutation screening do not identify 100% deleterious mutations. Complete sequencing of the *BRCA* genes identifies truncating mutations that are due to small-size or point alterations; however, large rearrangements may occur in 10–25% of *BRCA1* truncating mutations (Petrij-Bosch et al., 1997; Puget et al., 1999) and remain undetected. More commonly employed for genetics testing in genetics clinics are screening methods for detecting small-size or point mutations initially, such as single-strand conformation polymorphism (SSCP), conformation-sensitive gel electrophoresis (CSGE), denaturing gradient gel electrophoresis (DGGE), fluorescent-assisted

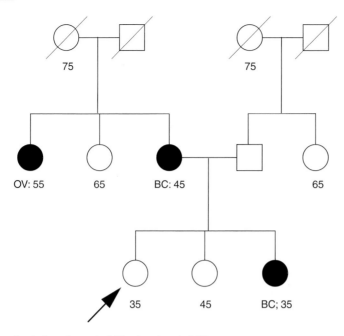

A priori carrier probability of proband: 0.36

A priori risk of breast cancer of proband: 0.32

A posteriori carrier probability of proband,
  given a negative genetic test and a sensitivity of 60%: 0.18

Risk of breast cancer (by 79 years), given disease free at age 35 years: 0.19

Figure 8.2   For a breast/ovarian cancer pedigree, the a priori carrier probability of the proband (according to Claus et al., 1994) as well as the a posteriori carrier probability and risk of breast cancer,
given a negative genetic test in the family and a genetic test sensitivity of 60%.

mutation analysis (FAMA), denaturing high-performance liquid chromatography
(DHPLC) and the protein truncation test (PTT), followed by direct sequencing of
detected sequence variants. These methods have lower levels of sensitivity. In
families with linkage evidence of disease due to *BRCA1*, standard mutation
screening methods were found to yield an estimated sensitivity of 63% (Ford et al.,
1998).

   Furthermore, all the predisposing genes for the disease may not have been
identified yet. Based on 237 families with at least four breast cancer cases aged less
than 60 years at diagnosis, collected by the Breast Cancer Linkage Consortium,
Ford et al. (1998) estimated that 80% of hereditary breast/ovarian cancer families
are attributed to *BRCA1* and 15% to *BRCA2*. For breast-cancer-only families,
BRCA1 and *BRCA2* contribute 28% and 37%, respectively, with 35% unexplained

by the identified genes. Since the majority of hereditary breast/ovarian cancer families are explained by the identified genes, *BRCA1* and *BRCA2*, the detection rate (or sensitivity) of genetic testing in such families will be higher than in breast-cancer-only families.

Is the calculated carrier probability valid for the prediction of mutations?

In most countries, a woman has to have a certain level of risk before testing for mutations in the *BRCA* genes is considered. Women from low-risk families rarely test positive due to the low prevalence of *BRCA* mutations in the population (Peto et al., 1999; Hopper et al., 1999); thus a negative test will not provide important information about the breast cancer risk. Some of the indications for carrying a *BRCA* mutation are: multiple early-onset breast cancer (under 50 years) in the family, ovarian cancer in addition to breast cancer in the family, breast and ovarian cancer in a woman, male breast cancer, and Ashkenazi ancestry.

We have shown that the complete pedigree could provide more valuable information; therefore, the carrier probability may be useful in the prediction of mutation. To evaluate this, we applied different models empirically to estimate the probability of carrying a breast cancer susceptibility gene for women with a family history of the disease, and compared these estimates with the outcome of mutation screening in a larger series of 618 families from eight collaborating centres in five European countries of the European Community demonstration project on familial breast cancer (Chang-Claude et al., 1999).

Screening for mutations in *BRCA1* was carried out in the affected proband or affected family member in each of the 618 families included in this study. Mutation screening in *BRCA2* was completed in 176 of these families. Different screening methods were employed in the different laboratories to detect sequence variants and included SSCP, CSGE, DGGE, FAMA and PTT. For other purposes of the study, only functionally relevant mutations were considered and individuals with missense mutations of unproven clinical significance were not considered 'positive' for germline pathogenic mutations (Durocher et al., 1996; Stoppa-Lyonnet et al., 1997).

For the individuals screened, carrier probability was calculated both using the penetrance parameters employed by both Easton et al. (1993) and Narod et al. (1995) for the analysis of the Breast Cancer Linkage Consortium data. Under the Easton model, breast cancer susceptibility is conferred by an autosomal dominant allele, with population frequency 0.0033, such that breast cancer risk is 67% by age 70 years. Under the Narod model, breast cancer susceptibility confers a breast cancer cumulative risk that is 71% by age 70 years and an ovarian cancer cumulative risk that is 42% by age 70 years.

For breast-cancer-only families, we observed a gradient of the proportion with *BRCA1* mutations with increasing carrier probability that appeared to be similar for carrier probabilities calculated according to the two genetic models. *BRCA1* mutations were detected in 34% or 26% (according to Easton or Narod model) of those who have a greater than 95% probability of carrying a mutant allele in a susceptibility gene, whereas mutations were found in about 5% among those with carrier probabilities of less than 40%. In the case of breast/ovarian families, *BRCA1* mutations were detected in 48% or 49% (according to Easton or Narod model) of those with carrier probabilities above 95%, and in 25% or 16% of those with carrier probabilities below 40%. Thus, for breast/ovarian cancer families (including ovarian-cancer-only families), the carrier probabilities calculated using the Narod model correlate better with the proportion of *BRCA1* mutations detected (Figure 8.3). *BRCA2* mutation analysis has not been completed for all families. Thus, although the largest proportion of mutations was detected in those who have carrier probabilities above 95%, the correlation with decreasing carrier probability is not clearly discernible.

Even solely in 97 families with four or more breast cancer cases diagnosed under the age of 60 years, regardless of the occurrence of ovarian cancer, there was clearly a correspondence between the proportion of mutations detected and the calculated carrier probability. The proportion of detected mutations was more than 40% in patients with carrier probabilities above 95%, less than 30% in those with carrier probabilities between 60% and 90%, and 0% for the nine families with carrier probabilities below 60%.

This data set was limited by the fact that mutation screening for *BRCA2* was not completed in all families. Nevertheless, the results indicate that estimation of the probability of being a carrier of a dominant breast cancer susceptibility gene, given the family history, provides a common measure for all types of families being counselled and gives a direct measure of the likelihood of detecting mutations in *BRCA1* and *BRCA2* if the contribution of these genes for the specific family type involved (breast-cancer-only or breast and ovarian cancer) is taken into account.

We also developed a maximum likelihood method for estimating the sensitivity of the genetic analysis based on this data set (Becher and Chang-Claude, 2002). Considering only families that were screened for *BRCA2* mutations when negative for *BRCA1* mutations, we estimated the sensitivity to be 65% for all families, 45% for breast-cancer-only families and 77% for breast/ovarian cancer families (unpublished data).

It is not possible to derive gene-specific risks using the LINKAGE software employed. Estimates of gene frequency of *BRCA1* and age-specific penetrance for *BRCA1* and *BRCA2* are available, and estimates of gene frequency of *BRCA2* are being generated from several population-based studies (Ford et al., 1995, 1998;

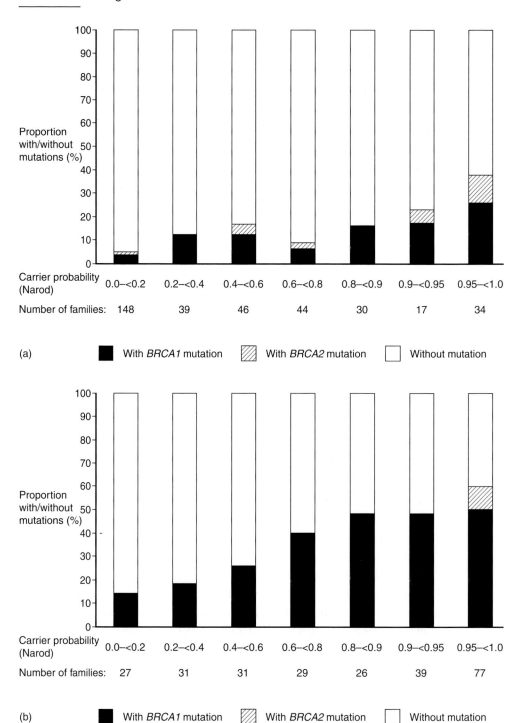

(a)   ■ With *BRCA1* mutation   ▨ With *BRCA2* mutation   □ Without mutation

(b)   ■ With *BRCA1* mutation   ▨ With *BRCA2* mutation   □ Without mutation

Figure 8.3   The proportion of (i) *BRCA1* mutation, (ii) *BRCA2* mutation and (iii) no mutation detected in screened patients from 358 breast-cancer-only families (a) and 260 breast/ovarian cancer families (b) in different ranges of carrier probability calculated using the genetic model according to Narod et al. (1995).

Fodor et al., 1998; Thorlacius et al., 1998; Antoniou et al., 2000). Bayesian prediction models have been proposed by Parmigiani et al. (1998) for determining carrier probabilities for breast cancer susceptibility genes *BRCA1* and *BRCA2*, requiring estimates of gene frequency and penetrances for the specific genes. It is also possible to use MENDEL to calculate gene-specific carrier probabilities based on genetic models that account for the two genes (Antoniou et al., 2000). Presently, it is not known whether the estimation of gene-specific carrier probabilities is useful in the clinical setting to prioritize mutation screening for one of the two *BRCA* genes. In the future, we shall be able to evaluate the usefulness of estimates of gene-specific risks for decision-making in genetic diagnosis.

Summary

For genetic counselling on familial breast cancer, an accurate evaluation is needed of the probability that a woman carries a mutation before any decisions are made regarding genetic analysis. One commonly employed model for estimating breast cancer risk, specifically for women with a family history of the disease, is based on the Cancer and Steroid Hormone (CASH) study data set. Claus et al. (1994) have used these data to construct detailed tables that provide an easy method of predicting the cumulative risk of breast cancer for a woman over a given time-interval, based on age at onset of one or two affected first- and/or second-degree relatives. A more sophisticated method of risk prediction considers the complete pedigree structure and allows the estimation of the proband's probability of carrying a susceptibility gene under a particular genetic model, given her family history. This provides a common measure for all types of families being counselled and gives a direct measure of the likelihood of detecting mutations in *BRCA1* and *BRCA2*.

Genetic analysis used to identify functionally relevant mutation in an affected woman in a high-risk family will permit differentiation between gene carrier and non-gene carrier status in family members tested for the identified mutation and thus more accurate quantification of risk for the unaffected family members. However, the sensitivity of genetic testing will be much less than 100% because of: (1) the sensitivity of the screening methods commonly employed for the genetic analysis of *BRCA1/2* in genetics clinics, and (2) the existence of further, as yet unidentified, predisposing genes for breast cancer, particularly for site-specific hereditary breast cancer. Therefore, women from families with an extensive family history who test negative for *BRCA* mutations will remain at a higher risk than the general population.

Acknowledgements

We would like to thank Maria Caligo, Diana Eccles, Gareth Evans, Neva Haites, Shirley Hodgson, Pål Møller, Brigitte Royer-Pokora, Dominique Stoppa-Lyonnet and Bernhard HF Weber for contributing pedigree, clinical and mutation data to the collaborative work presented, which was made possible by funding from the European Community. We also thank Christine Fischer for useful comments.

REFERENCES

Andersen TI, Borresen AL and Moller P (1996). A common BRCA1 mutation in Norwegian breast and ovarian cancer families? (letter) *Am J Hum Genet* **59**: 486–7.

Antoniou AC, Gayther SA, Stratton JF, Ponder BA and Easton DF (2000). Risk models for familial ovarian and breast cancer. *Genet Epidemiol* **18**(2): 173–90.

Becher H and Chang-Claude J (1996). Estimation of population specific individual disease risks for a given family history with an application to breast cancer. *Genet Epidemiol* **13**: 229–42.

Becher H and Chang-Claude J (2002). A note on estimating the sensitivity of a genetic test using gene carrier probability estimates and its application in genetic counselling. *J Epidemiol Biostatistics* (in press).

Berman DB, Costalas J, Schultz DC, Grana G, Daly M and Godwin AK (1996). A common mutation in BRCA2 that predisposes to a variety of cancers is found in both Jewish Ashkenazi and non-Jewish individuals. *Cancer Res* **56**: 3409–14.

Bondy ML, Lustbader ED, Halabi S, Ross E and Vogel VG (1994). Validation of a breast cancer risk assessment model in women with a positive family history. *J Natl Cancer Inst* **86**(8): 620–5.

Chang-Claude J, Becher H, Caligo M, et al. (1999). Risk estimation as a decision-making tool for genetic analysis of the breast cancer susceptibility genes. *Dis Markers* **15**: 53–65.

Claus EB, Risch N and Thompson WD (1991). Genetic analysis of breast cancer in the cancer and steroid hormone study. *Am J Hum Genet* **48**: 232–42.

Claus EB, Risch N and Thompson WD (1994). Autosomal dominant inheritance of early-onset breast cancer. *Cancer* **73**: 643–51.

Durocher F, Shattuck-Eidens D, McClure M, et al. (1996). Comparison of BRCA1 polymorphisms, rare sequence variants and/or missense mutations in unaffected and breast/ovarian cancer populations. *Hum Mol Genet* **5**(6): 835–42.

Easton DF, Bishop DT, Ford D, Crockford GP, et al. (1993). Genetic linkage analysis in familial breast and ovarian cancer: results from 214 families. *Am J Hum Genet* **52**: 678–701.

Easton DF, Ford D and Bishop DT (1995). Breast and ovarian cancer incidence in BRCA1-mutation carriers. Breast Cancer Linkage Consortium. *Am J Hum Genet* **56**: 265–71.

Easton DF, Steele L, Fields P, et al. (1997). Cancer risks in two large breast cancer families linked to BRCA2 on chromosome 13q12–13. *Am J Hum Genet* **61**(1): 120–8.

Fodor FH, Weston A, Bleiweiss IJ, et al. (1998). Frequency and carrier risk associated with common BRCA1 and BRCA2 mutations in Ashkenazi Jewish breast cancer patients. *Am J Hum Genet* **63**(1): 45–51.

Ford D, Easton DF and Peto J (1995). Estimates of the gene frequency of BRCA1 and its contribution to breast and ovarian cancer incidence. *Am J Hum Genet* **57**: 1457–62.

Ford D, Easton DF, Stratton M, et al. (1998). Genetic heterogeneity and penetrance analysis of the BRCA1 and BRCA2 genes in breast cancer families. *Am J Hum Genet* **62**(3): 676–89.

Frank TS, Manley SA, Olufunmilayo I, et al. (1998). Sequence analysis of *BRCA1* and *BRCA2*: correlation of mutations with family history and ovarian cancer risk. *J Clin Oncol* **16**: 2417–25.

Gail MH, Brinton LA, Byar DP, et al. (1989). Projecting individualized probabilities of developing breast cancer for white females who are being examined annually. *J Natl Cancer Inst* **81**(24): 1879–86.

Gayther SA and Ponder BA (1997). Mutations of the *BRCA1* and *BRCA2* genes and the possibilities for predictive testing. *Mol Med Today* **3**(4): 168–74.

Hopper JL, Southey MC, Dite GS, et al. (1999). Population-based estimate of the average age-specific cumulative risk of breast cancer for a defined set of protein-truncating mutations in BRCA1 and BRCA2. *Cancer Epidemiol Biomarkers Prev* **8**: 741–7.

Johannesdottir G, Gudmundsson J, Bergthorsson JT, et al. (1996). High prevalence of the 999del5 mutation in Icelandic breast and ovarian cancer patients. *Cancer Res* **56**: 3663–5.

Lange K and Weeks D (1988). Programs for pedigree analysis: MENDEL, FISHER, and dGENE. *Genet Epidemiol* **5**, 471–2.

Lathrop GM, Lalouel JM, Julier C and Ott J (1984). Strategies for multilocus linkage analysis in humans. *Proc Natl Acad Sci USA* **81**: 3443–6.

Malone KE, Daling JR, Thompson JD, O'Brien CA, Francisco LV and Ostrander EA (1998). BRCA1 mutations and breast cancer in the general population: analyses in women before age 35 years and in women before age 45 years with first-degree family history. *JAMA* **279**(12): 922–9.

Miki Y, Swensen J, Shattuck-Eidens D, et al. (1994). A strong candidate for the breast and ovarian cancer susceptibility gene BRCA1. *Science* **266**: 66–71.

Narod SA, Ford D, Devilee P, et al. (1995). An evaluation of genetic heterogeneity in 145 breast–ovarian cancer families. *Am J Hum Genet* **56**: 254–64.

Newman B, Mu H, Butler LM, Millikan RC, Moorman PG and King MC (1998). Frequency of breast cancer attributable to BRCA1 in a population-based series of American women. *JAMA* **279**(12): 915–21.

Parmigiani G, Berry D and Aguilar O (1998). Determining carrier probabilities for breast cancer-susceptibility genes BRCA1 and BRCA2. *Am J Hum Genet* **62**(1): 145–58.

Peto J, Collins N, Barfoot R, et al. (1999). Prevalence of BRCA1 and BRCA2 gene mutations in patients with early-onset breast cancer. *J Natl Cancer Inst* **11**: 943–9.

Petrij-Bosch A, Peelen T, van Vliet M, et al. (1997). BRCA1 genomic deletions are major founder mutations in Dutch breast cancer patients. *Nat Genet* **17**(3): 341–5.

Puget N, Stoppa-Lyonnet D, Sinilnikova OM, et al. (1999). Screening for germ-line rearrangements and regulatory mutations in BRCA1 led to the identification of four new deletions. *Cancer Res* **59**(2): 455–61.

Schmidt S, Becher H and Chang-Claude J (1998). Breast cancer risk assessment: use of complete pedigree information and the effect of misspecified ages at diagnosis of affected relatives. *Hum Genet* **102**: 348–56.

Stoppa-Lyonnet D, Laurent-Puig P, Essioux L, et al. (1997). BRCA1 sequence variations in 160 individuals referred to a breast/ovarian family cancer clinic. Institut Curie Breast Cancer Group. *Am J Hum Genet* **60**(5): 1021–30.

Stratton MR (1996). Recent advances in understanding of genetic susceptibility to breast cancer. *Hum Mol Genet* **5**: 1515–19.

Struewing JP, Hartge P, Wacholder S, et al. (1997). The risk of cancer associated with specific mutations of BRCA1 and BRCA2 among Ashkenazi Jews [see comments]. *N Engl J Med* **336**(20): 1401–8.

Thorlacius S, Struewing JP, Hartge P, et al. (1998). Population-based study of risk of breast cancer in carriers of *BRCA2* mutation. *Lancet* **352**: 1337–9.

Wooster R, Bignell G, Lancaster J, et al. (1995). Identification of the breast cancer susceptibility gene BRCA2 [see comments]. *Nature* **378**: 789–92.

Part 2

Screening

9

Developing a cancer genetics service: a Welsh model

Jonathon Gray

University Hospital of Wales, Cardiff, UK

Although genetic mechanisms have long been recognized as central in the causation of cancer, the practical importance of genetic and familial aspects has only now been widely appreciated. In the past, clinical genetics services were involved only in rare Mendelian cancer genetic disorders in which the risks were clear and intervention or surveillance was possible. It has recently become clear that in some of the more common cancers, notably breast, ovarian and colon cancer, there is a Mendelian subset in which the genetic risks are also extremely high. This subset is considerably more common than the combined incidence of the rarer, single-gene familial cancer syndromes.

The discovery of mutations and specific genes conferring a high risk of colorectal, breast or ovarian cancer means that comparable genetic approaches are now potentially applicable to this subset of common tumours. It is increasingly possible to distinguish family members who carry such genes from those who do not. As a result, surveillance and management resources can be directed towards family members who carry the predisposing gene, and those who do not carry such a gene can avoid the often uncomfortable diagnostic procedures and the possibility of surgical intervention.

A further influence on service demand has been intense media publicity and the high scientific profile of recent discoveries in breast cancer. Concerns are inevitably raised by such stories, and not just in families in which the genetic risk is high. The challenge is to develop a service that adequately reassures inappropriately worried individuals (remembering that they retain the population risk of cancer) and identifies those at high risk who require further information and management. In the UK, such services have been developed, albeit on an ad hoc basis, but many still rely on research funding.

Background

Recommendations have recently been made for a core service in cancer genetics (Genetics and Cancer Services Working Group, 1996). This chapter discusses some of the main issues and conclusions that can be taken from this report, and how they have been implemented on a practical level. We have attempted to place the recommendations of the central report in the context of an evolving cancer genetics service that is currently under evaluation in Wales.

Recommendations

Primary care

Primary care is identified as the principal focus for clinical cancer genetics services, particularly for referrals or enquiries that are likely to represent a low risk. This follows the general pattern for cancer services recommended in the Calman Hine report. Education initiatives for general practitioner trainees, practice nurses, health visitors and other key nursing staff must be established with the help of specialist nurses in cancer genetics. Information technology initiatives (e.g. provision of computer-based information, risk estimation programmes, etc.) should be developed and evaluated. Establishment of referral guidelines is essential to allow those in primary care to recognize the important minority who require specialist referral. Initial steps to implement these recommendations have already been taken, but ensuring that primary care services as a whole are equipped with the facilities required is a major challenge.

Cancer units

Cancer units have an important role in the provision of clinics for patients at intermediate levels of risk. The need for genetic involvement may be less certain in these individuals, but primary care staff may feel unable to deal alone with such cases. There should be a clear management plan that is comparable between the cancer units and enables recognition of which referrals from primary care are best dealt with at this level and which require direct involvement with a cancer centre and a specialist consultant in cancer genetics. Such plans must be agreed at all levels of the service. Each cancer unit could have a designated staff member to coordinate cancer genetic referrals and clinic activities; with appropriate training, this individual could be an existing nurse specialist within the locally based genetics or oncology service. Full-time cancer genetics staff are unlikely to be required at cancer unit level, and the costs would be high given the large number of such units. Whilst clinicians and other staff working in district hospitals and future cancer units will not have extensive expertise in genetic aspects of cancer, so education initiatives and genetic risk-estimation programmes will be as important as personnel at this level and in primary care. Once trained, existing cancer unit staff will form an important link in the chain of expertise linking primary care, cancer units and other cancer centres.

Cancer centres

Cancer centres require a partnership between medical genetics and oncology services. A specialist cancer genetics clinic should form the foundation of the clinical cancer genetics service; it should principally see patients and family members at high risk of inherited syndromes, and those in whom a common cancer is clearly genetic in origin. A consultant in cancer genetics should work in each centre. Training of such consultants should cover relevant aspects of medical genetics and oncology, and their role should include the development and coordination of management policies, referral guidelines and educational programmes for cancer units and primary care staff.

Genetic databases are an important part of the comprehensive system for identifying relatives at high risk of familial cancers, and should form an integral part of clinical cancer genetics services. Pre-symptomatic genetic testing is feasible in an increasing number of familial cancers. There are clear benefits in identifying gene carriers among individuals at high risk and in avoiding investigations and surveillance in some forms of inherited cancer, but the value of this approach in much lower risk situations remains unproven. Pre-symptomatic genetic testing should be undertaken only in conjunction with the provision of appropriate information, genetic counselling and support, and specific consent must be obtained. Because this form of genetic testing is often complex, laboratories undertaking pre-symptomatic genetic testing for familial cancers must be appropriately experienced and accredited, and must liaise closely with clinical cancer genetics staff. Genetic testing should form part of the overall cancer genetics services.

Evaluation of services

Evaluation of all new and existing services is essential because current evidence on efficacy is limited. It is recommended that services established without means of evaluation should not be funded. Coordination of such service implementation and data collection across the UK is required in order to allow key questions to be answered. Evaluation should include not only clinical effectiveness and acceptability, but also health economics and assessment of psychosocial aspects of healthcare provision.

The developing service in Wales

How can traditional medical genetics services cope with the demand generated by members of the public who are worried about a possible family history of cancer? What role does clinical genetics have in the increasing number of common conditions for which Mendelian genetic subtypes have been identified? Cancer genetics service models may provide a test. Whilst implementing the above recommendations in an all-Wales service, there have been many challenges. Some of the achievements and challenges are discussed in the remaining part of this chapter. Resources are finite, the current medical training programmes fail to deliver the required number of appropriately trained cancer genetics consultants, and the large potential demand for information on familial cancer risk forces us to look at service models that can practically be implemented in a resource-efficient way, capitalizing on an extended nurse/counsellor model of service delivery.

Our approach involves a triage or 'filtering' system, in which all referrals are received by the local counsellor (be that nurse or MSc trained genetic counsellor). Questionnaires are sent to all appropriate referrals on receipt, allowing pedigrees to be drawn using the Cyrillic-based pedigree system, cancer diagnoses are confirmed, and then risk assessment can be calculated. The outcome of this is the defining of low- (not significantly raised above population risk), moderate- and high-risk groups. Low-risk individuals are referred back to primary care, hopefully reassured (an area of active research). High-risk individuals attend the genetics clinics in cancer centres. Moderate-risk individuals are dealt with at cancer units with coordination of their screening and follow-up. The success of this programme depends on the cancer genetics counsellor input and an effective working relationship with primary care.

Primary care in the cancer genetics service for Wales

Guidelines were drawn up and distributed to all GPs in Wales by the National Assembly for Wales (Box 9.1). Crucially, the guidelines were developed in a multidisciplinary fashion – initially in conjunction with the cancer lead clinicians, public health representatives, voluntary groups, patient groups and GPs. Multiple meetings were required over an 18-month period and all decisions were taken to and endorsed by the Royal College of General Practitioners, the GP committee of the BMA, and the appropriate government committees. Key to our work with the GPs was a series of focus groups, as outlined in Box 9.2, giving a real sense of ownership to the primary care groups.

Box 9.1   **Referral guidelines**

Breast cancer
- 1 first-degree relative diagnosed at 40 years or younger
- 2 first-degree relatives diagnosed at 60 years or younger (on same side of family)
- 3 first- or second-degree relatives any age (on same side of family)
- 1 first-degree relative with male breast cancer
- A first-degree relative with bilateral breast cancer

Note: breast cancer can also be inherited through the *paternal* side of the family

Breast/ovarian cancer
- Minimum: 1 of each cancer in first-degree relatives
  (If only 1 of each cancer, the breast cancer diagnosed under 50 years)
- A first-degree relative who has *both* breast and ovarian cancer

Ovarian cancer
- 2 or more ovarian cancers, at least 1 first-degree relative affected (on same side of family)

Colon cancer
- 1 first-degree relative diagnosed at age 40 years or younger
- 2 first-degree relatives diagnosed at 60 years or younger (on same side of family)
- 3 relatives, all on same side of family (at least 1 should be a first-degree relative)
- Familial adenomatous polyposis
- Hereditary non-polyposis colorectal cancer (revised Amsterdam criteria)

Other cancer syndromes
- Patient from a family with a known single-gene cancer syndrome (e.g. von Hippel–Lindau disease, multiple endocrine neoplasia, retinoblastoma)
- 'Related cancers'. There are some rare cancer syndromes (e.g. Li–Fraumeni syndrome and Cowden syndrome) where a variety of different cancers occur within a family. Where there is a high index of suspicion, the possibility of referral should be discussed on an individual basis.

Evaluation of the service

The Cancer Genetics Service for Wales is one of the first services of this type to be established in the UK; therefore there is a particular responsibility to carry out adequate evaluation. Evaluation of the service is an independent exercise designed to assess aspects of acceptability, effectiveness and cost. The evaluation would be based on three established principles: (1) addressing a focus set of questions, (2)

Box 9.2   **General practitioner focus groups**

A pair of sequential focus groups met to explore the reactions of GPs to the triage system and associated referral guidelines. The participants were provided with reading material concerning cancer genetics and the proposed service. Existing studies had revealed that GPs were not acquainted with this clinical area and we chose to ensure that the participants became better informed over time and had the opportunity to consider the issues covered. It is recognized that initial reactions are often unrepresentative and we therefore designed a method where information provision and group interaction facilitated insights that were the outcome of a *reflective* process.

Participants and focus groups meetings

Over three-quarters of the Welsh population live in urban areas. Practitioners from Swansea and neighbouring areas were chosen for this study because the city represents an urban population that is distant from a tertiary genetics specialist centre.

We therefore convened two groups of GPs. The first group consisted of purposively selected doctors who had part-time educational roles in a university-based department of postgraduate education (age range 38–54 years). We chose this sample in order to represent the views of practitioners who had responsibilities for maintaining the professional development of their colleagues and an increased motivation to monitor the impact of clinical developments. The second group of practitioners was randomly selected from a list of all those who worked in the area, provided that they had no academic or educational roles. Prior to their attendance at the focus groups, and at the end of the series, each participant was asked to complete a short questionnaire that assessed their views on genetics generally and specifically on the new cancer genetics service.

Each participant was given reading material in advance of every meeting, which contained background articles on cancer genetics. During the focus groups, participants engaged in case study discussions and were given risk information and assessment tools and examples of patient information leaflets.

Topics

Focus group 1
- Impact of the 'new' genetics on general practice
- The new Cancer Genetics Service for Wales

Focus group 2
- The referral guidelines
- Who should manage patients at 'low risk'?

Focus group 3
- How acceptable is the triage system?
- How should the service supply information to primary care?

Box 9.2   **(cont.)**

> **Data collection and analysis**
>
> The interviews were tape-recorded, transcribed and analysed. The moderator studied the transcripts repeatedly, explored meanings and ascribed the main themes. First, the moderator checked the themes with each of those interviewed independently and obtained agreement by discussion. Second, a report was sent to the participants after each focus group had met, describing the process and listing relevant transcript excerpts under emergent themes. Third, by postal consultation, agreement was achieved that this account represented an accurate analysis of the discussions.

marrying questions to active goals and objectives, and (3) objectivity in the evaluation process.

Aims of the cancer genetics service for Wales

The Welsh Office and Macmillan Cancer Relief initially implemented the funding for the all-Wales service in 1998 as a model system with an evaluated framework. Initially, the main aims of the cancer genetics service were:

1 To filter referred patients before they reach hospital clinics, e.g. genetics, surgical and gynaecological outpatient clinics;

2 To extend the traditional role of nurse specialists (and MSc trained genetic counsellors), increasing their areas of expertise and creating skill mixes with the less traditional (in the UK) non-nursing genetics associate role;

3 To prevent individuals whose risk is not significantly greater than that of the general population from entering the hospital system. This avoids submitting these patients to further investigations and reduces the clinical load on the specialties.

Steering group

In committing the initial funding required for the first elements of the Cancer Genetics Service for Wales, the National Assembly required the establishment of a steering group, with representation from public health, primary care, surgery and cancer service coordination and the Chief Scientific Officer, to oversee the ongoing development, evaluation and roll-out of the new Wales service. Such a high level steering group has been of immense importance both in aiding the direction the service development has taken and also in giving high-level access to the government so that it may deal with issues and problems as they have occurred.

Evaluation group

An external evaluation group was seen as essential to assess the service development over its first 3 years, and advise on progress, failures and the relative benefits of future funding options.

Health service evaluation objectives

1 To describe the development of the new service
2 To study staff and referring agencies in order to find out about their perceptions of the service and the nature of consultation
3 To collate and analyse the routinely collected information so that the quality and equity of the service may be assessed
4 To follow three groups of patients and one group of non-users, and collect data on:
   - the impact of the service on uptake, decision making, perception of risk, family communication, health and psychosocial well-being
   - experience and perceptions of the service
   - use of other health and social services

Health economics objectives

1 From an NHS perspective – to identify and measure the direct costs from consumables, laboratory administration, overheads, capital charges and other expenditures of the service
2 To establish the main cost of genetics services for patients at high, medium and low risk of a range of cancers
3 To elicit the value placed by patients on the service

Development of benchmarks for the regional cancer genetics service

Benchmarks can be appropriate indicators of value in monitoring, understanding and predicting what improves the performance of the service. Agreement needs to be reached on what constitutes 'good' and 'poor' quality, and therefore performance, for a given indicator. The services need to be aware of the appropriate comparators, deciding appropriate local regional or national levels against which to compare performance. We have to be very aware of the potential inconsistency or conflict between the measures and determine which measures are reported internally and externally to stake holders in the wider community. We particularly wanted to look for performance indicators that related to both short-term achievements or progress towards stated targets, and that reflected evidence-based anticipated changes that we believe will be important to achieve the longer

Box 9.3   **Benchmarks being piloted for cancer genetics service provision**

Objective met by indicator	Indicator
F	Average time to given risk
F	Average time to clinic
EQ	Consultant/million total population
EQ	Cancer genetics clinics per million
EQ	Admin staff per million
EQ	Clinics per million
EQ	New families referred per million
EQ/A	Referrals per million cancer type
	Referrals by type/region
EQ/A	Waiting time – risk
EQ/A	Waiting time – clinic
EQ/A	Proportion of all referrals getting home visit
	Proportion of all referrals getting telephone counselling
A	Proportion of referrals getting a clinic appointment with a counsellor/at a cancer genetics clinic
A	Proportion of referrals getting follow-up (by letter or other means)
EF	Proportion of all referrals (high/moderate/low/inappropriate)
EF/EQ	Referral sources (GP/surgeon/O & G/Oncology)
EF	Ratio of attenders/non-attenders
EF	Proportion of new/follow-up
EF	Numbers seen in clinic (e.g. cancer genetics clinic)
P	Complaints to the service
P	Thank-you letters to the service

Laboratory services used (accredited? Y/N)

EV	*BRCA1/2* turnaround time
EV	Sensitivity of test (versus what gold standard)?

Journal club frequency/year

EV	Attendance at journal club as a proportion of total staff

Audit of protocol efficacy

QA	Appropriate/inappropriate referrals per million

Audit of risk assessment

QA	Proportion of positive mutation searches in high-risk group

Audit of clinical notes (% of satisfactory records)

QA	Satisfactory content

Box 9.3 *(cont.)*

Audit of lectures/talks given (number given per year)

QA	Consultant
QA	CGC
I	Talks given per month (total) (counsellor/cancer genetics clinic)

A, accessible; EF, efficient; EQ, equitable; EV, evidence based; F, fast; I, information; P, patient centred; QA, quality audit.

term outcomes. We looked for quantifiable targets within the agreed time-scale of yearly monitoring, and tried to reflect regional and national policies. In identifying precise indicators we felt it important to discuss them in relation to the service remit strategy, and within the agreed monitoring framework of our steering panel. It was important to identify what data were currently available and could be accessed and combined to produce these indicators.

In keeping with much of the work nationally on indicators in the NHS, we felt they needed to be relevant (relating directly to the objectives set), unambiguous (clear-held changes in the indicator reflect changes in the service or performance), cost effective (the costs of collecting and monitoring the information should not exceed the benefits), simple (what is measured and why it is important should be understandable), and output- and outcome-orientated (focusing on what we are trying to deliver). Box 9.3 shows a small sub-sample of the benchmarks that are currently being used by the service and piloted with other regional genetics services in the UK.

Service delivery and information technology

As referrals and interest increase in genetics, and the implications for families are recognized, there is an increasing pressure to develop service provision in relevant ways. The Government has laid out a programme of reform for the NHS that is intended to improve the quality of care. A key element in that strategy involves increasing the efficiency and effectiveness of healthcare professionals. Information technology is seen as playing a crucial role by its ability to improve communication and sharing of information across professional boundaries. We have explored three elements of such a high-level information and management technology strategy:

Box 9.4   **Development of a team website**

Website development

      Website provision has been developed and evaluated across Wales.

The website contributes positively to the areas of:

      (a) effectiveness – the goals of the intended users being supported by the website can be identified as being met;

      (b) efficiency – retrieval exercise undertaken assured that the users can perform a wide range of tests;

      (c) satisfaction – all the usability tests showed an overwhelming and positive attitude by users.

The website design guidelines:

      (a) make the users the focus,

      (b) make content paramount,

      (c) develop an iterative approach,

      (d) make updates frequently,

      (e) keep pages simple,

      (f) keep layout and navigation consistent,

      (g) give users training.

---

1 Development of an all-Wales team website (Box 9.4)

2 Development of a web-based all-Wales data entry system (Information System for Clinical Organizations) (Fig 9.1)

3 Videoconferencing ('telegenetics') to improve team communication between distanced centres, and also to allow the counselling of patients across Wales (Box 9.5).

Looking to the future

There have been many other essential components in developing and taking the first few faltering steps of this Cancer Genetics Service for Wales. One of the other crucial elements to our successful first few years has been the key input from our cancer genetics research team. Within our research strategy we targeted several key areas, including information technology, education and psychological interventions, within novel service structures. A key element within our research strategy has been our 'crystal ball gazing' attempts, looking ahead perhaps 10 years to the future and trying to predict what important developments are likely, and what may be needed. After many enjoyable sessions gazing into the future, we felt that we would share with you one such session in the form of the scenario outlined in Box 9.6.

Box 9.5   **Videoconferencing**

A pilot study of telegenetics

Videoconferencing ('telegenetics') is used to:

- Provide specialized healthcare advice to remote clinical sites.
- Meet the increasing demand for specialized service provision.
- Expand our capacity to give information at sites distant from the main specialist centre.
- Standardize technology.

In addition:

- Evaluation showed a high level of patient and doctor satisfaction, and a reduced level of nurse satisfaction.
- Work has to be done regarding the doctor/nurse counselling process at it alters the roles of the individuals involved. Telegenetics is an innovative and potentially cost-effective means of increasing contact with distant sites that require specialist service provision.
- Comments from patients:

'I found the experience very reassuring and would certainly recommend this method'. 'Initially, you are aware of the TV but afterwards forgot about it.' 'As TV is a medium that I am used to, it is quite usual to receive information from the television'. 'I do prefer this method of consultation as I do not like going to hospitals and sitting in overcrowded waiting rooms with many sick people, for an indeterminate length of time.'

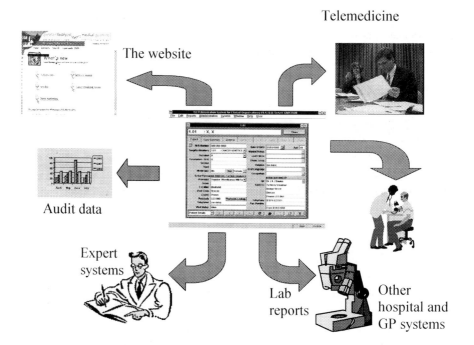

Figure 9.1   Development of a web-based data entry system across Wales.

Box 9.6   **One possible future!**

Scenario – Cardiff 2010

It all started just after we moved house and I had to register with the Virtual Health Centre down the road. Every new patient registering must submit a blood sample (which, of course, is stored for possible DNA analysis) and is also required to complete a detailed family history, even to the extent of submitting the details of any relatives' Virtual Health Centres too. It means they can all hook up electronically and send our family histories to and fro – which is common sense I suppose.

I had a number of cancer concerns when I went to the Virtual Health Centre for the first time. I had a bit of a family history of breast and colon cancer, but what *really* made me worry was all the scare stories in the media about brain cancer and 'mobile dementia', which was caused by the last generation of mobile phones you know, stories about breast cancer being caused by roll-on deodorants, cancer-causing electricity pylons, and so on and so on. When I went first, my intention was to ask to be referred to someone who could test me and tell me if I was *definitely* going to get cancer when I got older.

The Virtual Health Centre has a state-of-the-art link-up with the Cancer Genetics Centre (CGC) in Cardiff. It is the main cancer genetics centre in Wales now, though there are skeleton services available in west and north Wales. Cancer genetics used to be part of the Institute of Medical Genetics, but after the completion of the Human Genome Project in 2003 and the subsequent discovery of a whole range of cancer genes, including *BRCA3*, *BRCA4*, *OV7*, *OV8*, *PROST45* and *PROST57*, the demand for cancer genetics services really escalated and it made sense to separate cancer genetics from the rest of the rare genetic conditions that the Institute deals with.

This link-up from primary care to the CGC all started in 2005 when the government decided that everyone should be equipped with the latest technology – a laptop computer for every member of the primary healthcare team, all referrals to specialists be done by e-mail, and every specialist to develop their own website dedicated to 'clinical management' with links back to primary care.

The CGC website has information about the entire cancer genetics team. There are about 20 people working there already and they seem to be a mixed bag of nurses, psychologists, sociologists, IT people and lawyers. With shared decision-making all the rage these days, my GP and I looked at all their personal profiles and eventually chose the one I thought I would be most compatible with as my key worker. The rest was easy then and we simply e-mailed, requesting a referral.

Before our referral was accepted, we were directed to the section of the website that deals with family history and risk assessment. All sorts of risk tools are now up on the CGC's website and they are each ranked according to how quickly they assess risk, the reliability of the data they use, and how useful others have found them. My doctor and I went through my family history together to see if I was at significantly increased risk for any of the main cancers, and to see what genetic tests were available. We decided that I was at moderate risk for these cancers compared with the rest of the population. That really worried me, but luckily there was another bit of the website that did psychology – employing various techniques and even giving us access to real-time on-line counselling.

Almost immediately after my doctor and I e-mailed the CGC, we received an appointment for a video link-up with the genetic nurse for the next morning. It's great not having waiting lists any more! Most of the video-link appointment involved going through my completed family history forms and double-checking for errors. Obviously, they asked whether I had thought through the implications of having a test and what I would do if I discovered that I did actually have one of the *BRCA* or *COLCANCER* genes. They had to warn me about the insurance and employment implications too.

Box 9.6   **(cont.)**

Even though the Genetic Discrimination Act has been in force for many years now, most insurance companies do everything they can to find out about your predispositions. Most employers realize that the chances of their employees getting some form of cancer are huge but they have to cover themselves in case there is an environmental (i.e. workplace-induced) connection too. After the initial video-link discussion, I opted for a home visit to be 'blooded' – for those of you who don't know, the nurses still use this traditional term even though they collect saliva and hair now. The discovery that breast cancer could be diagnosed with a hair sample revolutionized the perception of genetic testing.

When I finally got an appointment to actually go to the CGC, I was assigned a code. They said every new patient needed a code because of the huge number of research studies that were running with people referred into the service. I was only allowed to be admitted into three research studies while I was a patient, but they said that once I had been discharged from their system, there could be an unlimited number of requests to take part in retrospective studies. Increasingly, researchers have to pay patients to participate in their studies, so I hadn't realized this would be quite so lucrative. In fact, I needn't have bothered applying for *Big Brother 2011* – now in its tenth year and with prize money of £1 million – if I knew I could get a bit of extra cash just by having a few cancer concerns. Anyway the research projects I chose were: (a) analysing non-verbal communication during the counselling process, (b) improving my coping strategies and, of course, (c) telegenetics.

The telegenetics project means that I get to see extra people to talk about my concerns, though obviously not face-to-face. They now hook you up remotely with each member of staff – the nurse, the psychologist, the lawyer, etc. – to go through the issues from every possible perspective. Admittedly you are accompanied by a specialist genetics nurse at each stage so you have that 'continuity of care'. Ever since an earlier research project showed that nurses do it just as well, most specialist services are trying to cut back on their consultants. It's just like maternity services now – you never see a consultant until something goes wrong. Still, the nurses have more experience, it feels like they really know what they are talking about, and it's nice to have their company throughout the different sorts of counselling.

Anyway, I've had my genetic counselling – both face-to-face and by teleconsultation. I've talked to every possible professional there is about the implications of having a genetic test. I have learnt about coping strategies and all sorts of distraction techniques. I've filled in piles of surveys and participated in every focus group going. I think I'm ready. I'll do the test.

Acknowledgements: With thanks to Rachel Iredale for producing the scenario.

REFERENCES

Genetics and Cancer Services Working Group (1996). *Working Group for the Chief Medical Officer on Genetics and Cancer Services.* London: Department of Health.

10

Referral criteria for cancer genetics clinics

Diana M. Eccles

Princess Anne Hospital, Southampton, UK

Introduction

Setting criteria for referral to a clinic requires a clear view of the purpose of the clinic for which the criteria are being set. This chapter will review the current approaches to assessing and managing breast cancer risk and will attempt to put these approaches into the context of the available evidence regarding clinical effectiveness.

Background

Primary care and breast cancer units have found themselves besieged by women who are worried about their risk of breast cancer. The origins of this worry may be media driven, family driven or physician driven and may be appropriate (in those at high genetic risk) or inappropriate. In response to public demand for risk management options, many 'family history' clinics have sprung up throughout western Europe, offering breast screening to women who present with concerns about breast cancer risk, usually in this circumstance based on a family history of the disease. Breast screening mammograms with or without physical examination are the measures usually aimed at early breast cancer detection. There are no large scale *randomized* trials of breast screening in women who are under 50 years of age and at increased genetic risk of breast cancer. There are a small number of reported cohort studies involving relatively small numbers that indicate that breast cancer can be successfully detected at early stages in women under 50 who undergo regular screening examinations (Kollias et al., 1998; Lalloo et al., 1998; Møller et al., 1998; Kerlikowske et al., 2000; Tilanus-Linthorst et al., 2000). Heightened awareness may facilitate earlier detection and diagnosis of interval cancers. Psychological morbidity related to false-positive screening results and the ensuing investigations need to be considered (Rimer and Bluman, 1997). The mortality reduction claimed for mammographic screening in the general population aged

50–64 years, and to a lesser extent 40–49 years, together with the earlier stage at detection observed in women screened because of a family history of breast cancer, has encouraged investigators to speculate that an earlier stage at detection in the family history group is likely to translate into a longer term reduction in mortality. Methodological flaws and small numbers mean that current studies are unlikely to be able to demonstrate convincing gains in mortality in the short term. There is some emerging evidence of a survival benefit for screening mammography in the 40–49 year age group in the general population, but this is smaller than the reduction in mortality found in the 50–64 year age group (Tabar et al., 1996; Bjurstam et al., 1997), and there are a number of studies showing that survival in *BRCA1* gene carriers with breast cancer may be worse than for matched controls (Foulkes et al., 1997; Pharoah et al., 1999; Stoppa-Lyonnet et al., 2000).

In the UK, a working party was required by the government to study the provision of healthcare services to individuals concerned about a genetic risk of cancer in the family (Harper, 1998). This working party recommended that, in broad terms, individuals should be defined as 'low', 'moderate' or 'high' genetic risk. In the NHS these could conveniently be dealt with by the primary care team if low risk, the cancer unit (hospital specialist for cancer screening) if moderate risk, and by both the hospital specialist for cancer screening and the regional genetics service for genetic investigation and family follow-up where the genetic risk is high. Further, the recommendation within this document was for cancer genetics specialists to be a part of the multidisciplinary approach to cancer treatment.

Thus, a framework is emerging in the UK and in many centres in mainland Europe where risk is assessed first by the patient and/or the primary care physician (GP) (Harper, 1998), and second, by the secondary care (hospital-based) team, with the genetics assessment being reserved in the main for moderate- and high-risk women. The level of risk at each level depends to a large extent on local resource and interest (often research interests).

Guidelines

Implementation of evidence-based guidelines may limit choices for doctors, for commissioners of health care and, most importantly, for patients. Implications for resources and the real effect of proposed strategies must be evaluated thoroughly if guidelines are to be of value (Haycox et al., 1999). Thus, guidelines for referral to cancer genetics clinics need to be interpreted in the context of methods for assessment of risk, evidence for benefit from intervention and the available local resources. Such guidelines will need to be regularly updated in the light of new scientific discoveries – for example newly recognized patterns of disease with potential genetic implications, or newly discovered strategies for intervention. In addition, mammographic screening, genetic testing and any other form of real or proposed intervention requires constant audit of outcomes to ensure that patients and their doctors are aware of the strength of evidence on which such management options are advocated.

Breast cancer

In the scheme proposed for managing varying levels of genetic risk, guidelines might be aimed at the primary care team to ensure that the GP can be confident in reassuring low-risk women (de Bock et al., 1999; Evans and Eccles, 2000). In the hospital-based screening clinic, guidelines and a working knowledge of the relevant literature should allow both patient and clinician to feel confident that a more thorough review of the family tree can help inform a more detailed assessment of risk (The BASO Breast Specialty Group, 1998; Armes et al., 1999) and, if higher risk, in addition to screening, this information can result in onward referral to the genetics specialist. The genetics specialist will use additional information to ensure appropriate use of genetic testing (Couch et al., 1997; Eccles et al., 1998). This, in turn, will allow many of those who appear at first look to be at moderate risk to be reassured that, on closer scrutiny, they appear unlikely to have a significant component of genetic risk. Those deemed at moderate risk may be unlikely to benefit from detailed genetic investigations at present but may benefit from early cancer detection strategies. This group may be eligible for trials of chemoprevention and approaches to identification of new, perhaps lower, penetrance genes that increase breast cancer risk to a lesser extent than the currently identified high-risk genes (Bishop and Hopper, 1997; Easton, 1997). In addition, guidelines at this level should allow clinicians both to select those at high genetic risk who may benefit from additional input from the cancer genetics service and to provide access to this service (BASO Breast Specialty Group, 1998; Eccles et al., 2000).

Ovarian cancer

Ovarian cancer is 10 times less common than breast cancer in the general population. Despite advances in new chemotherapeutic agents such as platinum and the taxanes, the outlook following this diagnosis is usually poor due to presentation at a late stage of the disease. Ovarian screening is of unproven efficacy and is dealt with in detail elsewhere. In view of this fact, guidelines for referral are less well developed than for breast cancer. Criteria have been developed for inclusion in the UK Familial Ovarian Cancer Screening Study. As part of the risk assessment process, ovarian cancer is weighted rather like a younger case of breast cancer (breast cancer under 40 years of age is 10 times less common than breast cancer over 60 years of age in the general population). In addition, there is a recognized association between breast and ovarian cancer in *BRCA1* and *BRCA2* families, such that the combination of breast and ovarian cancer occurring in four or more family members is a good predictor of a *BRCA1* (usually) or *BRCA2* (less frequently) gene mutation (Easton et al., 1993; Chang-Claude et al., 1999) . The inclusion of ovarian cancer in the higher risk groups in the breast cancer guidelines therefore seems reasonable, but development of similar ovarian cancer referral guidelines for primary and secondary care awaits the outcome of ovarian screening trials.

Guidelines cannot always be interpreted without some background knowledge of a subject, and misinterpretation can easily lead to confusion and conflicting advice. Cancer genetics specialists are well placed to provide the basic training required to interpret available guidelines, and one of the remits with which the cancer genetics services is charged is the education of healthcare professionals (Harper, 1998).

Risk assessment

Methods

Breast cancer is common in the general population. The greatest risk factors in that setting are increasing age and being female. Family history has been identified as a significant risk factor, the magnitude of which varies according to the strength of family history. Assessment of breast cancer risk, in the absence of a comprehensive molecular genetic test, might approach the problem from a genetic viewpoint using data from segregation analyses to provide parameters of inheritance (such as gene frequency) and penetrance on which to base a modified Bayesian calculation (Claus et al., 1994) or conventional epidemiological risk factors may be used to gauge risk (Gail and Rimer, 1998).

Where genetic status is known, gene-specific parameters are more appropriate. In all models and methods there are inherent inaccuracies due to uncertainties about key inputs. Predictions using epidemiological risk factors may be more accurate for women with a low component of genetic risk. For women with a high genetic risk, there are as yet no clear data to allow incorporation of conventional epidemiological risk factors into a general genetic model; however, there are studies suggesting an interaction between conventional epidemiological risk factors and penetrance in *BRCA1* gene carriers (Andrieu and Demenais, 1999; Rebbeck et al., 1999).

The various methods of risk estimation need to be validated in prospective studies but, for the time being, can provide a useful means of standardizing risk estimation and selecting only women at a moderate or high genetic risk for breast screening studies or trials of intervention such as chemoprevention.

Molecular genetic testing

Many studies have now been reported where *BRCA1* and *BRCA2* mutations have been sought and found in groups of patients ascertained through diverse strategies (Couch et al., 1996; Fitzgerald et al., 1996; Phelan et al., 1996; Stoppa-Lyonnet et al., 1996; Couch et al., 1997; Rebbeck et al., 1997; Eccles et al., 1998). These reported studies give a framework on which the application of genetic testing can be rationalized such that sensitivity (the chance of finding a mutation) is maintained at a reasonable level. This is particularly important given the high cost of genetic analysis and the unproven health benefits if testing is offered as part of a comprehensive healthcare plan. The pick-up rate for mutations in breast cancer populations is strikingly age dependent, decreasing rapidly as a proportion of all samples with increasing age (Peto et al., 1999).

For patients where the chances of the family history being due to a high-risk gene are strong (therefore those in the highest risk category), referral to the genetics clinic for further assessment is appropriate. The approach of the genetics team is to undertake detailed family studies initially by constructing a complete family tree and verifying key data. Using these data, a modified genetic risk can be estimated. Individuals referred to the genetics clinics need to be informed that molecular genetic testing may not be possible in every case. In many cases there are no suitable DNA samples available from affected family members; in others, detailed scrutiny of the family history and investigation to confirm diagnoses may reveal a lower chance of a genetic predisposition than originally thought. In addition, some women elect not to have genetic testing, and prior to testing it is imperative that the individual has an understanding of the limitations and potential disadvantages of genetic testing in addition to any potential benefits.

Molecular genetic diagnostic testing (particularly pre-symptomatic testing) should only be carried out by the clinical genetics service using a quality-assured diagnostic laboratory or as part of research protocols. However, the availability of a commercial test may encourage more widespread use, which could have an adverse effect on individuals receiving a test without adequate preparation (Cho et al., 1999).

Mutation testing throughout Europe has been offered in many centres as part of research projects. Diagnostic molecular genetics laboratories in many European countries, including the UK, Holland, France, Germany, Norway and Sweden, now offer routine mutation analysis and predictive testing in selected families, but current debates surrounding patenting of these genes may limit the availability of such tests due to high cost and currently limited evidence of the universal clinical utility of such tests.

It is only in a small proportion of those families in whom mutation analysis is possible that a mutation is found and therefore that a test can be offered to other family members. The likelihood of detecting a mutation depends on the criteria for selection of families, and on the sensitivity of the techniques used for mutation detection. Neither of these parameters can be readily estimated at the present time as techniques vary widely – mostly aimed at detection of small deletion or insertion mutations.

If a mutation is detected that is clearly causing the cancer predisposition, predictive (pre-symptomatic) testing can be offered to any family member by the genetics service. Pre-symptomatic testing involves, in most cases, a session to disclose all the relevant information and explore the individuals' expectations and concerns, and then a further session with a minimum of a 4-week 'cooling off' period prior to the test sample being taken. The result is given ('disclosure') usually face to face, and further follow-up is arranged thereafter according to the result and the needs of the individual. Current experience is that the number of men and women proceeding with predictive testing is substantial and may help to inform decisions about prophylactic surgery (Meijers-Heijboer et al., 2000).

However, even where genetic testing is not possible, many women will be eligible for studies in chemoprevention and screening that can be coordinated either by the genetics team or by the breast unit, or preferably by both in collaboration. In addition, these families may be suitable for genetic research to identify other breast cancer predisposition genes. Quantification of an individual's risk (often lower than they thought) (Burke et al., 2000) and information about screening and clinical trials are usually helpful both to the patient and to the referring doctor, and the level at which this is provided varies at present, depending on local resources and interests. Appropriate collaboration with the regional cancer genetics specialist will ensure referral of appropriate cases for formal genetics assessment within the regional genetics service. Women need information about level of risk and risk management options in order to make informed choices about their own health care. Current evidence indicates that risk counselling does improve knowledge and is not associated with increased anxiety (Burke et al., 2000).

Summary

Referral criteria for cancer genetics clinics have developed in various settings and vary according to the principal goal of the clinic (research or service, screening or genetic testing). Agreed methods of risk estimation with which to effectively triage individuals into risk categories are needed. Prospective cohort studies to audit the accuracy of currently advocated risk estimation methods are essential. Prospective studies (wherever possible randomized controlled trials) of early breast and ovarian cancer detection strategies, chemoprevention agents and prophylactic surgery are needed. At the very least we need a structure for gathering data in all cases where a genetic risk is likely and leads to medical intervention at any level such that in the future we may have evidence of benefit in addition to the wealth of expert opinion that informs current practice.

REFERENCES

Andrieu N and Demenais F (1999). Interactions between genetic and reproductive factors in breast cancer risk in a French family sample. *Am J Hum Genet* **61**: 678–90.

Armes JE, Trute L, White D, et al. (1999). Distinct molecular pathogenesis of early-onset breast cancers in BRCA1 and BRCA2 mutation carriers: a population based study. *Cancer Res* **59**: 2011–17.

Bishop DT and Hopper J (1997). AT-tributable risks? *Nat Genet* **15**: 226.

Bjurstam N, Bjorneld L, Duffy SW, et al. (1997). The Gothenburg breast screening trial – first results on mortality, incidence, and mode of detection for women aged 39–49 years at randomization. *Cancer* **80**(11): 2091–9.

Burke W, Culver JO, Bowen D, et al. (2000). Genetic counseling for women with an intermediate family history of breast cancer. *Am J Med Genet* **90**(5): 361–8.

Chang-Claude J, Becher H, Caligo M, et al. (1999). Risk estimation as a decision-making tool for genetic analysis of the breast cancer susceptibility genes. EC Demonstration Project on Familial Breast Cancer. *Dis Markers* **15**(1–3): 53–65.

Cho MK, Sankar P, Wolpe PR and Godmilow L (1999). Commercialization of BRCA1/2 testing: practitioner awareness and use of a new genetic test. *Am J Med Genet* **83**(3): 157–63.

Claus EB, Risch N and Thompson WD (1994). Autosomal dominant inheritance of early onset breast cancer. *Cancer* **73**(3): 643–51.

Couch F, Farid LM, DeShano ML, et al. (1996). BRCA2 germline mutations in male breast cancer cases and breast cancer families. *Nat Genet* **13**: 123–5.

Couch F, DeShano ML, Blackwood MA, et al. (1997). BRCA1 mutations in women attending clinics that evaluate the risk of breast cancer. *N Eng J Med* **336**: 1409–15.

de Bock GH, Vliet Vlieland TP, Hageman GC, Oosterwijk JC, Springer MP and Kievit J (1999). The assessment of genetic risk of breast cancer: a set of GP guidelines. *Fam Pract* **16**(1): 71–7.

Easton D, Bishop DT, Ford D, Crockford GP and the Breast Cancer Linkage Consortium (1993). Genetic linkage analysis in familial breast and ovarian cancer: results from 214 families. *Am J Hum Genet* **52**: 678–701.

Easton D (1997). Breast cancer genes – what are the real risks? *Nat Genet* **16**: 210–11.

Eccles DM, Engelfield P, Soulby MA and Campbell IG (1998). BRCA1 mutations in Southern England. *Br J Cancer* **77**(12): 2199–203.

Eccles DM, Evans DGR, Mackay J and UK Cancer Family Study Group (2000). Guidelines for using genetic risk to advise women with family history of breast cancer. *J Med Genet* 203–9.

Evans DGR and Eccles DM (2000). Genetic testing for breast cancer – who, when, where and why? *Pulse* (June 24): 65–6.

Fitzgerald MG, MacDonald DJ, Krainer M, et al. (1996). Germ-line BRCA1 mutations in Jewish and non-Jewish women with early-onset breast cancer. *N Engl J Med* **334**: 143–9.

Foulkes W, Wong N, Brunet JS, et al. (1997). Germ-line BRCA1 mutation is an adverse prognostic factor in Ashkenazi Jewish women with breast cancer. *Clin Cancer Res* **3**(12): 2465–9.

Gail M and Rimer B (1998). Risk-based recommendations for mammographic screening for women in their forties [see comments] [published erratum appears in *J Clin Oncol* (1999) 17(2): 740]. *J Clin Oncol* **16**(9): 3105–14.

Harper P (1998). Working party on Cancer Genetics Services in the UK. *DHSS discussion document.* Raising concerns about family history of breast cancer in primary care consultations: prospective, population based study. *Br Med J* **322**(7277): 27–8.

Haycox A, Bagust A and Walley T (1999). Clinical guidelines – the hidden costs. *Br Med J* **318**: 391–3.

Kerlikowske K, Carney PA, Geller B, et al. (2000). Performance of screening mammography among women with and without a first-degree relative with breast cancer. *Ann Intern Med* **133**(11): 855–63.

Kollias J, Sibbering DM, Blamey RW, et al. (1998). Screening women aged less than 50 years with a family history of breast cancer. *Eur J Cancer* **34**(6): 878–83.

Lalloo F, Boggis CRM, Evans DGR, Shenton A, Threlfall AG and Howell A (1998). Screening by mammography, women with a family history of breast cancer. *Eur J Cancer* **34**(6): 937–40.

Meijers-Heijboer EJ, Verhoog LC, Brekelmans CTM, et al. (2000). Presymptomatic DNA testing and prophylactic surgery in families with a BRCA1 or BRCA2 mutation. *Lancet* **355**(9220): 2015–20.

Møller P, Maehle L, Heimdal K, et al. (1998). Prospective findings in breast cancer kindreds: annual incidence rates according to age, stage at diagnosis, mean sojourn time, and incidence rates for contralateral cancer. *Breast* **7**(1): 55–9.

Peto J, Collins N, Barfoot R, et al. (1999). Prevalence of BRCA1 and BRCA2 gene mutations in patients with early-onset breast cancer. *J Natl Cancer Inst* **91**(11): 943–9.

Pharoah PD, Easton DF, Stockton DL, Gayther S and Ponder BA (1999). Survival in familial, BRCA1-associated and BRCA2-associated epithelial ovarian cancer. United Kingdom Co-ordinating Committee for Cancer Research (UKCCCR) Familial Ovarian Cancer Study Group. *Cancer Res* **59**(4): 868–71.

Phelan CM, Lancaster JM, Tonin P, et al. (1996). Mutation analysis of the BRCA2 gene in 49 site-specific breast cancer families. *Nat Genet* **13**: 120–2.

Rebbeck TR, Couch F, Kant J, et al. (1997). Genetic heterogeneity in hereditary breast cancer: role of BRCA1 and BRCA2. *Am J Hum Genet* **59**: 547–53.

Rebbeck TR, Levin AM, Eisen A, et al. (1999). Breast cancer risk after prophylactic oopherectomy in BRCA1 mutation carriers. *J Natl Cancer Inst* **91**(17): 1475–9.

Rimer BK and Bluman LG (1997). The psychosocial consequences of mammography. *J Natl Cancer Inst Monogr* (22): 131–8.

Stoppa-Lyonnet D, Fricker JP, Essioux L, et al. (1996). Segregation of two BRCA1 mutations in a single family. *Am J Hum Genet* **59**: 479–81.

Stoppa-Lyonnet D, Ansquer Y, Dreyfus H, et al. (2000). Familial invasive breast cancers: worse outcome related to BRCA1 mutations. *J Clin Oncol* **18**(24): 4053–9.

Tabar L, Larsson LG, Anderson I, et al. (1996). Breast-cancer screening with mammography in women aged 40–49 years. *Int J Cancer* **68**(6): 693–9.

The BASO Breast Specialty Group (1998). The British Association of Surgical Oncology Guidelines for Surgeons in the management of symptomatic breast disease in the UK (revision). *Eur J Surg Oncol* **24**: 464–76.

Tilanus-Linthorst M, Bartels C, Obdeijn A and udkerk M (2000). Earlier detection of breast cancer by surveillance of women at familial risk. *Eur J Surg Oncol* **36**(4): 514–19.

11

Guidelines for the development of cancer genetics services

Neva E. Haites, Shirley V. Hodgson and the Scottish Office Working Group
on Cancer Genetics

University of Aberdeen, UK

Most countries now have services for familial cancer genetics, but these vary considerably (Harris, 1998; Hodgson et al., 2000). There are, broadly, three potential approaches for developing a clinical service in response to the growing evidence of the links between inherited genetic factors and the risks of developing breast and ovarian cancers:

1 An ad hoc system of providing advice to patients, i.e. 'demand led'
2 The development of a selective system of screening patients who are estimated to be at relatively high genetic risk of developing these cancers
3 The establishment of systems of population screening to identify patients at increased risk

Over the last few years, many clinics worldwide have been providing advice to patients with a family history of cancer through clinics in an ad hoc and uncoordinated manner, funded largely through 'soft money'. The resources available have not kept pace with the rapid growth in demand, and this is reflected in the sharp increase in waiting times for appointments in recent years.

Only 5% of breast and ovarian cancers are thought to be due to a strong inherited susceptibility. A process of selection of individuals who are estimated to be at high risk on the basis of their family history for screening for cancer is a more pragmatic approach than screening the general population. However, it is important to demonstrate clearly the benefit of such surveillance programmes before this can be advocated on a large scale (Scottish Office Home and Health Department, 1998).

Identification of individuals with a genetic predisposition to cancer

The basic aims of genetic management for breast and ovarian cancer risks are:

- To identify individuals who are at a significantly increased genetic risk of inherited cancer
- To provide advice and counselling to individuals about their risks of developing cancer
- To establish evidence-based protocols for the surveillance and management of individuals and families at increased risk, which will reduce morbidity and mortality rate from these diseases
- To provide patients affected with cancer that is associated with a genetic predisposition with appropriate genetic counselling and management

Primary care

Given the growing awareness and demand for advice on familial aspects of cancer and the limited resources available to meet this demand, primary care and breast clinics should be provided with guidelines to resolve enquiries relating to inherited aspects of common cancers. The specialist services should be reserved for known familial forms of the more common cancers (only a minority of the total caseload), for other high-risk situations, and for cases where primary care professionals themselves consider specialist referrals to be desirable (Emery et al., 1999a).

The main roles of primary care or breast clinics for patients with a family history of cancer would ideally be as follows:

- To record relevant family history information concerning clinical conditions, including cancer, as part of a new patient registration, using computer-based systems as appropriate
- To hold (or to be able to obtain rapidly) information concerning the current clinical management policy for cancer genetics in each region, including the feasibility and availability of genetic testing
- To be able to use agreed guidelines to identify individuals at low, moderate and high risk of inherited cancer
- To convey to individuals, especially those at low risk, accurate risk information in a sensitive and supportive manner (low risk individuals can be reassured and moderate risk individuals referred for appropriate advice)
- Where genetic risks are likely to be high, to refer individuals to specialist cancer genetics teams, especially those individuals with rare familial cancer syndromes
- To provide ongoing support to individuals who are significantly distressed by their cancer family history, and refer them for specialist help if necessary

- To form a partnership between primary care and breast clinics and the specialist genetics clinics, to ensure that referral guidelines are locally appropriate and that educational material is relevant for all members of the primary healthcare team

However, at present in many primary care settings, there is insufficient manpower to administer such a system efficiently. This role could also be provided by the family history clinics in cancer units with such clinics, which are staffed by experienced/trained genetic counsellors who would maintain links with the genetics centres. National guidelines would need to be provided to enable primary care staff to identify the minority of individuals who will require specialist referral, to arrange appropriate management/referral for moderate-risk individuals and to reassure those at low risk.

Genetic counsellors/genetic nurses

Genetic counsellors (or genetic nurses) can play a key role in linking the work of primary care staff with the cancer genetics centres, and would be trained in the clinical genetics centres and would maintain close links with them. They would provide advice and expertise to primary care staff on the use of computer-based information systems and risk estimation programmes, and would also contact patients to assess their family history. Genetic counsellors often have a science background and may therefore be better placed to discuss the genetic aspects of cancer. However, the wide experience that genetic nurses have in dealing with patients may also make them suitable for this work. Genetic counsellors may have obtained an MSc in genetic counselling and may have followed training or a module in cancer genetics and pedigree risk evaluation. Career structures and training for genetic counsellors is being developed (Skirton et al., 1998).

In some centres, genetic counsellors from the genetic centres undertake clinics in regional centres and train nurses in pedigree taking and evaluation. Subsequently, those local nurses who use standardized family history forms and recognized risk-evaluation flow diagrams may run such clinics. They can then refer high-risk individuals to the genetics centres, discharge low-risk individuals and maintain moderate-risk individuals on audited surveillance protocols in their unit, with facilities for centralized computerized follow-up of outcomes. Any problematic cases are referred to the genetics centres.

Guidelines for risk estimation in individuals with a family history of cancer

Calculation of risk of breast cancer

In families where there is no clear-cut Mendelian genetic predisposition, empirical risks for breast cancer may be calculated based on the age at diagnosis of breast

Table 11.1. Importance of genetic predisposition to breast cancer

	Age at onset of cancer (years)	Percentage due to genetic susceptibility	Percentage due to other factors
Isolated cases	25	40	60
	35	25	75
	45	12	88
	55	8	92
	65	4	96
With two affected sisters	35	90	10
(mean age in years)	45	62	38
	55	38	62
	63	13	83

From Murday (1994).

cancer in first-degree relatives in studies carried out by Houlston et al. (1991) in the UK and by Claus et al. (1996) in the USA. Where more than one relative is affected various studies have produced figures for the relative risks to individuals (Table 11.1; Murday, 1994).

Computer-aided risk estimation

Many geneticists and clinicians collect and analyse data using pedigree drawing software with tools for managing genetic data concerning patients with inherited diseases or disorders. Programs such as Cyrillic provide unique tools for many aspects of working with genetic data. It facilitates the entering of individual and family data, creating family trees, displaying genetic data and making risk calculations. However, it is far too complicated for use by most GPs and provides inaccurate risk estimations in some types of family history.

For the majority of individuals with a family history of cancer, no specific gene mutations will have been identified as being causative. In such cases, data from epidemiological studies must be used to calculate the risks to relatives of those affected with cancer. Where a single relative is affected with breast cancer, data from the Claus et al. (1996) study may be used to calculate the risk to first-degree relatives, and similar studies allow estimation of the probability of a cancer susceptibility gene being involved when two first-degree relatives are affected with breast cancer, depending on the mean age at diagnosis. Such data can then be combined using a Bayesian calculation to determine the residual risk to the consultand based on their age, etc.

To expedite such calculations and to allow comparative methods to be utilized in different centres for the calculation of risk, various computer programs have been developed for calculating risk of breast cancer based on a range of family histories, e.g. the RAGS program (Emery et al., 1999b). However, many individuals in primary care and cancer units may find it impractical to use computer-aided techniques and prefer broader guidelines.

As it is likely that many referrals to clinics will, in the future, be made via the family doctor, it would be useful to have programs of varying complexity. Such programs have the potential to allow guidelines for referrals based on the availability of local resources to be distributed to family doctors, providing them with the information to ensure that their referrals are appropriate for the local clinic.

Guideline-based risk estimation

In Part 2, Chapters 5 and 6, other models of risk estimation are discussed. Those given below in Tables 11.2–11.6 are from the approach taken in Scotland (Tables 11.2–11.8) and in Guy's Hospital, London (Tables 11.9, 11.10), where a guideline-based approach with regular audit has been implemented. This approach is based on evidence for both risk categorization and best practice, as evidence for management is accumulated. In Scotland, previous guidelines were produced for the management of breast cancer and these included recommendations for the management of high-risk individuals. As a result, the current guidelines as presented in Tables 11.2–11.8 are based on these (Scottish Office Home and Health Department, 1998; Emery et al., 1999b; Hodgson et al., 2000a).

Genetic counselling of 'at risk' individuals and families

Genetic counselling may be described as the process of determining the occurrence, or risk of occurrence, of a genetic disorder within a family, communicating the results of the pedigree and risk assessment and providing appropriate non-directive information and advice about future courses of action.

Effective genetic counselling rests upon the establishment of a careful, detailed family history, recorded in the form of a pedigree chart in order to determine assessment of risk. The likelihood of a genetic susceptibility can be calculated with reference to published data on risk assessment and information on the number and age of affected individuals. The risk to the patient is dependent upon their relationship to the affected family members and their own age at interview.

Genetic counsellors should educate and support 'at risk' individuals within families, encourage health promotion practices, reassure those who over-estimate risk, and monitor psychological adjustment, referring to a psychiatrist if necessary.

Table 11.2. Patient management: a 5-step process

Step 1 Referral process	Step 2 Confirmation of family history	Steps 3 and 4 Risk stratification and counselling	Step 5 Management
• Referrals of individuals with family/personal history of cancer may come from GPs or other clinicians. • Most referrals will come direct to the RGU and this is the preferred route to prevent inappropriate referrals to clinics such as the symptomatic breast clinic. • Where possible, the genetic counsellors should preview the referral letters and apply the guidelines, classifying low, medium and high risk as appropriate. • Referrals falling outside the current guidelines but possibly suggestive of a high-risk situation should be discussed with the consultant in charge of the RGU.	• Genetic counsellors should contact referred individuals prior to their first full appointment to obtain a full history with details of cancer cases in the family. • Where possible, deceased case diagnoses should be confirmed using an appropriate source such as the Scottish Cancer Registry. • Consent should be sought from living affected relatives, to confirm and specify diagnosis, and a full pedigree produced with risk calculation by a standard genetic analysis (CYRILLIC 3) for audit purposes.	• Specific guidance on risk stratification and counselling for breast, ovarian and colorectal cancer is set out in Tables 11.1–11.3, identifying individuals who should be classified as: (1) low risk (not fulfilling a category within the guidelines), (2) medium or high risk (fulfilling the criteria). *Notes* 1. Clearly, as family history evolves and is confirmed or refuted, individuals may move from apparent high risk to medium or low, and vice versa. 2. It is also important that families are encouraged to re-contact the RGU if the family history changes following initial counselling.	• Specific guidance on the management of low-, medium- and high-risk individuals for breast, ovarian and colorectal cancer is set out in Tables 11.4–11.6. • The management of all high-risk individuals is carried out through a process of gene testing and screening. • For high-risk individuals, surgical management may be considered. *Notes* 1. It is anticipated that cancer-managed clinical networks will include individuals with specific expertise in the surgical management of cancers in high-risk individuals.

RGU, regional genetics unit.
Tables 11.2–11.8 = Scottish guidelines.

Table 11.3. Risk stratification and counselling for breast cancer

Low risk	Medium risk	High risk
Risk stratification		
• Anyone not fulfilling medium- or high-risk criteria	• One first-degree relative with bilateral breast cancer • One first-degree relative with breast cancer at <40 years or, male at any age • Two first-degree relatives or first- and second-degree relative with breast cancer diagnosed under 60 years or ovarian cancer at any age on same side of family • Three first- or second-degree relatives with breast cancer or ovarian cancer on same side of family (at least one first-degree relative unless history via father)	• Women with a family history that predicts a likelihood greater than 60% that a predisposing cancer gene of high penetrance is operative • Gene carriers (e.g. *BRCA1*, *BRCA2*, p53, *PTEN*) • Untested first-degree relatives of gene carriers • Women with first-degree relative (or second-degree via intervening male relative) in a family with four or more relatives affected with breast cancer (bilateral breast cancer being counted as two) or ovarian or male breast cancer in three generations • Women with one first-degree relative (or second-degree via intervening male relative) with breast and ovarian cancer
Counselling Individuals deemed at low risk will be informed either by: • Communication with referring doctor, who can reassure the patient; • Telephone consultation with the genetic nurse associate, followed by letter with a copy to the GP; *or* • Face-to-face consultation with the genetic nurse associate, followed by letter to the patient and the GP; • Individuals deemed to be too low risk may be offered a single appointment for breast examination by a surgeon in certain centres, and again the effect of the intervention on level of satisfaction will be assessed as above.	• Individuals deemed to be at medium risk will be counselled by the genetic counsellor, who will discuss with them appropriate information.	• Individuals deemed to be at high risk will be counselled by the clinical genetic physician in the genetics centre.

Table 11.4. Management of breast cancer

Low risk	Medium risk	High risk
• Reassurance • Healthy lifestyle advice • Return to GP care • Advise to report any symptoms or changes in family history promptly • If family history of breast cancer, letter and leaflet about breast awareness for female patients	Mammogram (and ultrasound as appropriate) at breast screening centre, as follows: • Every 2 years intervals for women aged 35–40 years • Annually for women aged 40–50 years • Thereafter, women enter the national screening programme and are screened at 3-yearly intervals until 64 years of age Physical examination by breast clinician annually for women aged 35–50 years (*Screening from 5 years younger than the youngest case but not younger than 35 years, or older than 40 years, as indicated*)	Mammogram (and ultrasound as appropriate) at breast screening centre as follows: • Every 2 years for women aged 35–40 years (or possibly earlier) • Annually for women aged 40–50 years • Every 18 months for women aged 50–64 years, through a breast screening programme • Every 3 years for women aged over 65 years Physical examination by breast clinician annually for women aged 25–64 years (*Screening from 5 years younger than the youngest case but not younger than 25 years, or older than 35 years*) *Gene testing* Following counselling by a clinical genetics physician, gene testing should be available to all high-risk families and predictive testing offered to all at-risk individuals within these families.

Surgical management of high-risk individuals

• In unaffected women, continued screening will probably be the preferred option, but prophylactic surgery may be considered in particularly high-risk cases.
• Affected individuals are offered the range of surgical and other therapeutic options, as appropriate. These include: lumpectomy followed by radiotherapy or chemotherapy, mastectomy with preservation of nipple and subsequent adjuvant therapy, reconstructive surgery, contralateral prophylactic surgery, and prophylactic oophorectomy.
(It is anticipated that cancer-managed clinical networks will include individuals with specific expertise in the surgical management of cancers in high-risk individuals.)

Table 11.5. Risk stratification and counselling for ovarian cancer

Low risk	Medium risk	High risk
Risk stratification • Anyone not fulfilling medium- or high-risk criteria • Individuals with a single first-degree or second-degree relative by their father, who have presented at any age, are not appropriate for screening.	• Two or more first or first- and second-degree relatives with ovarian cancer at any age • Two first or first- and second-degree relatives with ovarian cancer at any age or breast cancer diagnosis under 50 years (i.e. one of each type of cancer) • One ovarian cancer and two breast cancers diagnosed under 60 years on same side of family in first-degree relatives or second-degree relatives via a male • Two first- or second-degree relatives with colorectal cancer and an endometrial cancer and one ovarian cancer • One affected relative with ovarian cancer and HNPCC family history	• Women in a family where *BRCA1, BRCA2, hMLH1, hMSH2* or other predisposing gene has been identified • Untested first-degree relatives of gene carriers • A woman with at least one first-degree relative with breast and ovarian cancer
Counselling Individuals deemed at low risk will be informed either by: • Communication with the referring doctor, who can reassure the patient; • Telephone consultation with the genetic nurse associate, followed by letter with a copy to the GP; *or* • Face-to-face consultation with the genetic nurse associate, followed by letter to the patient and the GP.	• Individuals deemed to be at medium risk will be counselled by the genetic counsellor, who will discuss with them appropriate information.	• Individuals deemed to be at high risk will be counselled by the clinical genetic physician in the genetics centre.

Table 11.6. Management of ovarian cancer

Low risk	Medium risk	High risk
• Reassurance • Healthy lifestyle advice • Return to GP care • Advise to report any symptoms or changes in family history promptly	Screening is performed from 35 years of age or 5 years younger than the youngest affected member of the family. This should include: • Appointment with a gynaecological oncologist • Yearly transvaginal ultrasound • Yearly CA125 estimation • Discussion of prophylactic oophorectomy • Entry into UKCCCR Trial (if women have a history of both breast and ovarian cancer, or a family history of ovarian cancer only, or family history consistent with HNPCC with ovarian cancer in the family) (*The limitations of ovarian screening should be explained to all women in this category.*)	Such women are screened as for medium risk. Screening is performed from 35 years of age or 5 years younger than the youngest affected member of the family. This should include: • Appointment with a gynaecological oncologist • Yearly transvaginal ultrasound • Yearly CA125 estimation • Discussion of prophylactic oophorectomy • Entry into UKCCCR Trial (if women have a history of both breast and ovarian cancer, or a family history of ovarian cancer only, or family history consistent with HNPCC with ovarian cancer in the family) • Possible screening of other organs depending on family history (*The limitations of ovarian screening should be explained to all women in this category.*) *Gene testing* Following counselling by a clinical genetics physician, gene testing should be available to all high-risk families and predictive testing offered to all at-risk individuals within these families.

Surgical management of high-risk individuals

• In unaffected women, continued screening will probably be the preferred option, but prophylactic surgery may be considered in particularly high-risk cases.
• Affected women are treated along conventional lines, as for best management of sporadic ovarian cancer.
(It is anticipated that cancer-managed clinical networks will include individuals with specific expertise in the surgical management of cancers in high-risk individuals.)

Table 11.7. Risk stratification and counselling for colorectal cancer

Low risk	Medium risk	High risk
Risk stratification		
• Anyone not fulfilling medium- or high-risk criteria	• One first-degree relative with colorectal cancer diagnosed under 45 years • Two affected relatives (one affected under 55 years and one a first-degree relative) of subject • Three affected relatives with colorectal or endometrial cancer who are first-degree relatives of each other and one a first-degree relative of subject • Two affected first-degree relatives (one affected under 55 years)	• Gene carriers of HNPCC mutation • Untested first-degree relatives of gene carriers • People with a family history compatible with HNPCC
Counselling Individuals deemed at low risk will be informed either by: • Communication with the referring doctor, who can reassure the patient; • Telephone consultation with the genetic nurse associate, followed by letter with a copy to the GP, *or* • Face-to-face consultation with the genetic nurse associate, followed by letter to the patient and the GP.	• Individuals deemed to be at medium risk will be counselled by the genetic counsellor, who will discuss with them appropriate information.	• Individuals deemed to be at high risk will be counselled by the clinical genetic physician in the genetics centre.

Table 11.8. Management of colorectal cancer

Low risk	Medium risk	High risk
• Reassurance • Healthy lifestyle advice • Advise to report any symptoms or changes in family history promptly • Return to GP care	Screening comprises: • A single colonoscopy at 30–35 years; if findings are normal this need not be repeated until 55 years of age. • Incomplete colonoscopy should be followed by a barium enema, preferably at same hospital attended.	Screening comprises: • Colonoscopy every 2 years from age 30 years of age or 5 years younger than the youngest affected member of the family, until 70 years of age. • Discussion of prophylactic surgery, if recurrent polyps are identified; total colectomy, with rectal sparing and ileorectal anastomosis, is the best option. • Consideration needs to be given to screening for other cancers that may occur in specific families and that are part of the HNPCC spectrum. *Gene testing* Following counselling by a clinical genetics physician, gene testing should ideally be available to all high-risk families and predictive testing offered to all at-risk individuals within these families.

Surgical management of high-risk individuals

• In unaffected individuals, continued screening will probably be the preferred option, but prophylactic surgery may be considered in particularly high-risk cases where recurrent polyps are identified on repeat screening.
• Affected subjects should undergo resection of tumour with a major portion of contiguous bowel to decrease the risk of other tumour recurrence. Adjuvant therapy may subsequently be used and regular surveillance of any remaining large bowel is essential.
(It is anticipated that cancer-managed clinical networks will include individuals with specific expertise in the surgical management of cancers in high-risk individuals.)

Management of patients with established colorectal cancer (high risk)

These individuals require more extensive resection to reduce the risk of metachronous tumours. Colonic tumour is best treated by colectomy with ileorectal anastomosis; surgery for rectal cancer usually comprises extensive left hemi-colectomy with anterior resection.

Consideration also needs to be given to screening for other cancers that may occur in specific families and that are part of the HNPCC spectrum. Details of these are given in Table 11.9.

Table 11.9. Other cancers in HNPCC families

Endometrial and ovarian cancer

Discuss annual gynaecological screening. There is no established method for endometrial cancer screening and no available data on efficacy. Some centres offer clinical examination, transvaginal ultrasound and endometrial biopsy. Experience in familial ovarian cancer indicates that ovarian screening is of doubtful efficacy. There is a good case for the avoidance of screening outside of research studies.

Discuss prophylactic hysterectomy and bilateral oophorectomy. This should be done by a gynaecologist and a full-operative discussion of surgical risks/potential benefits is essential. There is no clear evidence of benefit, but surgery may be preferable to pelvic screening for women who are past reproductive age, particularly if there is no history of gynaecological cancer in the family.

Gastric cancer

Offer 2-yearly upper GI endoscopy, contemporaneous with colonoscopy: aged over 50 years or 5 years younger than the first case in the family. There are no available data on benefit, so this is a good case to recommend the avoidance of screening outside of trials.

Management of patients in medium- and high-risk categories

Having identified those patients who are at medium or high risk of developing breast or ovarian cancer, the next issue to consider is their appropriate management (Burke et al., 1997). This is considered in greater detail in Part 3.

For patients in the high-risk group – a relatively small number – regional genetics clinics would provide counselling about the potential for predictive testing, the availability of systematic surveillance, and other potential forms of management and their relative advantages and disadvantages (Eeles, 1996; Goldgar et al., 1996; Stratton et al., 1997).

Patients who are carriers of the genetic mutations that are known to be associated with a significantly increased lifetime risk of breast or ovarian cancer may wish to consider prophylactic surgery in addition to systematic surveillance.

Screening for breast and ovarian cancer has not been proven to prevent the occurrence of cancers, although preliminary evidence is accumulating to support the benefit of such screening (Kerlikowske et al., 1996; Møller et al., 1999).

Any estimates of cost-effectiveness take into account the potential saving in lives and the costs of regular screening. Clearly there are other considerations that would also have to be taken into account in a full assessment of the costs and benefits of screening people with a family history of breast, colorectal or ovarian cancer:

- In so far as screening enables cancers to be detected at an earlier stage, there are benefits to patients who may receive less radical treatment than would otherwise have been required. This may also reduce the costs of treatment.

- There are usually some risks associated with screening methods. In the case of breast and ovarian cancers, the risks associated with screening may be quite small. However, false-positive results may lead to investigative intervention, which in itself may carry a morbidity and mortality rate, albeit small, that is related to the accompanying anxiety provoked.

- The genetics clinics and the regular screening programmes may provide reassurance to patients. Although screening programmes may sometimes raise anxiety levels in patients, it should be borne in mind that the reason for referring patients to genetics clinics is that they are already likely to have raised anxiety levels because of their knowledge of their family history.

The individual and the individual's extended family

Any assessment of the genetically determined risk of cancer for an individual will inevitably require the assembly of detailed information about that individual and their extended family. In this context, information contained in the Cancer Registration and Scottish Morbidity Records Schemes and the Registrar General's mortality data archives provides an invaluable resource for the construction of family histories. Exploitation of these national data banks and other local data collections is now much more readily achievable because of the viability of sophisticated computer technology and record linkage techniques (Stratton et al., 1997). These allow rapid systematic search and retrieval of personal and family information.

However, the availability of such techniques carries both benefits and risks. Their use raises not only confidentiality and legal questions but also has ethical implications. The latter require a sensitive but balanced approach. It is essential to protect the interests of the individual and members of their extended family who may not know or wish to know that they are considered to be at risk. On the other hand, imposition of excessively rigid constraints on the use of this information may deny potential benefits to individuals and society.

Costs and benefits

The types of costs and benefits associated with proposed screening programmes are presented in Table 11.12.

The costs of screening people with a family history of cancer include the resources required for the education and training of primary care staff, the costs of the genetics clinics and the screening procedures, and the costs of treating cases identified as a result of screening. The costs of screening also include any increase

Table 11.10. Cancer family history clinics: referral guidelines (Guy's Hospital, London)

The genetic clinic provides risk estimation, genetic testing and advice on cancer screening and prevention (if appropriate), and research studies.

The local breast unit may be able to arrange screening.

In general (but not always), for genetic testing to be offered, a living affected relative is tested prior to offering testing to unaffected relatives.

Relationship of patient to affected relatives in family: The family history should be in blood relatives and can be through either the maternal or the paternal side.

First-degree relative = mother, father, brother, sister, daughter or son.

Refer if patient is an affected individual or if patient is FDR of an affected relative (unless in family history of female cancers, there is an intervening male relative between your patient and the family history).

Number of affected people in family	Ancestry	Type of cancer (ca)	Age of diagnosis (Dx) in affected individual(s) (years)	Refer to genetics clinic	Refer to local breast unit for screening
Breast cancer families					
1	Jewish	Breast ca	Under 45	Yes	Yes
	Any	Breast ca	Dx at <40	No	Yes
	Any	Male breast ca	Any age	No (unless family history of other associated cancers)	Yes
2 or two breast cancer primaries in one individual	Jewish	Breast ca	One Dx at <50, other Dx at any age	Yes	Yes
	Any	Male breast ca and breast ca in another relative	• Any ages	Yes	Yes
	Any	Breast ca in 2 close relatives	Dx between 50 and 60	No	Yes
	Any	Breast ca in 2 close relatives	Both Dx at <50	Yes	Yes
3	Any	Breast ca in 3 close relatives	Dx at <60	Yes	Yes
4 or more	Any	Breast ca in 4 close relatives	Any age	Yes	Yes

Ovarian cancer families

1	Jewish	Ovarian ca	Any age	Yes	—
	Other	Ovarian ca	Any age	No	—
2	Any	2 close relatives with ovarian ca	Any age	Yes	—
3 or more	Any	3 close relatives with ovarian ca	Any age	Yes	—

Breast and ovarian cancer families

1	Any	Breast and ovarian ca	Any age	Yes	—
2	Any	Male breast ca and ovarian ca in close relative	Any age	Yes	—
	Any	Ovarian cancer and breast ca	Ovarian ca Dx at any age, breast ca Dx at <60	Yes	—
3	Any	Breast/ovarian ca in 3 close relatives	Any age	Yes	—

Other cancers

- History of rare cancers, e.g. sarcomas, gliomas, several relatives with pancreatic cancer, CNS haemangioblastomas, retinal angiomas, phaeochromocytomas and renal cell cancers
- A family history of conditions that can predispose to cancer, e.g. multiple basal cell carcinoma, Cowden disease, juvenile polyposis, Peutz–Jeghers syndrome

Table 11.11. Guidelines for referral to Guy's Hospital colorectal cancer family history clinic

Number of affected[1] people in family related to the proband	Relationship to the proband	Type of cancer	Age of relative	Risk group	Screening required	Type of screening	To be seen at specialist genetics clinic?
1	One FDR	CRC[I] or HRC[II]	>45 years	Low	No	None	No – reassure. Advice on diet and bowel awareness
	One FDR	CRC	≤45 years	High/moderate	Yes	First colonoscopy at 45 years or when patient presents (whichever is later). Repeat every 5 years until 75 years	In some cases
2	Two SDRs	CRC or HRC	>45 years	Low	No	None	No – reassure. Advice on diet and bowel awareness
	One FDR + One SDR (on same side of family)	CRC or HRC	≤70 years ≤70 years	Low/moderate	Yes	Single colonoscopy at 55 years or when patient presents (whichever is later)	No
	Two FDRs	CRC		High/moderate	Yes	First colonoscopy at 45 years or when patient presents (whichever is later). Repeat every 5 years until 75 years	Yes
	Both parents affected	CRC		Low/moderate	Yes	Single colonoscopy at 55 years or when patient presents (whichever is later)	No
3	Two FDRs + One FDR or SDR (but Amsterdam[2] negative)	CRC or HRC		High/moderate	Yes	First colonoscopy at 45 years or when patient presents (whichever is later). Repeat every 5 years until 75 years	Yes

One FDR + Two FDRs or SDRs (but Amsterdam² negative)	CRC CRC or HRC	High/moderate	Yes	First colonoscopy at 45 years or when patient presents (whichever is later). Repeat every 5 years until 75 years	Yes
A family history of a known hereditary colorectal cancer syndrome, or multiple colorectal polyps (polyposis coli). E.g. FAP, AFAP, PJS, FJP or HNPCC (by fulfilment of modified Amsterdam criteria²)		High	Yes	FAP: according to current accepted practice (to be formalized) Attenuated FAP: on an individual/family basis, similar to HNPCC PJS and FJP/JPS: according to current accepted practice (to be formalized) HNPCC: first colonoscopy at 25 years or when patient presents (whichever is later). Repeated every 2 years until 75 years	Yes

FDR, first-degree relative; SDR, second-degree relative.

¹An affected individual is one diagnosed with the following tumour types at any age:

I

• Colorectal cancer (CRC) or
• >3 adenomatous polyps or
• 1 adenomatous polyp at <60 years, if it is >10 mm, or villous, or severely dysplastic

II

• an HNPCC-related cancer (HRC), i.e. endometrial, ovarian, small bowel, ureter or renal pelvis

An individual (relative or proband) affected with two tumours of the same type or one of each (as per I or II), either on different occasions or at the same time, will count as two relatives.

²Modified Amsterdam criteria

At least three separate relatives with CRC or two CRCs and one HRC. One must be a FDR of the other two. At least two successive generations affected. At least one cancer diagnosed at under 50 years. FAP excluded in CRC case(s). Tumours pathologically verified.

Dual primary does not count as two affected relatives.

or

Known mismatch repair gene mutation, or clinicopathological diagnosis after discussion with genetics department.

In all cases, increase the frequency of colonoscopy if adenomas are detected.

The above guidelines were proposed by the Public Health Genetics Unit (Eastern Region), with some modifications.

Table 11.12. Evaluation of process

Costs	Benefits
Education and training for primary care staff, and health information leaflets for patients	Provision of information that reassures patients
Genetics clinics	Savings in life years
Raised anxiety levels in patients	Improvements in quality of life
Management protocols	Treatment for advanced cancer avoided
Risks associated with screening methods, including false-positives and subsequent investigations	
Treatment	

in anxiety levels in patients and the risks of morbidity and mortality caused by the screening procedures.

The benefits of screening include reductions in morbidity and mortality, savings in treatment costs because of the prevention of cancers or their detection at an earlier stage, and reassurance provided to patients.

The likely uptake and compliance with screening programmes is uncertain. There is some evidence concerning the effectiveness of such screening programmes in detecting or preventing cases of cancer in people with a family history; however, there is no evidence at present about the effect of screening on longer term mortality rates. The resource implications of these screening programmes are also uncertain (Caulfield, 1995).

Genetic testing

The principle of informed consent

The decision as to whether or not genetic testing should be carried out in individual cases does not lie solely with the responsible clinician. The final decision must rest upon the informed consent of the individual.

This means that patients must receive sufficient information, in a way that they can understand, concerning the proposed management, the possible alternatives and any risks. The information must be given in a non-directive manner, so that they themselves can make a balanced judgement. They must be allowed to decide whether they will agree to the treatment, and they may refuse or withdraw consent at any time.

The principle of informed consent requires not only full counselling before genetic screening, but also public education in human genetics, to counteract media or commercial over-simplification of the issues involved.

Apart from the entitlement to sufficient information, it has to be borne in mind that in many cases individuals being offered genetic screening are not 'patients', as normally understood by that term. They are probably healthy people who may well not have previously been aware of the possibility of future serious disease for themselves and/or their families beyond the normal awareness of age-related disease/infirmity.

The key ethical principles of a genetic counselling service, as described in the Nuffield report (Nuffield Council on Bioethics, 1993), emphasize:

- the voluntary nature of genetic testing, and the freedom and responsibility of the individual or couple to decide;
- the importance of ensuring that the individual (or others) who is offered genetic testing understands the purpose of the test and the significance of a positive result;
- an assurance of confidentiality in the handling of results, coupled with an emphasis on the responsibility of individuals with a positive (abnormal) result to inform partners and family members; and
- the fact that consent to genetic testing, or to a subsequent confirmatory test, does not imply consent to any specific treatment, or to the termination of a pregnancy.

The report also stresses the need for special safeguards in certain instances where truly informed consent may not be possible, viz:

- in the case of minors;
- in the case of the mentally ill and those with severe learning difficulties;
- in cases where the individuals do not speak English. In this instance, the importance of the availability of interpreters is emphasized.

Many of the key ethical principles discussed by the Nuffield Council are reiterated in the Report of the Select Committee on Science and Technology (Shaw, 1995). The committee made specific mention of two issues of considerable importance in relation to the diagnosis of late-onset disorders:

1 People coming forward to be tested for a late-onset condition must first be given extensive counselling concerning both the medical and social implications of a positive result. There must be adequate provision for follow-up counselling and support.

2 Children should not have a genetic diagnosis for a late-onset disorder. Such a diagnosis is only justifiable if those requesting it have fully considered all its implications.

The impact of cancer genetic counselling and testing on mental health is not well known to date but reported reactions to cancer risk assessment include denial, low self-esteem, guilt and anxiety. The impact on families is even less well documented but it is possible to infer from other genetic programmes, such as Huntington's disease, that the implications may be considerable in terms of psychological morbidity.

Disclosure of test results

An individual that has consented to genetic screening has a right to know the outcome and the attendant implications. In considering disclosure of information, those responsible should analyse very carefully the anxieties attached to the particular situation. In some instances, positive results may not necessarily indicate clinical implications and disclosure could lead to needless worry on the part of the individual concerned. In other cases, disclosure of results may not necessarily be covered by the informed consent itself, for example when unexpected results are obtained that were not foreseeable at the time of primary counselling on the advisability of genetic screening. Failure to disclose information obtained, as it were 'accidentally', and for which specific informed consent had not been obtained, raises another ethical dilemma.

Another aspect of this particular situation is where samples are stored, perhaps for re-testing, for research purposes for future diagnostic requirements. The Nuffield report (Nuffield Council on Bioethics, 1993) is quite specific both as to the requirement to obtain an individual's consent for such uses and on the need for effective methods of security and confidentiality of stored genetic material.

Because ethical and practice problems may arise from the future testing of stored specimens, for example as new tests become available, it is essential that very careful consideration is given as to how such stored genetic material is to be used. Again, the confidentiality and security of stored samples is of paramount importance.

Harper (1993, 1995) has devised a proposed code of conduct for the use of research samples from families with genetic disease. When offering genetic testing services to individuals and their families, all of these aspects would have to be taken into full consideration, in advance, and would form part of the accompanying counselling and a truly informed consent from the individual(s) concerned.

The possible effect on marital and family relationships must also be considered. The genetic consequences for children – born or unborn – may have serious repercussions on marriage and other family relationships. Such families may often require extensive support to help prevent the breakdown of relationships and its consequences.

Individuals who are tested (with a positive outcome) at a time of life when they have still to make decisions about parenthood face the added dilemma of making difficult choices against the background of the genetic risks now known to them.

Once positive results have been obtained, individuals facing the problems of increased personal anxiety about their future health have the added worry of deciding whether or not to give consent for disclosure to other members of their families.

The ethical dilemmas inherent in this situation are daunting. The main issues that need to be addressed are:

- What information should be shared with other family members who may be at risk?
- With whom does the responsibility lie for imparting information?
- Who should initiate the appropriate investigation and counselling of these individuals?

Such decisions require careful consideration. Any benefits to members of the family being given such information and the 'right to know' must be weighed in the balance against the disadvantages to them of being given information that may cause anxiety and that they did not seek in the first place. Disclosure also carries with it the loss of confidentiality (of the individual's personal medical information) and an attendant loss of his/her rights to personal privacy, as outlined in Article 8(1) of the European Convention on Human Rights.

The implications of positive results for other members of the family should always be discussed with the individual tested. The potentially serious implications of such results for a family pose difficult ethical problems in, on the one hand, applying the long-standing principle of confidentiality between the professional and the individual concerned against, on the other, the need to disclose genetic information that may be vital to the well-being or future of other family members.

Ethical issues

For the individual, the ethical implications arising from the ability of technology to provide genetic test information about late-onset and disease-susceptibility disorders are more complex than those arising from early-onset single-gene disorders. Much depends on the likelihood and time-scale of events. This, in turn, depends on many as yet unknown or inherently unpredictable factors, only some of which are genetic.

Key considerations are:

- the individual and individual's extended family – their needs and confidentiality issues
- equity of access
- the legal protection of genetic information
- employment issues
- insurance issues
- stigmatization
- the implications of testing by commercial organizations

Equity of access

The general public should have equity of access to all genetic testing, counselling and surveillance programmes agreed and established nationally. Such programmes must also be supported by the provision of adequate treatment and follow-up services.

Cancer genetics services should be subject to a full and regular evaluation, which includes an assessment of equity of provision to the target population.

In the UK, confidentiality and security of genetic information is covered by:
- the common law of patient confidentiality
- the Data Protection Act (1984)
- the Access to Health Records Act (1990)
- professional codes of conduct, including guidance from the General Medical Council

However, the duty of confidentiality placed upon all employees in the NHS may, in exceptional circumstances and if it is felt to be in the public interest, be overridden on a case-by-case basis by medical practitioners.

Employment issues

The Nuffield report (Nuffield Council on Bioethics, 1993) states that the use of genetic screening by employers in the UK has so far not given any cause for concern. However, there may be special circumstances in which occupational risks may endanger health.

Insurance issues

Predictive cancer genetic testing plays an extremely small part in life insurance assessment. Only if there is a strong positive family history and/or a known mutation in key genes (e.g. *BRCA1*, *BRCA2* or *TP53*) would insurers seek to charge higher premiums or to decline insurance. In February 1997, the Association of British Insurers (ABI) in the UK made a public announcement that for 2 years' life insurance, which was to be used to cover a mortgage for the individual's own house (and for a sum less than £100 000), no genetic test results would be used, even if these were adverse. Insurers wished to hear of any abnormal test results, however, in order to audit and monitor this change. However, in the UK recently, the ABI has obtained consent for the use of genetic test results for Huntington's disease by insurers; other genetic conditions will be considered in this way in the future.

The Select Committee on Science and Technology (Shaw, 1995) urged those involved to find ways of regulating the use of genetic information in insurance so as to protect the interests of society and enable as many people as possible to obtain insurance, as well as to protect the insurance companies. The committee recommended that the insurance industry be given 1 year in which to propose a solution that was acceptable to all parties. Recently, the Genetics Advisory and Insurance Committee (GAIC) decided to allow insurers to use Huntington's disease test results in fixing life assurance premiums (Major, 2000).

Stigmatization

The avoidance of stigmatization arising from genetic screening programmes must form part of the debate on the way forward. Adequate safeguards covering confidentiality and security, soundly based informed consent, and careful monitoring of genetic testing and screening programmes should help in this respect.

However, consideration must also be given to raising the level of consciousness among the general population via appropriate health education measures.

Regulation of commercial testing facilities

A number of laboratories currently offer commercial genetic testing for certain disorders and telephone counselling direct to the public. This may lead to inappropriate tests and a lack of adequate counselling and follow-up. The Select Committee on Science and Technology called for these laboratories to be regulated through a process of protocol review and licensing (Shaw, 1995). The Advisory Committee on Genetic Testing has drawn up a code of practice and guidance on human genetic testing services offered direct to the public.

Education and training

Primary care staff have a key role to play in providing advice to patients who are concerned about familial risk and in identifying those patients who require the more specialized advice of genetics clinics. To assist primary care staff in carrying out this role, guidance and training would need to be provided about the criteria to be used for identifying those patients at increased risk of developing breast and ovarian cancers.

The costs of providing guidance and training for primary care staff have not been estimated. However, they are likely to be relatively small. They would include the costs of providing printed guidance on the criteria that should be used to identify patients at increased risk, the costs of carrying out training sessions for primary care staff, and the costs of providing information leaflets and letters for patients.

Similarly, training for nurses and counsellors could be dealt with by specific modules and clinical attachments for a few months, facilitating continuing liaison with genetics clinics to be offered ongoing support.

Implementation

If the screening programmes outlined earlier in this report are to be implemented successfully, there are a number of key tasks that need to be carried out. The main changes required for the implementation of these changes are as follows.

- Guidelines should be prepared on the criteria that should be used by primary care staff to assess whether individuals are at low, medium or high risk of developing breast, colorectal or ovarian cancer.
- Training should be provided to primary care staff on the use of criteria for assessing familial risk.
- Appropriate management protocols should be agreed for regular screening of people considered to be at medium or high risk of developing cancer.
- Funding should be identified and provided both for the genetics clinics and for the screening programmes required by people who are assessed at medium and high risk.
- Appropriate screening programmes should be implemented for people at medium or high risk of developing cancer.
- Patients should have access to appropriate counselling services.
- A database of families at increased risk should be maintained to facilitate evaluation and research.
- A programme to evaluate screening outcomes of individuals at increased risk should be established.

Evaluation

There are many uncertain aspects to the proposed system of screening people at significantly increased risk of breast and ovarian cancer, and it is essential that the clinical and cost-effectiveness of these services should be subject to thorough evaluation. A detailed and comprehensive programme of evaluation should be drawn up and implemented within an agreed national framework (Harper, 1995).

The main issues that need to be evaluated include the following:

- The effectiveness of the guidance and support provided to primary care or breast clinics. For many people who are at increased familial risk of cancer, the first point of contact will be with primary care or breast clinics, and it is important that the guidance and support provided to primary care staff enable them to make a proper initial assessment of risks and to avoid inappropriate referrals to genetics clinics.
- In some countries, the cancer care is separated into cancer units (secondary care) and cancer centres (tertiary care) facilities. The genetics clinic may work closely with the cancer centre while the cancer unit may be staffed by genetic

nurses and counsellors with additional training in the identification and care of high-risk individuals.

- The effectiveness of genetic counsellors (or genetic nurses) in providing appropriate support to primary care and in assessing the risk of referred individuals.
- The effectiveness of screening programmes in detecting cases of cancer. This will require monitoring of the number of cancers detected per 1000 patients screened, and the number of interval cancers occurring among the screened population, and the false-positive rate. This monitoring of information should be done within different age bands so that an assessment can be made of the appropriateness of the age ranges covered by the screening and the screening frequency. Computerized systems for audit of surveillance outcomes are essential for assessing the long-term efficacy of follow-up in relation to risk estimate.
- The appropriateness of the criteria used to assess people at medium or high risk on the basis of their family history. A relatively low detection rate (together with other criteria) may suggest that the family history criteria need to be reviewed.
- The risk of complications associated with the screening procedures, especially the risks associated with colonoscopy. In addition to the risks of procedures used for the diagnosis of cancer, there is also a risk from false-positive findings on screening.
- The effects of screening programmes on mortality rates. This is a crucial measure of the effectiveness of screening of individuals at increased risk of cancer.
- The effects of screening on anxiety levels in patients. It is important that the effectiveness of screening programmes in providing reassurance to people concerned about familial risks of cancer should be assessed.

The clinical and cost-effectiveness of the proposed screening programmes will need to be evaluated over a period of several years. Some aspects – for example, the effect on mortality rates – can only be evaluated over a long time-scale, but other aspects may be evaluated within a shorter time-scale. It would be appropriate for there to be a clear and agreed programme of evaluation established at the outset of any such programme so that proposed screening systems can be managed efficiently and effectively.

- In planning the development of services for people with a significant family history of cancer, it would be important to recognize that the major part of the extra costs in the medium term will consist of the screening programmes.
- Some individuals, who might have been enrolled onto surveillance protocols prior to genetic assessment, may be found to be at low risk after such assessment and may then be reassured, thus saving healthcare costs of surveillance.
- The estimated screening costs are based on the full average costs of the various screening methods. It is possible that some of these screening services could be

expanded at marginal costs, which are less than the full average costs. However, the projected levels of screening in the medium term represent a significant increase in workload, and the extra costs may not differ greatly from the full average costs.

• The healthcare costs of treating cancer will be reduced if surveillance detects cancers at an earlier, more treatable, stage.

Conclusion

The benefits of genetic counselling and testing for inherited cancer susceptibility in high-risk families are becoming very clear, particularly in conditions conferring susceptibility to colorectal cancer, such as familial adenomatous polyposis and HNPCC, and such management is well within the remit of clinical genetics services. The benefits of surveillance in families at moderate familial cancer risk are less proven as yet and require long-term evaluation of audit of a very large cohort of families. Working guidelines are now available for stratification of familial risks and for clinical surveillance of each risk group, and follow-up of these groups provides the information required for evidence-based management of these families in the future. This will inform health-service development in different countries in the future.

REFERENCES

Burke W, Daly M, Garber J, et al. (1997). Recommendations for follow-up care of individuals with an inherited predisposition to cancer: BRCAl and BRCA2. *JAMA* **277**: 997–l003.

Caulfield TA (1995). The allocation of genetic services: economics, expectations, ethics and the law. *Health Law J* **3**: 213–34.

Claus EB, Schildkraut JM, Thompson WD and Risch NJ (1996). The genetic attributable risk of breast and ovarian cancer. *Cancer* **77**: 2318–24.

Eeles R (1996). Testing for the breast cancer predisposition gene, BRCAl. *Br Med J* **313**: 572–3.

Emery J, Watson E, Rose P and Andemann A (1999a). A systematic review of the literature exploring the role of primary care in genetic services. *Fam Pract* **16**: 426–45.

Emery J, Walton R, Murphy M, et al (1999b). Computer support for interpreting family histories of breast and ovarian cancer in primary care: comparative study with simulated cases. *Br Med J* **321**: 28–32.

Goldgar DE, Stratton MR and Eeles RA (1996). Familial breast cancer. In *Genetic Predisposition to Cancer*, ed. R.A. Eeles, B.A.J. Ponder, D.F. Easton and A. Horwich. London: Chapman & Hall.

Harper P (1993). Research samples from families with genetic diseases: a proposed code of conduct. *Lancet* **341**: 1391–3.

Harper PS (1995). Genetic testing, common diseases and health service provision. *Lancet* **346**: 1645–6.

Harris R (1998). Genetic counselling and testing in Europe. *J R Coll Physicians Lond* **32**(4): 335–8.

Hodgson SV, Haites NE, Caligo M, et al. (2000a). A survey of the current clinical facilities for the management of familial cancer in Europe. European Union BIOMED II Demonstration Project. Familial breast cancer: audit of a new development in medical practice in European centres. *J Med Genet* **37**(8): 605–7.

Hodgson SV, Haites NE, Caligo M, et al. (2000b). Demonstration project. Familial breast cancer auditing of a new development in medical practise in European centres. *J Med Genet* **37**: 1–2.

Houlston RS, McCarter E, Parbhoo S, Scurr JH and Slack J (1991). Family history and risk of breast cancer. *J Med Genet* **29**: 154–7.

Hughes HE, Aldman JK, Krawzck M and Rogers C (1998). Contracting for clinical genetic services: the Welsh model. *J Med Genet* **35**(4): 309–13.

Kerlikowske K, Grady D, Barclay J, Sickles EA and Ernster V (1996). Effect of age, breast density, and family history on the sensitivity of first screening mammography. *JAMA* **276**: 33–8.

Major S (2000). UK allows insurers to use gene test for Huntington's disease. *Br Med J* **321**: 977.

Møller P, Evans G, Haites N, et al. (1999). Guidelines for follow-up of women at high risk for inherited breast cancer. Consensus statement from the Biomed II Demonstration Programme on Inherited Cancers. *Dis Markers* **15**(1–3): 207–11.

Murday V (1994). Genetic counselling in the cancer family clinic. *Eur J Cancer* **30A**: 2015–29.

Nuffield Council on Bioethics (1993). *Genetic Screening: Ethical Issues.* London: Nuffield Foundation.

Scottish Office Home and Health Department (1998). *Cancer Genetics Services in Scotland.* A report by the Priority Areas Cancer Team/Genetics Sub-Committee of the Scottish Cancer Co-ordinating and Advisory Committee.

Shaw G (1995). *Human Genetics: The Science and its Consequences,* The Science and Technology Select Committee. London: HMSO.

Skirton H, Barnes C, Guilbert P, et al. (1998). Recommendations for education and training of genetic nurses and counsellors in the United Kingdom. *J Med Genet* **35**(5): 410–11.

Stopfer JE (2000). Genetic counselling and clinical cancer genetic services. *Surg Oncol* **18**(4): 347–57.

Stratton JF, Gayther SA, Russell P, et al. (1997). Contribution of BRCAl mutations to ovarian cancer. *N Engl J Med* **336**: 1125–30.

12

Cultural and educational aspects influencing the development of cancer genetics services in different European countries

Shirley V. Hodgson

Guy's Hospital, London, UK

There is a rapidly increasing appreciation of the importance of familial cancer susceptibility and the potential for the identification and surveillance of at-risk individuals with a strong family history of cancer to reduce morbidity and mortality from the disease.

The development of healthcare strategies for the identification of individuals with a risk of familial cancer susceptibility, for stratifying their risk and for developing agreed surveillance protocols is dependent on many factors, which will differ in different countries. This service development requires a partnership between clinicians, service providers and purchasers, and healthcare planners. Evaluation of the cost-effectiveness of such a service is vital. In many countries this service was initially funded by research charities. However, funding is now being transferred to the public sector as the research questions are answered.

There is a good deal of inequality in the sophistication of cancer genetics services in different countries, and those countries initiating service development should be enabled to benefit from the experience of others with established services.

This type of service has several levels: (1) there is a need for ascertainment and prioritization of referrals at the primary care level; (2) there should be an agreed management care pathway for the surveillance of individuals at different degrees of estimated moderate risk; and (3) there should be provision for genetic counselling and testing of individuals from families in which there is a high chance of an inherited susceptibility to specific cancers. This includes the provision of molecular genetics tests in laboratories that have attained appropriate accreditation, and predictive test counselling for at-risk relatives. A detailed description of the organization of such a service is provided by the Harper report for the UK Department of Health (1998). This report describes a system based upon the three activities enumerated above, utilizing the concept of primary care referrals being prioritized and moderate-risk patients being referred to cancer units for surveillance, where the results of such surveillance can be monitored, and where only high-risk individuals would be referred to the genetics centre. A system by which healthcare providers can be educated to be able to prioritize individuals into the different risk categories is an important part of service delivery.

The factors that influence the development of cancer genetics services are those that influence all features of the above overview of the service. First and foremost must be the finance available to public health care in the country, since surveillance strategies of this kind may be perceived as a relative luxury compared with many other aspects of medical services. Their development will be driven partly by public awareness and demand for such a service, and partly by the demonstration of its efficiency in reducing morbidity and mortality from cancer.

There is some correlation between the gross national product of the country and the level of cancer genetics services. However, other factors also have an influence (Table 12.1). Such important factors include: existing primary health service structures, the presence of public and private sectors in the medical service and their mutual relationships, the existence of an established network of integrated genetics services, and the tradition of screening for other genetic conditions within the population, e.g. thalassaemia and sickle cell anaemia.

Standards

In order to ensure standards and regulate the development of the service, appropriate guidelines are needed, which can also promote uniformity of practice. The advisability of such guidelines is well recognized (Cancer Genetic Services in Europe, 1997). There is a very variable background in such legal guidelines in different European countries. Some countries already have statutory guidelines for various aspects of genetics services, such as Austria, Denmark, Belgium, Italy, the Netherlands, Finland, France, Germany, Norway, Sweden and the UK. No clear guidelines for genetic testing exist in Hungary, and few exist in Portugal and Greece as yet.

International organizations such as UNESCO, HUGO and WHO have published general guidelines on these issues, such as the WHO-proposed international guidelines on ethical issues in medical genetics and genetics (WHO, 1998). The Council of Europe Convention for the Protection of Human Rights and Dignity of the Human Being with regard to the application of biology and medicine (1997) is an international legal text with effect on those Council of Europe's member states that have ratified it. Belgium, Germany, Ireland and the UK have not yet signed the convention.

Table 12.1. Selected World Wide Web sites concerning cancer genetics issues

Subject	Remit	Website
What is genetic screening? Understanding gene testing	BIOSIS European Initiative for Biotechnology Education; resources for teaching aimed at students aged 16–19 years.	http://www.scicomm.org.uk/biosis/human/whatis/html http://134.225.167.114.8001/EIBE/preview/html
Advisory Committee on Genetic Testing Draft Code of Practice	BIOSIS	http://www.scicomm.org.uk/biosis/acgt/ACGT2/html
'The Gene Letter'	Internet-based newsletter, aiming to educate consumers and professionals about emerging medical, ethical, legal and policy dilemmas in this area. Established by the Shriver Centre with a grant from the US Dept of Energy/ELSI programme. Further discussions about this appear on the website given below.	http://www.geneletter.org
Cancer facts	(National Cancer Institute) supplies information for cancer patients, their families and the public, and backs this up with a telephone advice service.	w.graylab.ac.uk/cancernet/600349.html cancerweb@www.graylab.ac.uk

As part of the Cancer Genome Anatomy Project, funded by the NCI, Al Gore recently unveiled a website with the aim of having 'all the pieces together in the same place'.

Registries

Genetic and cancer registries provide a useful basis upon which to build cancer genetics services. These are well established in the UK, the Netherlands, Denmark, Belgium, Finland, Norway, Poland, Sweden and Denmark, and are being developed in Cyprus, Latvia, Hungary, Romania, Slovenia, Switzerland and the Ukraine.

The presence of cancer registries and registers of individuals with familial cancers such as familial adenomatous polyposis (FAP) sets a useful framework for the establishment of similar registries for familial cancer. Denmark and the UK were the first countries to set up FAP registries, but other countries, such as the Netherlands and Poland, have set up similar registries, and have developed these for hereditary non-polyposis colorectal cancer (HNPCC) and hereditary breast/ovarian cancer. This greatly facilitates the ascertainment of at-risk individuals and the monitoring of the efficacy of surveillance in high-risk individuals. However, genetic registers are considered to be unethical in Germany and Austria. New registers are being developed in Greece, Latvia and Portugal. The Finnish register for HNPCC has provided initial comprehensive information regarding the results of long-term follow-up of screened and unscreened individuals from HNPCC families (Jarvinen et al., 2000), and provides crucial evidence about the efficacy of surveillance in HNPCC. This information is applicable throughout Europe and can be utilized when negotiating for service funding. The tradition of audit of medical services in general is important in facilitating such exercises and crucial for providing evidence for service efficacy and the development of evidence-based healthcare policies.

Financial constraints still hamper the development of cancer genetics services in many of the Eastern European countries, where cancer genetics is not a priority. Where research funding is not available to initiate the service and thereby provide evidence for its cost-effectiveness, the experience from other countries with established services and audit of outcomes can be used to inform healthcare planners in countries that are initiating them.

Healthcare structure

The structure of health care, and the presence of networks of peripheral care services in the country, are important, allowing the funding for service to be defined and negotiated appropriately. Thus, in the UK there is a model of contracting for clinical genetics services that provides a basis for negotiation for new services when they are being proposed to purchasers (Hughes et al., 1998).

Competition and non-communication between public and private healthcare systems could be a potential impediment to the co-ordination of service development.

Genetics is still not a recognized specialty in Belarus, Croatia, Cyprus, the Czech Republic, Greece, Slovenia or Spain, and this may hamper service development. The education of medical students and doctors is improved in countries where the discipline is recognized.

Cancer genetics services

A survey of cancer genetics services, particularly in relation to breast cancer, in 34 European countries was undertaken as part of a BIOMED II Demonstration Project – 'Familial Breast Cancer, an Audit of a New Development in Medical Practice in European Countries' – and the results have been published in detail (Hodgson et al., 1999, 2000). There was considerable variation between the current status of such services in the different countries. The UK, the Netherlands, Belgium and the Scandinavian countries were the first to develop these, profiting from relatively high levels of gross national product and healthcare funding. However, much of the initial funding was provided by research charities. Other countries with active service development are France, Austria, Italy and Germany, but in these countries genetic counsellors are not yet accepted as having a role in service development. Israel, Poland and Ireland are also actively developing these services, including the acceptance of genetic counsellors as part of the service.

Multidisciplinary regional genetics centres are well established in the UK, Belgium and the Netherlands, in particular, and are being developed in Poland and Italy, but less so in Eastern European countries, and are being actively developed in Spain, Portugal and Turkey.

In Poland, 16 new regions have been established with a consultant geneticist at each, to coordinate genetics services.

In the USA, a national network of cancer genetics services was proposed by the National Institutes of Health in 1996. Five years of funding was provided in 1997 to support collaborative investigation into inherited cancer susceptibility and how this knowledge could be translated into medical practice, and to address the associated psychosocial, ethical, legal and public health issues involved (Senior, 1998). However, there are difficulties in administering this in the absence of a well-established collaborative health service network in the USA. Common guidelines for the management of individuals with an inherited susceptibility to breast/ovarian and colorectal cancer have been drawn up, based on a task force from the National Human Genome Research Institute Consortium, organized by the National Human Genome Research Institute (Burke et al., 1997a,b). In the US, the role of genetic counsellors is well accepted as forming a part of the genetics services (Peters and Stopfer, 1996).

In Australia, despite the large, relatively underpopulated territory, attempts are being made to standardize the management of susceptible individuals throughout the country, according to agreed guidelines (Hopper, 1996).

Networks and discussion fora to enhance the standardization of cancer genetics services, and discussion of policy development, are being implemented in many countries, including the Cancer Genetics Group (CGG) in the UK, the Danish breast cancer collaborative group, the Netherlands' National Registry of Hereditary Breast Cancer Families, the French network known as the 'Genetics and cancer group from the Federation Nationale des Centres de Lutte Contre le Cancer' (FNCLCC), and similar networks in Italy and Germany, which are funded partly by government and partly by research. Thus, in France, the FNCLCC is supported by a French charity, the League against Cancer, whereas the Ministry of Health supports the Foundation for the Detection of Hereditary Tumours in the Netherlands, aiming to promote and guarantee surveillance in families with hereditary cancer, and to encourage research. In Germany, the Ministry of Health promoted and provided financial support for the establishment of a multicentre interdisciplinary network for the management of hereditary breast cancer, and advised the Deutsche Krebshilfe on its national research funding programme in this area. In Italy, the establishment of a network of the relatively autonomous regions involved in providing cancer genetics services is being coordinated from Milan by the National Cancer Institute, with research funding. In the UK, the CGG was initiated as the Cancer Family Study Group, with strong backing from the Imperial Cancer Research Fund (ICRF), as a forum for the development of collaborative research into this area. As part of the development of the British Society for Human Genetics (BSHG – an umbrella organization for cytogeneticists, molecular geneticists and clinical geneticists), the CGG has now been accepted as a part of the BSHG, in recognition of the increasing importance of cancer genetics.

Networks of cancer genetics centres exist in the UK and much of the service work is now government funded. The continuing audit of a group of cancer genetics clinics funded in part by the ICRF is being facilitated by a recent grant from the National Lottery Charities Board for the establishment of a common database that will record and correlate family history data, molecular and pathological information, and surveillance outcomes. Since cancer genetics services are, by their nature, multidisciplinary and imply a degree of cooperation between clinical centres and health service planners, they are dependent on the establishment of collaborative groups. This is also important to ensure the consistency of services offered throughout the country.

Genetic counsellors

As part of the delivery of cancer genetics services, with a potentially high volume of referrals for risk assessment prior to stratifying individuals for appropriate surveillance, there is an important role for trained genetic counsellors who can see and evaluate a large number of individuals who have a family history of cancer, in order to prioritize them into risk groups. Thus, low-risk individuals may require reassurance, moderate-risk individuals may be offered screening, and high-risk individuals may be referred to a genetics centre for discussion of possible predictive testing and prophylactic management. Such a service relies on the availability of large numbers of trained genetic counsellors who may not necessarily be doctors. The acceptance of such counsellors in the delivery of such a service is important, and they should have appropriate educational provision, supervision and career structure (Skirton et al., 1998). In some countries they are recognized as being part of service provision (e.g. the UK, the Netherlands, Israel and Denmark), whereas in others (France, Germany, Latvia and Spain) they are not.

Education

Postgraduate training in cancer genetics is well established in Scandinavian countries, France, Germany, the Netherlands, Belgium, the UK, Italy, Poland, Romania, Latvia and Lithuania.

Undergraduate training in genetics is of a higher profile in countries where genetics is a recognized specialty, but education in cancer genetics at undergraduate level is often scanty.

Cancer genetics courses are being developed in several centres in the UK and elsewhere, often as modular courses available for healthcare professionals, and there is an international course that is run annually at Sestri Levante. Many of these courses are available to train genetic counsellors and nurses in the discipline. For instance, in Israel there is such a course for genetic counsellors in the Hebrew University in Jerusalem, associated with the Hadassah University, Ein karem.

Information about cancer genetics is becoming available on the World Wide Web, including sites listed in the proceedings of the Biomed 2 project (Cancer Genetic Services in Europe, 1997; Hodgson et al., 1999; see Tables 12.1 and 12.2). The Web is becoming of increasing importance in the dissemination of knowledge about cancer genetics, and of particular relevance for the USA and potentially for developing countries (Edejer, 2000).

Training in genetics for the non-geneticist is being promoted in the UK and in Latvia, Turkey and Denmark, amongst others.

Table 12.2. Factors influencing the development of cancer genetics services

- The GNP of the country, and the proportion spent on health services; the availability of charity funding
- Health service structure and the relationship between public and private systems on the delivery of health care
- The tradition and network structure of primary health care and its relationship to other healthcare systems
- The recognition of genetics as an official specialty
- The presence of established networks of genetics services
- Cancer service networks and their relationship to the genetics services
- The existence of medical service audit systems
- The existence of cancer registries
- The prior existence of screening programmes for genetic disorders such as thalassaemia
- Education provision regarding cancer genetics for healthcare professionals
- The recognition of the role of genetic counsellors in service delivery
- Public awareness of genetics issues, especially cancer genetics
- The presence of active patient support groups for families with cancer, often through the cancer charities
- Perceptions of social and ethical problems surrounding genetic issues
- Agreed guidelines for service provision
- Quality control for laboratory and clinical services

Public awareness

The level of public awareness of cancer genetics, with consequent empowerment to drive demand-led services, is important, and is dependent upon background beliefs about the influence of genetic factors on disease development, and media promotion of such issues. The acceptance of clinical genetics as a discipline is relatively new in many countries, and political, ethical and social barriers to genetic concepts are also extremely important. Thus, genetics is only just becoming accepted in countries such as Austria and Germany subsequent to the backlash against eugenics.

Education of the public in issues about cancer genetics is largely media driven, and in all European countries there is rapidly increasing media coverage of these issues, although the extent of this coverage varies widely. Genetics centres tend to provide information to referred families using letters and leaflets. Some videos are also being developed. Wider promotion of education about this is transmitted through primary care, although this is relatively under-developed at the moment. There is only a moderate amount of information available to specific high-risk groups such as the Ashkenazi Jewish population, although some literature on the subject is provided by charities such as the Imperial Cancer Research Fund and Cancer Research Campaign, now amalgamated to form Cancer Research UK (CRUK). General educational material is being offered in some countries in museum exhibitions, such as those in the Science Museum and the Gene Dome in the UK, and in an exhibition on 'Mensch und Gene' ('Man and the Gene') in Bonn, Germany, in 1998. Websites are increasingly being consulted by members of the general public, but are more easily accessed by individuals from wealthier countries.

Conclusions

It is clear that, although cancer genetics services are developing rapidly, there are very different degrees of service development in different European countries, dependent on many factors. There is, therefore, great potential for those countries with more advanced development of such services to provide guidance and evidence-based information to facilitate the service planning for countries in which services are at an early stage of development.

REFERENCES

Burke W, Peterson G, Lynch P, et al. (1997a). Recommendations for follow-up care of individuals with an inherited predisposition to cancer. 1. Hereditary non-polyposis colon cancer. *J Am Med Assoc* **277**: 915–19.

Burke W, Daly M, Garber J, et al. (1997b). Recommendations for follow-up care of individuals with an inherited predisposition to cancer. II. BRCA1 and BRCA2. *J Am Med Assoc* **277**: 997–1003.

Cancer Genetic Services in Europe (1997). A comparative study of 31 countries by the concerted action group on genetic services in Europe. *Eur J Hum Genet* **5** (Suppl. 2): 1–220.

Council of Europe (1997). *Convention for the Protection of Human Rights and Dignity of the Human Being with Regard to the Application of Biology and Medicine.* Convention on Human Rights and Biomedicine. Council of Europe: European Treaty Series no. 164, Oviedo, 4 April 1997.

Department of Health (1998). Genetics and Cancer Services. Report of a working group for the Chief Medical Officer, Department of Health, UK. London: Department of Health.

Edejer TT (2000). Disseminating health information in developing countries: the role of the internet. *Br Med J* **321**: 797–800.

Harris R (1998). Genetic counselling and testing in Europe. *J R Coll Physicians Lond* **32**: 335–8.

Harris R, Lane B, Williamson P, et al. (1999). National confidential enquiry into counselling for genetic disorders by non geneticists: general recommendations and specific standards for improving care. *Br J Obstet Gynaecol* **106**: 658–63.

Hodgson S, Milner B, Brown I, et al. (1999). Cancer genetics services in Europe. *Dis Markers* **15**: 3–13.

Hodgson SV, Haites NE, Caligo M, et al. (2000). A survey of the clinical facilities for the management of familial cancer in Europe: details of the current status. *J Med Genet* **37**: 605–7.

Hopper JL (1996). Some public health issues in the current state of genetic testing for breast cancer in Australia. *Aust N Z J Public Health* **20**: 464–72.

Hughes HE, Alderman JK, Krawczac M and Rogers C (1998). Contracting for clinical genetics services: the Welsh model. *J Med Genet* **35**: 309–13.

Jarvinen HJ, Aarnio M, Mustonen H, et al. (2000). Controlled 15-year trial on screening for colorectal cancer in families with hereditary nonpolyposis colorectal cancer. *Gastroenterology* **118**: 829–34.

Peters JA and Stopfer JE (1996). Role of the genetic counsellor in familial cancer. *Oncology (Huntingt)* **10**(2): 159–66.

Senior K (1998). New US cancer genetics network announced. *Mol Med Today* **4**: 459–60.

Skirton H, Barnes C, Guilbert P, et al. (1998). Recommendations for education and training of genetic nurses and counsellors in the United Kingdom. *J Med Genet* **35**: 410–12.

World Health Organization (1998). *Proposed International Guidelines on Ethical Issues in Medical Genetics and Genetic Services.* Report of a WHO Meeting on Ethical Issues in Medical Genetics, Geneva, 15–16 December 1997. Geneva: WHO.

13

Screening, detection and survival patterns of breast and other cancers in high-risk families

Pål Møller and C. Michael Steel

The Norwegian Radium Hospital, Oslo, Norway

Background

Untreated inherited breast cancer is recognized as a lethal disorder. The first detailed description in modern literature is probably 'Family Z', reported by Broca in 1866. If interpreting 'liver cancer' as ovarian cancer with spread, Broca described a family with dominantly inherited breast/ovarian cancer syndrome causing early death, and concluded that the cause had to be genetic factors with sex-limited phenotypic expression. He also discussed the putative impact of modifying genetic and environmental factors on the penetrance and expression of the major mutations, which may be discouraging for those who claim to have discovered new insights lately. More than 100 years later, it was agreed that inherited breast cancer was not rare (Iselius et al., 1992). In this chapter, the term 'inherited' is used for monogenic inheritance with high penetrance. Recessive or X-linked inherited breast cancer has not been described. The postulated category of inherited breast cancer caused by more frequent mutations with lower penetrance has yet to be defined precisely, and is outside the scope of this chapter. Thus, 'inherited breast cancer' denotes dominant inheritance, as indicated by family history or demonstrated mutation. BRCA1, BRCA2, PTEN, TP53 and other genes do, when mutated, cause inherited breast cancer. All mutations proven to cause breast cancer also increase the risk of other cancer(s) (Lynch et al., 1997; Johansson et al., 1999; Chompret et al., 2000). In recent years it has been shown that there is geographical and ethnic variation, and average figures for prevalences of the genetic factors that cause inherited cancer should at the moment be considered with great caution. Prevalence figures from one area may not be valid for adjacent communities.

The above introduction is intended to stress that 'inherited breast cancer', even within narrow definition of the term, covers a heterogeneous group of disorders. Keeping this in mind, this chapter will discuss the strategies for treating and/or preventing inherited breast cancer on three levels: (1) considering inherited breast cancer to be an entity distinct from sporadic breast cancer; (2) considering putative differences between the subgroups (genetic syndromes) included in inherited breast cancer; and (3) considering the possibilities of curing/preventing associated cancers (other expressions of the underlying mutations) that are specific for each of the genetic syndromes.

While it is generally agreed that infiltrating breast cancer without spread may proceed to cancer with spread, it is not agreed that carcinoma in situ (CIS) may proceed to infiltrating cancer. Moreover, CIS is subclassified into ductal, lobular and other groups. Interestingly, lobular CIS, which is recognized as a marker of risk for bilateral invasive cancer, has not been found to be associated with either *BRCA1* or *BRCA2* mutations. Discussion of the subgroups of CIS is outside the scope of this chapter. The generic term 'CIS' will therefore be used.

There may be three approaches to breast cancer treatment: do nothing, try to cure the demonstrated disease, or try to prevent occurrence of the disease. Nobody will today advocate doing nothing. In general, cure rate is dependent upon early detection and effective treatment. This is not only a simple, mechanistic interpretation of the metastatic process. It is also in keeping with the concept of a time-dependent probability of acquiring the mutations that underlie both spread and resistance to available treatment, and with the concept of total tumour mass as a predictor of prognosis. In general, early treatment is encouraged by public education (breast awareness, self-examination, seeking your doctor in time). In addition, formal screening programmes for women more than 50 years of age have been implemented. All current activity aimed at early diagnosis of breast cancer is set on the somewhat precarious base of prevention policies for the general population. Controversies surrounding their effectiveness reflect, at least in part, the different social settings in which they have been conducted, including different public education programmes for breast awareness, variation in intensity of screening protocols for older women, and geographical as well as time-associated variation in treatment given to breast cancer patients.

A further consideration is that it is neither practically nor ethically possible to randomize high-risk women within a trial designed to withhold intervention (e.g. mammographic screening) for one group in order to demonstrate that it is effective in reducing mortality.

Early diagnosis

A decade ago, a number of centres independently set up clinics for the early diagnosis and treatment of inherited breast cancer. This was done before the underlying genes were cloned, and inclusion criteria were based on family history

Table 13.1. Outcome of prospective surveillance programmes of women at risk in breast cancer kindreds (findings according to stage at diagnosis)

	CIS	CaN0	CaN+
Møller et al., 1998	9	28	9
Lalloo et al., 1998	6	6	5
Kollias et al., 1998	6	15	8
Tillanus-Linthorst et al., 2000	5	16	5
Møller et al., 1999[a]	32	91	38
Total[b]	43	122	51

[a]Combined European series including Møller et al. (1998), Lalloo et al. (1998) and the majority of the prospective cases reported in a UK survey (Macmillan, 2000).
[b]Total excluding Møller et al. (1998) and Lalloo et al. (1998).

alone. Precise risk estimation from family history is difficult; commonly used statistical models may give conflicting results (McGuigan et al., 1996). Most centres used eligibility criteria and follow-up protocols that were similar (Vasen et al., 1998). In principle, all criteria selected sisters and daughters of affected women in kindreds with assumed dominant inheritance and/or early onset of disease. Most of these centres joined forces in a Biomed 2 project and pooled their results for analysis of efficacy of the programmes and a consensus statement on how to proceed.

There are several reports from prospective screening programmes in the high-risk groups concerning stage at diagnosis of breast cancer. They are compiled in Table 13.1. Most centres report a favourable stage distribution, indicating that most women were likely to have a favourable outcome. No centre had a randomized control group. All centres report some cancers with nodal spread, indicating that not all patients were cured. The reports include CIS. It is commonly agreed that CIS is a marker that the woman has a high probability of developing an invasive cancer, but it is still debated whether or not CIS is the pre-cancer itself. This controversy is crucial to the interpretation of the findings, if the goal is to identify and remove the pre-cancer. In addition, it has not been demonstrated that prognostic indices (based on stage at diagnosis, histological grade, etc.) derived from empirical data on sporadic breast cancers are valid for the group of inherited cancers.

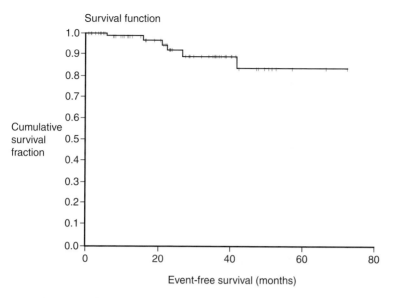

Figure 13.1 Event-free survival of the prospectively detected breast cancers reported by the Biomed 2 Demonstration Programme (Møller et al., 1999a).

Survival studies

Prospective studies

In 1999, seven of the collaborating centres in the Biomed 2 project updated the status of all patients who were prospectively diagnosed in their follow-up programmes to examine survival (Møller et al., 1999a). The results are presented in Figure 13.1: 5-year survival was 89% and 5-year event-free survival was 86%. The group, as a whole, followed the survival curve expected for sporadic breast cancer of comparable stage at diagnosis. Thus, the results indicated that survival was indeed improved by early diagnosis. The results also showed that patients with nodal spread at diagnosis fared worse and that those with CIS (but no invasive cancer) fared better than the average (5-year event-free survival 67% and 100%, respectively). As discussed in the report, CIS was found so frequently as to suggest strongly that CIS is indeed the pre-cancer. If so, the frequency of CIS and the event-free survival in all CIS cases after diagnosis indicate that the objective of early diagnosis and treatment was successfully achieved by reference to this subgroup alone. Again, however, the interpretation is influenced by whether or not CIS is the pre-cancer.

Reports on patients undergoing prophylactic surgery indicate that the contralateral breast in women with inherited breast cancer contains pre-invasive tumours in a high proportion of cases. In contrast, such lesions were not found in the contralateral breast in women with sporadic breast cancer (Kuhurana et al., 2000).

Retrospective studies

It is possible to define retrospective series of *BRCA1* or *BRCA2* mutation-carrying kindreds. These series, together with a number of other reports, indicate substantial differences between the distinct genetic syndromes included in inherited breast cancer. The *BRCA1* syndrome includes oestrogen-receptor-negative, high-grade tumours (Sobol et al., 1995; Verhoog et al., 1998; Lakhani et al., 2000). CIS is infrequently seen, and there may be indications that the infiltrating cancers do worse than stage at diagnosis would indicate (Johansson et al., 1998; Verhoog et al., 1998; Foulkes et al., 2000; Stoppa-Lyonnet et al., 2000). However, retrospective studies often include a number of methodological problems. In keeping with standards in evidence-based medicine, no hypothesis derived from retrospective studies alone should determine health care until confirmed in prospective series.

Combined interpretation

The combined information indicates that inherited breast cancer, taken as a whole, benefits from early diagnosis and treatment, but there may be substantial differences between subgroups. *BRCA1* cancers may not be detected at the pre-invasive stage with the diagnostic means employed so far, while other groups of inherited breast cancers may be diagnosed as CIS and cured. These are, at present, no more than hypotheses, but at the same time it is not possible to arrive at any conclusion in conflict with these hypotheses. If true, subgroups may need different follow-up regimens and different treatments. In that case, mutation testing may be indicated as a preoperative procedure in any breast cancer patient, and the demand for genetic testing may increase far beyond the level required to serve breast cancer kindreds alone.

Retrospective studies and descriptions of current patients may give answers to a number of the questions discussed above. Empirical data for long-time survival, however, take a long time to obtain. The ongoing studies already concluded to 5-year survival should, therefore, be continued as they will produce figures for long-time survival earlier than any study initiated today. However, numbers included in studies reported so far are insufficient and broader studies are needed, especially to distinguish between subgroups as discussed.

Population versus high-risk group screening

Population screening in women over 50 years of age, with mammography every second year, is beneficial, although cost-effectiveness is debated. The merit of such

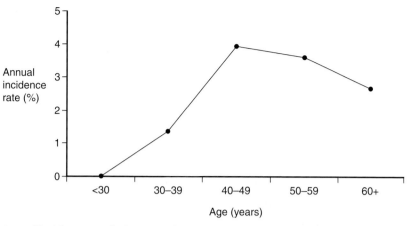

Figure 13.2 Annual incidence rate for breast and/or ovarian cancer for *BRCA1* mutation carriers.

screening before 50 years of age is controversial. Looking more closely at the effect of screening over the age of 50, the benefit seems to increase with age. In other words, screening with mammography seems effective after the menopause, but may have limited effect earlier. Moreover, the discussions on the effect of screening by mammography are statistical debates on whether or not it is beneficial to the group examined. Mammography every second year does not provide a guarantee against dying of breast cancer; the individual women examined may not feel safe. When dealing with one young *BRCA1*-mutation-carrying woman, the issues surrounding her need for health are quite remote from the population-based cost/benefit strategic thinking that underlies the screening programmes. Screening mammography may be very efficient at population level, but still inadequate for any given high-risk woman.

In breast cancer kindreds, the risk group is younger. Proven *BRCA1* and *BRCA2* mutation carriers are at risk and must be cared for from 30 years upwards. Up to half of these carriers will get cancer before they reach 50 years of age. Correspondingly, mean age at diagnoses in the combined prospective follow-up studies are close to 50 years. The observed annual incidence rate for breast cancer in families selected on the basis of family history alone is low – up to 30 years of age. From 40 years upwards, the annual incidence is about 0.75% in sisters and daughters of affected members (Møller et al., 1998). In *BRCA1* carriers, the annual incidence rate for contracting cancers rises from close to zero at 30 years of age, to about 3% per year at 40 years of age, and remains at this level for the rest of life (Dørum et al., 1999) (Figure 13.2). This contrasts with data for the general population where the risk is very low in young adulthood, and increases steadily up to 70+ years of age. (The exact age-related incidence curve for sporadic breast cancer is outside the scope of this chapter.)

When the breast cancer screening programmes today consider costs and benefits of screening women from 40 years upwards, the question is whether or not that will have a measurable effect. Within the breast cancer kindreds, the question is what we can do for each woman at risk. To demonstrate a slightly reduced risk of dying young is not good enough for the high-risk group.

Examination methods and interval between examinations

'Time in pre-clinical detectable stage' (also called 'mean sojourn time') is the time-window in which a breast cancer is asymptomatic but may be diagnosed by professional examination. Time in pre-clinical detectable stage is estimated at 1.25 years in sporadic breast cancer before 50 years of age and has been shown to be similar in inherited breast cancer (Tabàr et al., 1992; Møller et al., 1998). Re-evaluation of the Swedish mammography trials indicates that, for the age-group 50–59 years, time in pre-clinical detectable stage is shorter in inherited cancers than in sporadic cancers (Nixon et al., 2000). About one-quarter of inherited breast cancers are mammographically occult at diagnosis (Møller et al., 1999a; Tillanus-Linthorst et al., 2000). Together, these results indicate that an annual (or more frequent) interval(s) is necessary up to 60 years of age in women at high risk of inherited cancer, and that clinical examination is indicated in addition to mammography. In addition to clinical examination, other techniques for diagnosis by imaging are being assessed. Early reports on the efficacy of magnetic resonance imaging are promising (Kuhl et al., 2000). Ultrasonography is generally not considered as a screening tool, but it is useful for identifying possible lesions detected by other methods. The fear that the pressure for early diagnosis would lead to too many invasive procedures has proved false: three independent centres report similar and reasonable frequencies (4–7%) of fine-needle aspiration cytology, 11–17% of these resulting in diagnoses of cancer (Møller et al., 1999b).

In conclusion, it is agreed that clinical examination and mammography should be offered to the high-risk group annually from 30 to 60 years in centres capable of proceeding to invasive procedures whenever needed. Whether this is proved to be beneficial is not an immediate concern: nobody suggests that high-risk women should be offered substantially less. The subjects for debate are whether or not more frequent examinations are indicated, whether or not more sophisticated imaging techniques should be employed, and whether or not prophylactic measures are indicated and available.

Treatment

A full discussion of treatment is outside the scope of this chapter. The following outline is simply a grouping of modalities to provide a structure. There are three forms of treatment: surgery, ionizing radiation and chemotherapy (including anti-oestrogens). Tumours are removed surgically. Breast conservation surgery is combined with radiation to prevent local recurrence. Metastatic cancer is treated with radiation and chemotherapy (including anti-oestrogens) as indicated. Survival after diagnosis is a measure of treatment efficacy. Strictly speaking, the discussion above, relating survival to stage at diagnosis, is conceptually wrong. If treatment had no effect, the association between survival and stage at diagnosis would reflect nothing more than 'lead time' bias, the patients seeming to live longer because they had been diagnosed earlier. Given that the time in pre-clinical detectable stage is agreed to be about 1 year, the 'lead time' cannot be greater than this. Because the effect on survival discussed above is much more than that, it has to be attributable to the treatment (this remains true even when due allowance is made for the 'dilution' of true cancers with cases of CIS detected on screening). To assess the effect of treatment more rigorously, standardized protocols are needed. However, no centre with an established follow-up regimen for high-risk women has reported a special protocol for treatment of the cancers found. This means that the choice, for example between breast conservation surgery and mastectomy, will be an individual one, influenced by patient preference, but also reflecting differences in practice between countries, centres and surgeons. In addition, there are time-trends: treatment given today is likely to differ from that in standard use some years ago.

Strategies for treatment

There are two distinct strategies for treatment: one is to do as little harm as possible ('non-malefice'), the other is to maximize probability for long-term cure ('benefice').

In practical terms, this can be applied to breast conservation surgery versus mastectomy. The former is usually accompanied by ionizing radiation to the remaining breast tissue to avoid recurrence, as an alternative to removal of all breast tissue on the affected side. Because of the risk of contralateral breast cancer, bilateral mastectomies are performed in a number of cases. To the authors it is a logical mystery why ionizing radiation is considered to be an acceptable alternative to mastectomy for the remaining tissue in the diseased breast, while only surgical removal (and not ionizing radiation) is considered to minimize risk of tumour growth in the contralateral breast. We do need a debate on this subject. The balance between maximizing the prospects of cure, versus doing least possible harm, may be an individual question to be resolved by the patient. It is the common experience of counsellors, however, that patients do seek and actually follow advice. This is substantiated by the wide variation in uptake of prophylactic surgery among centres. It is not reasonable to assume that the differences in practice between centres arise purely from patient attitudes. There are reasons to believe that patient choice is influenced by the preferred policy of a given centre. Underlying this, however, are the social settings controlling both what doctors may regard as their 'professional advice', and what the patients may consider their 'free choice' (Julian-Reynier et al., 2000). Full discussion of these factors is outside the scope of this chapter, but the brief résumé may serve to highlight the complexities that surround the treatment of breast cancer in high-risk patients. At present, clarification of the arguments for constructive debate should be the priority.

Bearing in mind the stratification problems in the outcome analyses discussed above, it is reasonable to suggest that the centres should collaborate to provide the ground for evidence-based treatment. Whenever possible, handling of the high-risk group should accord with the general standards in evidence-based medicine. The general standard is to perform randomized trials when necessary and feasible.

Prophylaxis

Briefly, prophylactic measures may be surgical or chemical (as mentioned above, ionizing radiation for prophylaxis has not been suggested). Bilateral mastectomy provides protection against breast cancer, although not 100% (Hartmann et al., 1999). The discussion regarding treatment options re-emerges: complete ablation seems better than subcutaneous mastectomy, but complete ablation does more harm to the patients. Chemoprevention trials include anti-oestrogens and have side-effects. A specific form of chemoprevention, reported to reduce breast cancer risk in *BRCA1* carriers, is oophorectomy and subsequent hormonal replacement therapy (Rebbeck et al., 1999).

The point of mentioning prophylaxis in this chapter is to highlight the fact that, while surgical prophylaxis removes the breasts and makes them 'unavailable' for subsequent trials, early diagnosis strategies may be combined with chemoprevention trials. Moreover, prophylactic surgery may not answer the question of whether or not it was indicated, unless there is a suitable control group or an expectation of what would have happened without mastectomy. This returns us to the initial issue of establishing an agreed platform for basic healthcare provision for the high-risk group, and the feasibility of superimposing clinical trials on that platform. As discussed, we cannot use control groups to validate the basic level of provision for the high-risk group. Prophylactic trials, however, should include randomized controls.

Associated cancers

There are at least four dominantly inherited breast cancer syndromes where the underlying mutations are known. In genetic terminology, associated cancers would be called 'different (pleiotropic) expressions of the underlying mutations'. Ignoring infrequent or undocumented associations, prostate, pancreatic and other cancers are associated with inherited breast cancer. As there is no current agreement on either early detection strategies or benefit from early detection if that were possible, these cancers will not be discussed here.

The *BRCA1* syndrome is characterized by early-onset breast and ovarian cancer. Initial reports, influenced by mode of ascertainment of families (concentrating on breast cancer), may have under-estimated the relative frequency of ovarian cancer. Moreover, the families were ascertained by age of onset of cancer and, accordingly, mutations, when demonstrated, were correlated with very-early-onset disease (Easton et al., 1995). *BRCA1* mutation carriers may contract breast cancer two or three times as often as they contract ovarian cancer (Moslehi et al., 2000). However, studies in extended families exploring different and assumption-free models for estimating penetrance indicate that ovarian cancer may be as frequent as breast cancer in *BRCA1* kindreds. The discrepancies were initially attributed to statistical problems (including informative censoring) (Dørum et al., 1999). However, the findings have been replicated in another series and explained on the basis of ascertainment bias in the earlier work, taking account of factors that modify expression of *BRCA1* mutations (Antoniou et al., 2000). On the other hand, other reports do not support this conclusion (Anonymous, 2000; Moslehi et al., 2000). Penetrance of *BRCA1* mutations with respect to ovarian cancer therefore remains an open question.

The *BRCA2* syndrome is also characterized by ovarian cancer, but in *BRCA2* mutation carriers ovarian cancer is seen less frequently and tends to occur later in life. In addition, male breast cancer is seen in *BRCA2* kindreds, and associations with prostate and other cancers are known (Moslehi et al., 2000).

For both *BRCA1* and *BRCA2* carriers, the ovarian cancer is epithelial. Attempts at early diagnosis and treatment, so far, have failed. Within follow-up programmes, the frequency of cancers with spread is far too high to provide safety for the woman at risk. Virtually all inherited ovarian cancer seems to be explained by *BRCA1* and *BRCA2*; the epidemiological data do not allow for any additional genes with similar prevalence. As mentioned above, however, given the present state of knowledge, population data should not be projected from one geographical area to another. About 50% of *BRCA1*-associated ovarian cancers may be prevented by use of oral contraceptives (Narod et al., 1998). However, oral contraceptives may increase the penetrance for breast cancer in the same women.

No clear recommendation can thus be made for or against use of oral contraceptives in *BRCA1* carriers.

All reports agree that ovarian cancer in *BRCA1* carriers occurs only rarely before the age of 40 years and, in *BRCA2* carriers, rarely before 50 years. The French consensus statement – that suggesting oophorectomy to a woman under 35 years of age is unethical – has been generally adopted (Eisinger et al., 1998). Reports on ovarian cancer after prophylactic oophorectomy are not complete. In general, the prophylactic effect is considered good but prospective series to clarify the problem are not yet available. In conclusion, it is agreed that prophylactic oophorectomy will prevent most ovarian cancers and it is sufficient to raise this option at the end of the childbearing years. Perimenopausal oophorectomy with hormonal replacement therapy may have a substantial impact upon deaths from ovarian cancer. As mentioned above, the risk of breast cancer may also be reduced. The side-effects seem tolerable. More work has to be done to verify and quantify the outcome of this approach, but a mortality reduction of 50% may be hoped for.

A detailed description of the Li–Fraumeni (p53) and Cowden (*PTEN*) syndromes will not be given here. They are both multi-organ cancer syndromes with high penetrance for breast cancer in mutation-carrying women, assuming they do not die earlier from other cancers. Predictive genetic testing is complicated by disease manifestations in childhood, especially in the Li–Fraumeni syndrome. Testing in childhood is unethical if there is no clear benefit to the individual child. Informed consent from their parents may be compromised by complex intrafamilial conflicts of interest.

Possibly around half of all inherited breast cancer in northern Europe is caused by neither of the above-mentioned genes. We may call the residual syndrome *BRCAx*. The *BRCAx* syndrome is characterized by breast cancer with histopathological and clinical features, plus a pattern of associated cancers, that distinguish it from the other syndromes. Delineation of the *BRCAx* syndrome(s) may await uncovering of the causative gene(s).

Summary

Inherited breast cancer, taken as a whole, benefits from early diagnosis and treatment in a manner comparable with sporadic breast cancer. The group of inherited breast cancers is heterogeneous, with respect both to the breast tumours and to the associated cancers. Preventive strategies to avoid premature death include early diagnosis and treatment, both for breast cancer and for the associated cancers. Health care for any given patient has to take account of all aspects of the syndrome in question, not just the breast cancer risk.

For *BRCA1* and *BRCA2* cancer kindreds, it is agreed that prophylactic oophorectomy after childbearing age and follow-up, aiming at early diagnosis and treatment for breast cancer, should be implemented. In inherited breast cancer kindreds without demonstrated mutations and without cases of ovarian cancer, the suggested healthcare strategy is follow-up for breast cancer alone.

Chemoprevention studies may be added to the group enrolled in surveillance programmes for early diagnosis, without compromising (mandatory) evaluation of the effect of the follow-up protocols. Prophylactic mastectomy is incompatible with measuring effects of early diagnosis and chemoprevention. The conclusion is that early diagnosis and chemoprevention strategies should be proved inadequate before actively promoting prophylactic surgery. High-risk women should, however, have access to prophylactic mastectomy at their own request.

A number of methodological problems are apparent when considering the effect of early diagnosis and treatment. Among the most obvious are the requirement for standardized protocols, and the need to determine intermediate endpoints so that conclusions may be drawn within a reasonable time-span. The controversy surrounding interpretation of CIS (as the pre-cancer or not) is serious because it is crucial to interpretation of the initial results. If CIS really is the pre-cancer, and we fail to interpret it as such, we may achieve total protection by removing the pre-cancer but the result will be that we have no apparent result because nobody in the study group contracted the disease. In most settings this would have been clarified by comparison with a control group, but we do not have control groups. Moreover, there is no agreement regarding penetrance of the underlying mutations, leaving expectations (predicted numbers of cases) for the prospective programmes uncertain.

The rapid expansion of molecular testing capacity for *BRCA1* and *BRCA2* will clarify problems related to penetrance and expression of the mutations in population-based series. Long-term effects of prevention strategies (primary or secondary prevention, through early diagnosis and treatment) will only be determined within a reasonable time through broad international collaborative efforts. The Inherited Breast Cancer Demonstration Programme, funded by Biomed 2, concluded in May, 1999, with a conference in Heidelberg, Germany, attended by professionals from 37 European countries. A consensus report on how to proceed was agreed upon and published (Møller et al., 1999b) (see below).

Suggested guidelines

Definition of women at high risk of inherited breast cancer:
- A family history of two or more first-degree relatives (or second-degree relatives, though males) with early-onset (<50 years) breast cancer, and/or
- Multiple cases of breast cancers in the same lineage compatible with dominant inheritance in the family, and/or

- A combination of early-onset breast cancer and ovarian cancer in the family, and/or
- Family history that is suggestive of Li–Fraumeni syndrome (SBLA) or Cowden disease, and/or
- Demonstrated *BRCA1/2* truncating mutation or *TP53* or *PTEN* mutation.
- Males with *BRCA2* truncating mutation are also considered to be at risk.

Genetic counselling

Each woman at risk of inherited breast cancer should be entitled to genetic counselling by a specially trained doctor or genetic counsellor after validation of the family history and before risk estimates are finalized. The need for specially designed healthcare programmes should be determined and discussed in the course of such counselling. Predictive genetic testing should be carried out under strict quality control, with pre- and post-test genetic counselling by the responsible medical geneticist or associated genetic counsellor, and respecting the privacy and individual rights of each patient. Demonstrated high risk for inherited breast cancer should ensure access to the healthcare programmes suggested below, pending direct evidence of a survival benefit but on the assumption that this will emerge from pre-symptomatic detection of breast cancers.

Follow-up examinations

- Annual mammography and clinical expert examinations from 30 years of age (some centres modify starting age according to age of disease onset in affected relatives). From 60 years of age, mammography every second year (screening mammography) may be sufficient. Outside very-high-risk families (*BRCA1/2* carriers or clearly dominantly inherited disease in the kindred), more limited screening, such as annually from 35 to 50 years and every 18 months up to 60 years, may be appropriate.
- *BRCA1* mutation carriers (demonstrated or assumed by family history of two or more ovarian cancers and/or one relative with both breast and ovarian cancer) may benefit from mammography and clinical expert examinations twice a year and, where facilities permit, this option should be evaluated.
- Monthly self-examination or 'breast awareness' education should be encouraged.

Prophylactic surgery

- *BRCA1* mutation carriers (demonstrated or strongly indicated by two or more ovarian cancers and/or one with both breast and ovarian cancer in the family) may benefit from oophorectomy at 35–50 years of age. Those not choosing oophorectomy should be offered follow-up, including regular transvaginal ultrasound examination.

- *BRCA2* carriers (demonstrated, or strongly indicated by male breast cancer, plus other relevant cancers, in the family) may benefit from oophorectomy at menopause (45–50 years of age).
- Indications for prophylactic mastectomy are not considered here but should be subject to continuing evaluation.

Monitoring and evaluation of activity

To evaluate the effect of screening and preventive activities, it is of the utmost importance that they are carried out as prospective multicentre studies that are subjected to strict protocols and continuous evaluation. This is essential not only to establish the effect of such interventions, but also to generate data from which screening and/or intervention strategies can be matched more precisely to individual estimates of risk and to provide the background necessary for the assessment of new chemopreventive modalities in the near future.

REFERENCES

Anonymous (2000). Prevalence and penetrance of BRCA1 and BRCA2 mutations in a population-based series of breast cancer cases. *Br J Cancer* **83**: 1301–8.

Antoniou AC, Gayther SA, Stratton JF, et al. (2000). Risk models for familial ovarian and breast cancer. *Genet Epidemiol* **18**(2): 173–90.

Broca P (1866). *Traité des Tumeurs*. Paris, pp 151–5.

Chompret A, Brugieres L, Ronsin M, et al. (2000). P53 germline mutations in childhood cancers and cancer risk for carrier individuals. *Br J Cancer* **82**: 1932–7.

Dørum A, Heimdal, K, Hovig E, Inganäs M and Møller P (1999). Penetrances of BRCA1, 1675delA and 1135insA with respect to breast and ovarian cancer. *Am J Hum Genet* **65**: 671–9.

Easton DF, Ford D and Bishop DT (1995). Breast and ovarian cancer incidence in BRCA1-mutation carriers. *Am J Hum Genet* **56**: 265–71.

Eisinger F, Alby N, Bremond A, et al. (1998). Recommendations for medical management of hereditary breast and ovarian cancer: the French national ad hoc committee. *Ann Oncol* **9**: 939–50.

Foulkes WD, Chappuis PO, Wong N, et al. (2000). Primary node negative breast cancer in BRCA1 mutation carriers has a poor outcome. *Ann Oncol* **11**: 307–13.

Hartmann LC, Schaid DJ, Woods JE, et al. (1999). Efficacy of bilateral prophylactic mastectomy in women with a family history of breast cancer. *N Engl J Med* **340**: 77–84.

Iselius L, Litter M and Morton N (1992). Transmission of breast cancer – a controversy resolved. *Clin Genet* **41**: 211–17.

Johansson O, Ranstam J, Borg Å and Olsson H (1998). Survival of BRCA1 breast and ovarian cancer patients: a population-based study from Southern Sweden. *J Clin Oncol* **16**: 397–404.

Johansson O, Loman N, Möller T, et al. (1999). Incidence of malignant tumours in relatives of BRCA1 and BRCA2 germline mutation carriers. *Eur J Cancer* **35**: 1248–57.

Julian-Reunier C, Eisinger F, Evans G, et al. (2000). Variation in prophylactic surgery decisions. *Lancet* **356**: 1687.

Kollias J, Sibbering DM, Blamey RW, et al. (1998). Screening women aged less than 50 years with a family history of breast cancer. *Eur J Cancer* **34**: 878–83.

Kuhl CK, Schmutzler RK, Leutner CC, et al. (2000). Breast MR imaging screening in 192 women proved or suspected to be carriers of a breast cancer susceptibility gene: preliminary results. *Radiology* **215**(1): 267–79.

Kuhurana KK, Loosmann A, Numann PJ and Khan SA (2000). Prophylactic mastectomy: pathologic findings in high-risk patients. *Arch Pathol Lab Med* **124**: 378–81.

Lakhani SR, Gusterson BA, Jacquemier J, et al. (2000). The pathology of familial breast cancer: histological features of cancers in families not attributable to mutations in BRCA1 or BRCA2. *Clin Cancer Res* **6**: 782–9.

Lalloo F, Boggis CRM, Evans DGR, et al. (1998). Screening by mammography, women with a family history of breast cancer. *Eur J Cancer* **34**: 937–40.

Lynch ED, Ostermeyer EA, Lee MK, et al. (1997). Inherited mutations in PTEN that are associated with breast cancer, Cowden disease, and juvenile polyposis. *Am J Hum Genet* **61**: 1254–60.

Macmillan RD (2000). Screening women with a family history of breast cancer – results from the British familial breast cancer group. *Eur J Surg Oncol* **26**: 149–52.

McGuigan KA, Ganz P and Breant C (1996). Agreement between breast cancer risk estimation methods. *J Natl Cancer Inst* **88**: 1315–17.

Møller P, Maehle L, Heimdal K, et al. (1998). Prospective findings in breast cancer kindreds: annual incidence rates according to age, stage at diagnosis, mean sojourn time, and incidence rates for contralateral cancer. *Breast* **7**: 55–9.

Møller P, Reis MM, Evans G, et al. (1999a). Efficacy of early diagnosis and treatment in women with a family history of breast cancer. *Dis Markers* **15**: 179–86.

Møller P, Evans G, Anderson E, et al. (1999b). Use of cytology to diagnose inherited breast cancer. *Dis Markers* **15**: 206.

Møller P, Evans G, Haites N, et al. (1999c). Guidelines for follow-up of women at high risk for inherited breast cancer: consensus statement from the Biomed2 Demonstration Programme on Inherited Breast Cancer. *Dis Markers* **15**: 207–11.

Moslehi R, Chu W, Karlan B, et al. (2000). BRCA1 and BRCA2 mutation analysis of 208 Askenazi Jewish women with ovarian cancer. *Am J Hum Genet* **66**: 1259–72.

Narod SA, Risch H, Moslehi R, et al. (1998). Oral contraceptives and the risk of hereditary ovarian cancer. *N Engl J Med* **339**: 511–18.

Nixon RM, Pharoah P, Tabar L, et al. (2000). Mammographic screening in women with a family history of breast cancer: some results from the Swedish two-county trial. *Rev Epidemiol Sante Publique* **48**: 325–31.

Rebbeck TR, Levin AM, Eisen A, et al. (1999). Breast cancer risk after bilateral prophylactic oophorectomy in BRCA1 mutation carriers. *J Natl Cancer Inst* **91**: 1475–9.

Sobol H, Eisinger F, Stoppa-Lyonnet D, et al. (1995). *Hereditary Cancer, 2nd International Research Conference On Familial Cancer*, ed. H Müller, RJ Scott and W Weber, pp. 11–18. Basel: Karger.

Stoppa-Lyonnet D, Ansquer Y, Dreyfus H, et al. (2000). Familial invasive breast cancers: worse outcome related to BRCA1 mutations. *J Clin Oncol* **18**: 4053–9.

Tabàr L, Fagerberg G, Duffy SW, et al. (1992). Update of the Swedish two-county program of mammographic screening for breast cancer. *Radiol Clin North Am* **30**: 187–210.

Tillanus-Linthorst MMA, Bartels CCM, Obdeijn AIM and Oudkerk M (2000). Earlier detection of breast cancer by surveillance of women at familial risk. *Eur J Cancer* **36**: 514–19.

Vasen HF, Haites NE, Evans DG, et al. (1998). Current policies for surveillance and management in women at risk of breast and ovarian cancer: a survey among 16 European family cancer clinics. European Familial Breast Cancer Collaborative Group. *Eur J Cancer* **34**: 1922–6.

Verhoog LC, Brekelmans CT, Seynaeve C, et al. (1998). Survival and tumour characteristics of breast-cancer patients with germline mutations of BRCA1. *Lancet* **351**: 316–21.

14

Screening for familial ovarian cancer

Barnaby Rufford, Usha Menon and Ian Jacobs

St Bartholomew's and The Royal London School of Medicine and Dentistry, London, UK

Despite advances in surgery and chemotherapy, the overall prognosis for ovarian cancer remains poor. It has improved little over the last 30 years. The best way of improving outcome may be to detect the condition at an early stage through screening the population at risk. The high incidence of disease in those with a strong family history of ovarian cancer makes them particularly amenable to this strategy.

Why should we screen?

There are estimated to be approximately 50 000 women in the UK who have a significant family history of ovarian cancer with two or more affected close relatives. These women have an approximately ten-fold increased risk compared with the general population. This translates to an average lifetime risk of developing ovarian cancer of 15%.

The prognosis for ovarian cancer is generally poor, with an overall 5-year survival of about 30%. Seventy per cent of women are diagnosed with stage III or IV disease, with 5-year survivals of 15–20% and less than 5% respectively (Teneriello and Park, 1995). The lack of symptoms of early ovarian cancer results in women frequently presenting with advanced disease. This is due to the location of the ovaries within the peritoneal cavity, which results in minimal local irritation or interference with vital structures until ovarian enlargement is considerable, or metastasis occurs. Initial symptoms may be so vague that multiple consultations with a GP may occur before a gynaecological referral is initiated. Approaches that result in early diagnosis may impact on the significant mortality associated with the disease.

A screening programme should ideally be based on detection of a pre-malignant condition in order to lower disease incidence and maximise mortality reduction, as is the case with the cervical cancer screening programme. Although it has been suggested that inclusion cysts and benign and borderline ovarian tumours may be pre-malignant, this remains speculative. In the absence of confirmed pre-malignant change, screening for ovarian cancer is directed at present to the detection of pre-clinical disease. Disease detected at an earlier stage carries a significantly improved prognosis. In patients diagnosed with stage I disease, survival is above 80%, and above 90% in those with stage Ia disease (Nguyen et al., 1993). Successful detection of early-stage disease could therefore have a significant effect on mortality. Although no screening strategy has as yet been shown to reduce mortality, a randomized control trial in the general postmenopausal population has reported a significantly increased median survival (72.9 months) in women with ovarian cancer in the screened group, compared with the control group (median survival 41.8 months) (Jacobs et al., 1999).

Are there any reasons not to screen?

The most important reason is that screening has not yet been shown to reduce mortality in any population. Large studies are under way in the general population to address this. Screening relies on the presumption that stage I tumours would progress further if they were not identified and treated. Although unlikely, it is possible that they are a different disease entity, and if not discovered may remain at this stage, death eventually occurring from another cause, as occurs with many early prostatic cancers. Little is also known about the rate of disease progression, with obvious implications for screening frequency. In addition, primary peritoneal cancer is likely to be a variant of ovarian cancer, with a higher incidence in the high-risk population, and ultrasound and CA125 are not reliable in detecting this disease (Karlan et al., 1999).

Another key factor to consider is surgical morbidity in women with false-positive screening results. Definitive diagnosis can only be made at laparotomy or laparoscopy. In studies that gave details of diagnostic procedures, most women underwent laparotomy (Bell et al., 1998). There are few reports on morbidity arising as a result of screening. Muto et al. (1993) reported a woman suffering a bowel perforation. Extrapolating from reports for similar surgery in clinical series, between 0.5% and 1% of women undergoing oophorectomy – either by laparoscopy or laparotomy – may suffer a significant complication such as haemorrhage, infection, or bowel or bladder damage. Psychological sequelae resulting from the anxiety of being screened and potential false-negative results should also be considered (Wardle et al., 1993). Finally, there are also cost implications. It is possible that the higher incidence of ovarian cancer in the high-risk population may result in a lower cost per cancer detected than in the general population.

What do we need from a screening test?

A suitable screening test requires both high sensitivity and specificity. Women who have a positive screen require further investigation, often in the form of exploratory surgery. It is therefore imperative to maximize specificity in order to obtain a high positive predictive value, and to decrease the number of false-positive screens. In the general population, a specificity of 99.6% is required to achieve a positive predictive value of 10% (Jacobs and Oram, 1988). However, because of the much higher incidence of the disease in the familial group, a lower specificity may achieve the same positive predictive value. It is important to note, however, that, unlike in the general population, 60–75% of women undergoing screening for familial ovarian cancer are premenopausal. This results in an increased false-positive rate with both ultrasound and CA125 screening.

What screening tests are in use?

The ovaries are not easily accessible. Although vaginal examination is important in assessing symptomatic women, it lacks both the sensitivity and specificity required for a first-line screening test in asymptomatic women. Van Nagell et al. (1995) found that only 30% of women who had ovarian masses on transvaginal ultrasound had an abnormal pelvic examination.

Visualization or direct sampling to detect malignant disease, or perhaps in the future a pre-malignant condition, is being investigated in preliminary studies using office laparoscopy and cytological examination of brush samples from the ovarian surface in screening high-risk populations. The possibility of using optical methods, such as optical spectroscopy, is also being investigated. The accepted methods of screening include serum tumour markers and ultrasound.

Of the ovarian tumour markers, the most extensively studied is CA125. It is an antigenic determinant on a high-molecular-weight glycoprotein that is recognized by the mouse monoclonal antibody, OC125, developed using an ovarian cancer cell-line as an immunogen. CA125 was first discovered in 1981 (Bast et al.). Levels are raised in 50% of stage I ovarian tumours and in 90% of stage II ovarian tumours (Zurawski et al., 1988). CA125 levels may also be raised in a range of other physiological and pathological conditions, which may be gynaecological or non-gynaecological, benign or malignant (Table 14.1). This can cause particular problems in screening the high-risk population. Many of these women are premenopausal and the CA125 level may fluctuate with the menstrual cycle or may be elevated by such conditions as endometriosis. Specificity using CA125 as a screening tool can be improved using serial determinations over time (Einhorn et al., 1992). An algorithm has been developed in postmenopausal women from the

Table 14.1. Examples of conditions found in association with an increased CA125 level

Gynaecological conditions
Endometriosis
Fibroids
Haemorrhagic ovarian cysts
Menstruation
Acute pelvic inflammatory disease
Pregnancy (first trimester)

Gastrointestinal/hepatic conditions
Acute pancreatitis
Colitis
Chronic active hepatitis
Cirrhosis
Diverticulitis

Miscellaneous conditions
Pericarditis
Polyarteritis nodosa
Renal disease
Sjögren's syndrome
Systemic lupus erythematosus

Malignant conditions
Bladder
Breast
Endometrium
Lung
Liver
Non-Hodgkin's lymphoma
Ovary
Pancreas

general population that determines the risk of ovarian cancer based on CA125 profile with time (Skates et al., 1995). This is based on the observation that women with ovarian cancer have increasing levels of CA125, whereas women without ovarian cancer have static or decreasing levels, even if they remain above a cut-off point of 30 U/ml. The greater the rate of rise in CA125 levels, the greater the risk of ovarian cancer. The latest in a line of tumour markers that have been assessed is plasma lysophosphatidic acid, a bioactive phospholipid with mitogenic and growth-factor-like activities that may have a potential role in ovarian cancer screening (Xu et al., 1998). It is currently undergoing extensive testing in the USA.

Ultrasound has been studied as a screening test for ovarian cancer for more than a decade. Initially, transabdominal scanning lacked specificity, and in one of the early studies involving 5540 women, 50 underwent surgical investigation for each case of ovarian malignancy detected (Campbell et al., 1989). Specificity has improved with the introduction of transvaginal scanning, and the use of morphological scoring systems for interpreting scans has reduced the number of women undergoing surgical investigation to 10 for each case of malignancy detected (Van Nagell et al., 2000). Some authors have used colour-flow Doppler imaging to assess vasculature and blood flow characteristics in ovarian masses. Malignant masses have increased blood flow during diastole, helping to distinguish them from benign ones (Carter et al., 1995; Predanic et al., 1996). Bourne et al. (1993) reported the results of screening 1601 women with a positive family history of ovarian cancer who underwent transvaginal ultrasound examination with colour-flow Doppler imaging. As a result of positive scan findings, 61 women (3.8%) were referred for surgery, and six primary ovarian cancers were detected, five of which were stage I tumours. However, as a result of the subjective nature of Doppler imaging, it has failed to make the anticipated impact on reducing false-positive results in other screening trials. In the largely premenopausal group of women who undergo familial ovarian cancer screening, the increased incidence of benign and physiological ovarian lesions creates similar problems with false-positive rates as seen with CA125 testing.

What are the current screening strategies?

There are three main strategies: (1) an ultrasound approach based on primary screening with transvaginal ultrasound, with repeat testing after a fixed time interval if an abnormality is detected; (2) multimodal screening, which incorporates primary screening using a serum marker, usually CA125, with repeat assessment of the marker and transvaginal scanning (TVS) as a second-line test (CA125 results are interpreted using the risk of cancer algorithm previously alluded to); (3) a combined approach that uses both serum CA125 and TVS as first-line tests to maximize the detection rate. Its use is limited to screening the high-risk population. The optimal screening strategy is yet to be established.

What data are available regarding screening in high-risk women?

To date, eight prospective studies have reported on screening for familial ovarian cancer (Appendix 1 and 2). A total of 5100 women have been screened and 28 epithelial ovarian and primary peritoneal cancers detected using mainly a combined screening strategy. Criteria for interpreting the results were varied and screening protocols were not always clearly reported. Lack of follow-up data on screen negatives makes calculation of sensitivity difficult. Information on the ideal screening frequency is also scarce, with only two of the studies reporting on interval cancers, which presented 2–16 months (median 7) following the last screen (Bourne et al., 1994; Karlan et al., 1999). The limited data suggest that more frequent screening of the high-risk population should be investigated.

What is current practice?

Despite the lack of conclusive evidence that screening can reduce mortality, there has been widespread introduction of screening for familial ovarian cancer in women aged over 35 years (Vasen et al., 1998). This has led a number of groups (UK Committee for Co-ordinating Cancer Research, the French National Ad Hoc Committee, 1999, and the NIH Consensus Conference, 1995) to recommend the use of defined screening strategies for familial ovarian cancer within the context of clinical trials.

What are the current trials?

Although no conclusive evidence is available to prove that screening has an impact on ovarian cancer mortality, the adoption of annual screening as standard practice in the high-risk population makes it impossible to institute a randomized control trial with a control group who are not screened. In addition, unlike the situation in the general population, the performance characteristics of the screening strategies in use are unclear.

In order to develop an optimal screening strategy in the high-risk population, a multicentre Familial Ovarian Cancer Screening Study (UK-FOCSS) involving 5000 high-risk women is being set up in the UK. This is a prospective study using a standard screening protocol based on annual CA125 measurement and trans-vaginal ultrasound. The trial design includes two further blood samples a year, collected at 4-monthly intervals, for retrospective analysis of CA125 and other tumour markers. The intention is to document outcome at the end of 5 years following 17 000 woman years of screening. The study size should include suffi-cient cases of ovarian cancer to achieve a reliable estimate of sensitivity and positive predictive value of the screening strategy. Systematic data collection will allow the derivation of a familial risk of ovarian cancer (FROC) index, similar to the ROC index in use in the general population. In addition to longitudinal CA125 measurements and age, this will be based on pedigree analysis and molecular genetic information. To be eligible, an individual must be a first-degree relative of a high-risk family (Table 14.2). Exclusion criteria for the study include a past history of bilateral oophorectomy, age under 35 years and participation in other

Table 14.2. Criteria for defining high-risk families in the UK Familial Ovarian Cancer Screening Study

---

(1) Two or more first-degree[a] relatives with ovarian cancer.
(2) One first-degree relative with ovarian cancer and one first-degree relative with breast cancer diagnosed under 50 years of age.
(3) One first-degree relative with ovarian cancer and two first-degree relatives with breast cancer diagnosed under 60 years of age.
(4) An affected individual with one of the known ovarian cancer predisposing genes.
(5) Three first-degree relatives with colorectal cancer with at least one diagnosed before the age of 50 years and at least one first-degree relative with ovarian cancer.
(6) Criteria (1), (2) and (3) modified where paternal transmission is occurring; families where affected relatives are related by second degree through an unaffected intervening male relative who has an affected sister.

Family history of cancer should be confirmed by histopathology report or death certification or a documented mutation of an ovarian cancer predisposing gene.
[a]A first-degree relative is mother, sister or daughter.

ovarian cancer screening trials. Data addressing quality of life issues, morbidity and cost will be collected.

A similar trial is under way in the USA under the auspices of the Cancer Genetics Network of the National Cancer Institute. In this trial, high-risk women will be screened every 3 months using CA125 measurements. This will be in addition to any screening that they are already undergoing. The inclusion and exclusion criteria are similar to those for the UK trial. In this trial, CA125 results will be interpreted using a risk of ovarian cancer calculation similar to that in use in the older general population, and interventions will be undertaken based on these results.

Conclusions

Ovarian cancer most commonly presents as advanced-stage disease with a poor prognosis. In the absence of a known pre-malignant lesion, the ability to detect early-stage disease is clearly desirable. However, as yet, no conclusive evidence is available to prove that screening has an impact on ovarian cancer mortality. The adoption of annual screening as standard practice in the high-risk population makes it impossible to institute a randomized control trial with a control group who are not screened. This has led a number of professional groups to recommend the use of defined screening strategies for familial ovarian cancer within the context of trials. This would enable evaluation of the performance characteristics of the current screening strategies that are based on annual transvaginal ultrasound and serum CA125 assessments. Multicentre trials currently under way in the UK and USA should lead to the development of an optimal screening strategy for the high-risk population and provide data on screening frequency, morbidity, quality of life issues and cost.

Appendix 14.1. Prospective ovarian cancer screening studies in women with a family history of ovarian or other cancer or a personal history of breast cancer

Study	Population	Screening protocol	Criteria for primary test	Criteria for secondary test / Referral for diagnosis
Bourne et al., 1993	Aged > 17 yrs (mean 47) F/H of ov cancer	TVS then colour Doppler imaging First 1000 Second 601	Areas of hyper- or hypoechogenicity Areas of hyper- or hypoechogenicity	Persistent morphological change Unless vol. ↓ to <63% of initial vol. Pulsatility index <1 or morphological score ≥5
Weiner et al., 1993	P/H of br cancer	TVS and CDI	Vol. >20 ml, cyst, mass present Low-impedance intra-ovarian blood vessels	Persistent enlargement, complex mass or low-impedance blood flow
Karlan et al., 1993, 1999 USA	Aged >35 yrs F/H of ov, br, endo or colon cancer P/H br cancer	TVS, CDI and CA125 6-monthly until 1995, then annually	Adnexal mass ≥5 cm Abnormal morphology Resistance index <0.4 CA125 >35 U/ml	Persistent abnormality on scan
Muto et al., 1993 USA	Aged >25 yrs F/H of ov cancer	TVS and CA125	CA125 ≥35 U/ml Postmenopausal: any ovarian mass Premenopausal: complex ovarian mass or simple cyst >2 cm	CA125 doubled or >95 U/ml in 3 months Persistent abnormality on scan in 2–3 months

Study	Inclusion criteria	Screening	Abnormal result	Repeat/further
Schwartz et al., 1995 USA	Aged >30 yrs F/H of ov cancer	TVS, CDI and CA125	Resistance index <0.5 CA125 >35 U/ml Other abnormality	Not stated
Dorum et al., 1996, 1999 Norway	Aged >25 yrs (mean 43) Strict criteria for F/H of br/ov cancer	TVS and CA125	CA125 >35 U/ml Uni- or bilocular cyst Ovarian tumour: direct referral for diagnosis	Repeat CA125 >35 U/ml Persistent cyst
Menkiszak et al., 1998 Poland	Aged >20 yrs F/H of br/ov cancer	TVS and CA125 (6-monthly)	Not available	Not available
Belinson et al., 1995 USA	Aged >23 yrs (mean 43) F/H of ov cancer	TVS, CDI and CA125	CA125 ≥35 U/ml Abnormal morphology Abnormal resistance index Postmenopausal: vol. >8 ml Premenopausal: vol. >18 ml	Not stated

br, breast; endo, endometrial; F/H, family history; ov, ovarian; P/H, personal history. All volumes refer to ovarian volume.

Appendix 14.2. Prospective ovarian cancer screening studies in women with a family history of ovarian or other cancer or a personal history of breast cancer

Study	No. screened (premenopausal %)	No. of positive primary screens (%)	No. referred for diagnostic tests[a] (%)	No. of invasive EOC detected (borderline tumours)	Probability of ov cancers at diagnostic intervention PPV (%)	Cancers in screen-negative women	Outcome of diagnostic procedures
Bourne et al., 1993	1000 (60)	909 (56.8)	52 (5.2)	2 (1) 2 stage I	3.8	2 PPC (2, 8 mths)	Benign 48
	601		9 (1.5)	1 (2)	11.1	3 EOC (24–44 mths)	No abnormality 7
Weiner et al., 1993	600	Not clear ?146	12 (3)	3 1 stage I	25	Not stated	Benign 8 Malignant 1
Karlan et al., 1993, 1999	597[b] (75)	115 (19.2)	10 (1.7)	0 (1)	—	Not stated	Benign 8
	1261	Not stated	Not stated	1 EOC, 3 PPC (2) 1 stage I	Not stated	4 PPC (5,6,15,16 mths)	Malignant 1 —
Muto et al., 1993	384 (85.4)	89 (23.2) scans 42 (10.9) CA125	15 (3.9)	0	—	Not stated	Benign 13 No abnormality 1 Malignant 1
Schwartz et al., 1995	247	Not clear	1 (0.4)	0	—	Not stated	Benign 1
Dorum et al., 2000	180[b]	Not clear	16 (8.9)	4 (3)	25	Not stated[c]	Benign 9
	803	Not clear	Not stated	16 (4)	Not clear	Not stated	Not stated

Menkiszak et al., 1998	124	Not available	Not available	1 (3)	Not available	Not available	Benign 5
Belinson et al., 1995	137	Not clear	2 (1.5)	1	50	Not stated	Not stated
Total	5157	—	—	28	—	—	—

EOC, epithelial ovarian cancer; PPC, primary peritoneal cancer; PPV, positive predictive value.

[a]Following positive secondary screens.

[b]Not included in total as there are more recent updates on the trial.

[c]A further 13 women underwent oophorectomy for breast cancer; two had ovarian cancer not detected by TVS.

REFERENCES

Bast R, Klug TL, St John E, et al. (1981). Reactivity of a monoclonal antibody with human ovarian carcinoma. *J Clin Invest* **68**: 1331–7.

Belinson JL, Okin C, Casey G, et al. (1995). The familial ovarian cancer registry: progress report. *Cleve Clin J Med* **62**(2): 129–34.

Bell R, Luengo S, Petticrew M and Sheldon T (1998). Screening for ovarian cancer: a systematic review. *Health Technol Assess* **2**(2): 1–84.

Bourne TH, Campbell S, Reynolds KM, et al. (1993). Screening for early familial ovarian cancer with transvaginal ultrasonography and colour blood flow imaging. *Br Med J* **306**: 1025–9.

Bourne TH, Campbell S, Reynolds K, et al. (1994). The potential role of serum CA 125 in an ultrasound based screening programme for familial ovarian cancer. *Gynecol Oncol* **52**(3): 379.

Campbell S, Bhan V, Royston P, et al. (1989). Transabdominal ultrasound screening for ovarian cancer. *Br Med J* **299**: 1363–7.

Carter JR, Lau M, Fowler JM, Carlson JW, Carson LF and Triggs LB (1995). Blood flow characteristics of ovarian tumours: implications for ovarian cancer screening. *Am J Obstet Gynecol* **72**: 901–7.

Dorum A, Kristensen GB, Abeler VM, Trope CG and Møller P (1996). Early detection of familial ovarian cancer. *Eur J Cancer* **32A**(10): 1645–51.

Dorum A, Heimdal K, Lovslett K, et al. (1999). Prospectively detected cancer in familial breast/ovarian cancer screening. *Acta Obstet Gynecol Scand* **78**(10): 906–11.

Einhorn N, Sjovall K, Knapp RC, et al. (1992). Prospective evaluation of serum CA 125 levels for early detection of ovarian cancer. *Obstet Gynecol* **80**: 14–18.

Jacobs I and Oram D (1988). Screening for ovarian cancer. *Biomed Pharmacother* **42**: 589–96.

Jacobs IJ, Skates SJ, MacDonald N, et al. (1999). Screening for ovarian cancer: a pilot randomised controlled trial. *Lancet* **353**: 1207–10.

Karlan BY, Raffel LJ, Crvenkovic G, et al. (1993). A multidisciplinary approach to the early detection of ovarian carcinoma: rationale, protocol design, and early results. *Am J Obstet Gynecol* **169**(3): 494–501.

Karlan BY, Baldwin RL, Lopez-Luevanos E, et al. (1999). Peritoneal serous papillary carcinoma, a phenotypic variant of familial ovarian cancer: implications for ovarian cancer screening. *Am J Obstet Gynecol* **180**(4): 917–28.

Menkiszak J, Jakubowska A, Gronwald J, Rzepka-Gorska I and Lubinski J (1998). Hereditary ovarian cancer: summary of 5 years of experience. *Ginekol Pol* **69**(5): 283–7.

Muto MG, Cramer DW, Brown DL, et al. (1993). Screening for ovarian cancer: the preliminary experience of a familial ovarian cancer center. *Gynecol Oncol* **51**: 12–20.

Nguyen NH, Averette HE, Hoskins W, et al. (1993). National survey of ovarian carcinoma. VI. Critical assessment of current International Federation of Obstetrics and Gynaecology staging system. *Cancer* **72**: 3007–11.

Predanic M, Vlahos N, Pennisi JA, Moukhtar M and Aleem FA (1996). Color and pulsed Doppler sonography, gray-scale imaging and serum CA 125 in the assessment of adnexal disease. *Obstet Gynecol* **88**: 283–8.

Schwartz PE, Chambers JT and Taylor KJ (1995). Early detection and screening for ovarian cancer. *J Cell Biochem Suppl* **23**: 233–7.

Skates SJ, Xu FJ, Yu YH, et al. (1995). Toward an optimal algorithm for ovarian cancer screening with longitudinal tumor markers. *Cancer* **76**(10 Suppl.): 2004–10.

Teneriello M and Park RC (1995). Early detection of ovarian cancer. *CA Cancer J Clin* **45**: 71–87.

Van Nagell JR, Gallion HD, Pavlik EJ, et al. (1995). Ovarian cancer screening. *Cancer* **6**: 2086–91.

Van Nagell JR Jr, DePriest PD, Reedy MB, et al. (2000). The efficacy of transvaginal sonographic screening in asymptomatic women at risk for ovarian cancer. *Gynecol Oncol* **77**(3): 350–6.

Vasen HF, Haites NE, Evans DG, et al. (1998). Current policies for surveillance and management in women at risk of breast and ovarian cancer: a survey among 16 European family cancer clinics. European Familial Breast Collaborative Group. *Eur J Cancer* **34**(12): 1922–6.

Wardle JF, Collins W, Pernet AL, Whitehead MI, Bourne TH and Campbell LS (1993). Psychological impact of screening for familial ovarian cancer. *J Natl Cancer Inst* **85**: 653–7.

Weiner Z, Beck D, Shteiner M, et al. (1993). Screening for ovarian cancer in women with breast cancer with transvaginal sonography and color flow imaging. *J Ultrasound Med* **12**(7): 387–93.

Xu Y, Shen Z, Wiper DW, et al. (1998). Lysophosphatidic acid as a potential biomarker for ovarian and other gynecologic cancers. *J Am Med Assoc* **280**: 719–23.

Zurawski V, Orjaseter H, Andersen A, et al. (1988). Elevated serum CA 125 levels prior to diagnosis of ovarian neoplasia: relevance for early detection of ovarian cancer. *Int J Cancer* **42**: 677–80.

Part 3

Management

15

Management of *BRCA1/2* mutation carriers

Pierre O. Chappuis[1] and William D. Foulkes[1,2,3]

[1]McGill University Health Centre, Montreal, QC, Canada
[2]Sir M.B. Davis-Jewish General Hospital, McGill University, Montreal, QC, Canada
[3]McGill University, Montreal, QC, Canada

Introduction

The application of predictive genetics in oncology offers the opportunity, through a simple blood draw, to identify asymptomatic individuals carrying a predisposition to develop certain cancers. Specific recommendations regarding prevention and surveillance can be proposed to these individuals. Concomitantly, family members who are identified as non-carriers of the predisposing gene can be reassured. These persons are no longer considered 'at high risk' and return to the cancer risks of the general population. They can be withdrawn from often demanding screening protocols and can be reassured regarding the absence of risk of transmission of the predisposition to their children.

Here, we provide an overview of the options and issues in the management of women identified as being at high risk of developing breast or ovarian cancer, based on their personal and familial history, or through the identification of a germline *BRCA1* or *BRCA2* mutation.

Breast and ovarian cancers combined account for about one-third of all incident cancers in Canadian women, and for about one-fourth of all cancer deaths (Table 15.1). Primary care for survivors of sporadic breast cancer has been recently reviewed (Burstein and Winer, 2000), but women carrying genetic predisposition to breast/ovarian cancer have unique health issues. Approximately 3% of all breast cancer and 5–10% of all ovarian cancer is caused by germline mutations in breast/ovarian cancer susceptibility genes. The most important of these genes are *BRCA1* and *BRCA2*, which were identified in 1994 and 1995 respectively (Rahman and Stratton, 1998; Welcsh et al., 1998). Many hundreds of different mutations have been found in these two genes. Penetrance (the proportion of individuals who show the mutation-associated phenotype) of germline *BRCA1* or *BRCA2* mutations is variable and cannot be precisely estimated (Blackwood and Weber, 1998; Gauthier-Villars et al., 1999). Women with a family history of breast or ovarian cancer who carry an alteration in *BRCA1* have up to an 85% lifetime risk

Table 15.1. Epidemiological data for breast and ovarian cancer in Canada (2001)[a]

	Breast cancer	Ovarian cancer
Number of new cases per year	19 500	2500
Number of deaths per year	5500	1500
Cumulative risk of developing cancer	10.6%	1.5%
Cumulative risk of dying of cancer	3.9%	1.1%
Estimates of the *BRCA1*- and *BRCA2*-related cases	600 per year (~3%)	200 per year (~7.5%)

[a]Source: http://www.cancer.ca

of developing breast cancer and about a 40–50% lifetime risk of developing ovarian cancer. Men who carry an altered *BRCA1* gene may have up to a three-fold increased risk of developing prostate cancer, but this remains controversial. Mutations in *BRCA2* predispose men to breast cancer and women to breast and ovarian cancer and probably to other types of cancers (prostate, pancreatic, stomach, head and neck, melanoma) (Breast Cancer Linkage Consortium, 1999; Risch et al., 2001). Recent studies suggest that up to age 70 years, women carriers of *BRCA2* mutations have a risk of developing breast cancer that is similar to carriers of *BRCA1* mutations. However, depending on the mutation site in *BRCA2*, the risk for ovarian cancer may be lower than for *BRCA1* mutation carriers (Thompson and Easton, 2001). Men who carry an altered *BRCA2* gene have a risk of about 6% for developing breast cancer by age 70 years. Many questions are still open regarding the exact evaluation of the risks in the presence of a given *BRCA1* or *BRCA2* mutation, particularly if we take into account the fact that the penetrance and expressivity is variable within a family. Not all women harbouring a *BRCA1* or *BRCA2* mutation will develop a cancer or, if they do, it is frequently at different ages or sites. This individual variability of the cancer risks is being studied with the aim of clarifying the role of environmental and genetic factors such as the influence of the location and type of mutations within the *BRCA1/2* genes or the implication of modulator genes (Narod et al., 1995; Narod, 1998; Dunning et al., 1999; Nathanson et al., 2001).

Prevention (Table 15.2)

Reducing the risk of first primary breast cancer
Lifestyle modification

Based on the abundant literature (and contradictory conclusions) on a plethora of environmental factors that have been evaluated as potential risk factors for breast

Table 15.2. Preventive strategies for breast and ovarian cancer in *BRCA1/2* mutation carriers

	Preventive strategies for breast cancer	Preventive strategies for ovarian cancer
Premenopausal women	Tamoxifen Prophylactic mastectomy Prophylactic oophorectomy (±HRT up to age 50 yrs) + general guidelines for overall health	Oral contraceptive Tubal ligation Prophylactic oophorectomy (±HRT up to age 50 yrs)
Postmenopausal women	Tamoxifen ± HRT Tamoxifen vs raloxifene (NSABP-P2 trial) Prophylactic mastectomy + general guidelines for overall health	Prophylactic oophorectomy

Note: None of these recommendations have been proved to be effective in prospective studies (see text for detail).

HRT, hormone replacement therapy.

cancer, it is very difficult to advocate particular lifestyle modifications in at-risk patients. We should discuss how useful it is for overall health, and a fortiori for cancer prevention, to follow some general guidelines such as a low-fat, fibre-rich diet, smoking abstinence and to regular exercise. Despite repeated requests of many mutation carriers, it is difficult to go far beyond these general recommendations if we wish to base our decisions on currently available scientific data (Chlebowski, 2000; Vogel, 2000). Indeed, very few of the well-accepted, although relatively modest, risk factors for breast cancer (i.e. age at menarche and menopause, family history of breast/ovarian cancer) are accessible to lifestyle modification. Interestingly, some risk factors for breast cancer may have a different significance among *BRCA1/2* mutation carriers. Thus, pregnancy, which is associated with a reduction in the incidence of subsequent breast cancer in the general population, appears to increase the risk of early-onset breast cancer in *BRCA1/2* mutation carriers (Jernström et al., 1999). Moreover, in a provocative retrospective study, Brunet et al. (1998) showed that cigarette smoking was associated with a decrease in breast cancer risk among women with *BRCA1/2* mutations. This result should be confirmed in other studies, as although the incidence of other hormonally sensitive cancers, such as endometrial cancer (Lesko et al., 1985) and thyroid cancer (Rossing et al., 2000), are also inversely related to cigarette consumption, the effect observed in the study of Brunet et al. was based on rather low levels of consumption and small differences between cases and controls (mean number of pack-years of cigarette smoking in cases, 4.5; controls, 6.1; $P = 0.04$).

The issue of hormone replacement therapy (HRT) in *BRCA1/2* mutation carriers is particularly difficult. HRT in the general population has been reported to be associated with a moderate, but significant, increase in breast cancer risk, particularly with a long period of use. A prospective cohort study of 37 105 women found a relative risk (RR) for breast cancer of 1.81 and 2.65 for women who had used HRT for 5 or less years, or more than 5 years, respectively (Colditz et al., 1990). But not all large, prospective, cohort studies are concordant with an increased risk of breast cancer associated with HRT use (Schuurman et al., 1995; Willis et al., 1996). The most recent collaborative re-analysis of data from 51 epidemiological studies of 52 705 women with breast cancer and 108 411 women without breast cancer found that the probability of having breast cancer diagnosed is increased by 2.3% (95% confidence interval (CI), 1.1–3.6%) per year of HRT use, or a 31% increase in breast cancer incidence for long-term HRT users (Collaborative Group on Hormonal Factors in Breast Cancer, 1997). Of note, in the Royal Marsden study that showed no significant preventive effect with tamoxifen (Powles et al., 1998), the use of HRT at randomization was a risk factor for breast cancer development (RR = 1.9; $P < 0.04$) compared with women not receiving HRT.

HRT users develop breast cancer at a younger age than non-users, supporting the hypothesis that oestrogens accelerate the growth of pre-existing tumours (Bilimoria et al., 1999; Cobleigh et al., 1999). Moreover, the issue of an increased breast density associated with HRT is particularly worrisome in a high-risk subgroup (Laya et al., 1996; Ursin et al., 1998; Chlebowski and McTiernan, 1999; Kavanagh et al., 2000). The impact of combined oestrogen and progestin on the risk of breast cancer has been controversial (Verheul et al., 2000), but the evidence that the addition of progestins to oestrogens increases the risk of breast cancer is strong (Schairer et al., 2000; Willett et al., 2000), possibly because the combination increases the breast density and thus reduces the sensitivity and specificity of the mammographic screening. The impact of the combined hormonotherapy on breast cancer risk among *BRCA1/2* mutation carriers is unknown.

Despite the absence of early evidence that HRT has significant effect on breast cancer recurrence in women previously treated for breast cancer (Col et al., 2001), it is probably recommendable to avoid a 'routine' prescription of HRT among women with *BRCA1/2* mutations. Decision analysis suggests that the absolute benefit of HRT falls as the risk of breast cancer increases (Armstrong et al., 2000). Indications for HRT, such as the treatment of debilitating symptoms due to oestrogen deprivation (e.g. hot flushes, mood disturbances, sexual dysfunction) or the prevention of chronic diseases, based on a personal or family history of osteoporosis or coronary heart disease, should be carefully distinguished and investigated, as should the alternative treatments for each situation (Chlebowski and McTiernan, 1999; Willett et al., 2000). For example, tamoxifen or raloxifene prescription is a good option for preventing osteoporosis without increasing (and possibly even decreasing) the risk of breast cancer development. HRT may also be prescribed for a restricted period of time, for example after prophylactic oophorectomy performed during the premenopause until age 50 years (Eisen et al., 2000b; Rebbeck, 2000), but there are no convincing data to support this recommendation. The combination of HRT with tamoxifen has been proposed as an alternative for hormone deficiency symptom relief, but no data are yet available in terms of effect on breast cancer risk, particularly in high-risk women. Interestingly, in the Italian prevention trial with tamoxifen (Veronesi et al., 1998), there was one case of breast cancer in the tamoxifen + HRT group compared with eight in the placebo + HRT group ($P = 0.02$), suggesting a particular efficacy of tamoxifen in the context of exogenous oestrogen use. Such a difference was not seen in the UK tamoxifen prevention trial (Powles et al., 1998). For women with an intact uterus, raloxifene might counter the increased risk of endometrial cancer observed with oestrogen replacement therapy, without increasing the risk of breast cancer, which might be observed if a progestin were to be added in its place.

Medical intervention (chemoprevention)

Evidence that implicates both endogenous and exogenous oestrogens in the development and growth of breast cancer has been recently reviewed (Clemons and Goss, 2001). A series of experimental data, although incomplete, support the hypothesis of a close interaction between oestradiol and BRCA1 or BRCA2 pathways (Gudas et al., 1995; Marquis et al., 1995; Marks et al., 1997; Rajan et al., 1997; Fan et al., 1999; Hilakivi-Clarke, 2000).

Tamoxifen – a non-steroidal anti-oestrogen synthesized in 1966 – was the first anti-oestrogen to be approved for the treatment of breast cancer in 1973 (Jordan, 2000). Initially used in the treatment of advanced stages, it was rapidly used as an effective adjuvant treatment in oestrogen receptor (ER) positive cases. In the meta-analysis performed by the Early Breast Cancer Trialists' Collaborative Group (EBCTCG) (1998), a gain of 2–5 years' survival could be attributed to tamoxifen as an adjuvant hormonal agent. The same analysis also confirmed that women who had received tamoxifen for 5 years had a 47% reduction in new primary breast cancer occurring in the 10 years after treatment initiation ($P < 0.00001$) (Early Breast Cancer Trialists' Collaborative Group, 1998). Based on these observations, several multicentre, randomized trials have been initiated to assess the efficacy of tamoxifen as an agent for the prevention of breast cancer (Cuzick, 2000).

The National Surgical Adjuvant Breast and Bowel Project (NSABP) P1 study or the Breast Cancer Prevention Trial enrolled 13 388 women between 1992 and 1997 (Fisher et al., 1998). The eligible women should have had an increased risk of breast cancer based on a modified version of the Gail model (Gail et al., 1989). The risk of developing breast cancer should be at least equivalent to a 5-year risk of an average 60-year-old woman (1.67%). Women with concurrent HRT were excluded. This large, randomized, double-blind study was terminated early after a median follow-up of 4.7 years by an independent data monitoring committee, as women in the tamoxifen arm demonstrated a significant reduction in invasive (89 events vs 175; odds ratio (OR) = 0.51; 95% CI, 0.39–0.66; $P<0.0001$) and non-invasive (35 events vs 69; OR = 0.50; 95% CI, 0.33–0.77; $P<0.002$) breast cancer incidence (Fisher et al., 1998). The risk reduction was seen in all age and family history risk groups, but was greater in women aged 60 years (55%) than in women aged 49 years or younger (44%). Of note, ER-positive, but not ER-negative, breast cancers were prevented and a reduction of the breast-cancer-specific mortality was not found among women taking tamoxifen, but the median follow-up was probably too short to adequately evaluate this end-point. A significant reduction in the incidence of bone fractures to the hip, radius and spine was also noted, probably due to the maintenance of bone mineral density. With these findings, the US Food and Drug Administration approved tamoxifen (20 mg/day for 5 years) for breast cancer risk reduction in high-risk women, similarly defined as in the NSABP-P1 trial.

Data are just emerging that hoped to answer the question of great relevance to *BRCA1/2* mutation carriers: can tamoxifen prevent primary breast cancer in *BRCA1/2* mutation carriers? Mary-Claire King recently presented the preliminary results from *BRCA1/2* mutation analysis of 288 women who developed breast cancer during the P-1 study (King et al., 2001, presented at ASCO, 13 May). Nineteen mutation carriers (11 *BRCA2*, 8 *BRCA1*) were identified. Among affected *BRCA2* mutation carriers, three had been randomized to tamoxifen and eight to placebo. For *BRCA1*, the numbers were five and three respectively. This result suggests that women with *BRCA1* mutations are unlikely to benefit from tamoxifen, whereas *BRCA2* mutation carriers may gain benefit. Interestingly, of the seven *BRCA1*-related breast tumours with known ER status, six were ER negative, whereas for the nine evaluable *BRCA2*-related cancers, six were ER positive. These data fit with both the findings and interpretation of Karp et al. (1997) who, on observing that *BRCA1*-related tumours were more likely to be ER negative than *BRCA2*-related cancers, wrote: 'Tamoxifen use has been considered to be a preventive strategy for women with inherited risks for breast carcinoma.

The current data show that this strategy may be appropriate for BRCA2 carriers, but raise concern that . . . BRCA1 carriers . . . may not be susceptible to antiestrogenic measures'. It is therefore of some interest that two prospective European studies that also assessed tamoxifen (20 mg/day) as a breast cancer preventive drug were unable to reproduce the NSABP-P1 results (Table 15.3). Could this be because there were substantial numbers of *BRCA1* mutation carriers in these two studies?

Between 1986 and 1996, the randomized Royal Marsden Hospital Tamoxifen Chemoprevention Trial enrolled 2471 healthy women aged 30–70 years with an increased risk of breast cancer that was strictly based on family history; 26% of them were taking HRT (Powles et al., 1998). After a median follow-up of 5.8 years, an interim analysis showed that the overall frequency of breast cancer was similar in women in the tamoxifen or placebo arm (34 vs 36 events; RR = 1.06, 95% CI, 0.7–1.7; $P = 0.80$). Thirty-six per cent of all participants and more than 60% (44/70) of those developing breast cancer had a greater than 80% probability of carrying a BRCA1 or BRCA2 mutation, but early data on mutation frequency do not suggest that this many mutations will in fact be identified in this cohort of women (R. Eeles, personal communication) and, in particular, there is no evidence that *BRCA1* mutation carriers are more prevalent than are *BRCA2* mutation carriers. The authors have therefore argued that oestrogen promotion, which is counteracted by tamoxifen, may not be important in the aetiology of clinical breast cancer in carriers of mutations in highly penetrant genes, including those that remain undiscovered.

An increased risk of breast cancer was not a criterion for women to be eligible in the Italian Tamoxifen Prevention Study (Veronesi et al., 1998). This study was restricted to hysterectomized women, and a past history of oophorectomy was noted in 48% of the participants. Between 1992 and 1997, 5408 women aged 35–70 years were randomized to receive either tamoxifen or placebo for 5 years, and HRT was allowed. This study was stopped early 'because of the number of women dropping out'. After a median follow-up period of 3.8 years, the frequency of breast cancer was the same in the tamoxifen and the placebo groups (22 vs 19 events, respectively; $P = 0.64$) (Veronesi et al., 1998). There was a statistically significant reduction of breast cancer among women receiving tamoxifen who also used HRT during the trial.

Interpretation of these conflicting data have been widely discussed (Eeles and Powles, 2000; Fisher et al., 2000; Jordan, 2000; Mamounas, 2000; Vogel, 2000). No clear reasons for the lack of effect seen in the UK study have emerged, and despite the suggestion that the criteria for entry in the UK study were biased towards those more likely to carry mutations in highly penetrant genes, mutations in *BRCA1/2* do not appear to be common in the UK study (R. Eeles, personal

Table 15.3. Selective oestrogen receptor modulators (SERMs) as chemopreventive agents for breast cancer (prospective randomized studies)

Study	Population studied	n	SERM	Invasive breast cancer risk			
				SERM	Placebo	RR	P
NSABP-P1 (Fisher et al., 1998)	5-year risk of breast cancer ≥1.7% (Gail model)	13 888	Tamoxifen	89	175	0.51	<0.00001
Italian study (Veronesi et al., 1998)	Prior hysterectomy	5408	Tamoxifen	19	22	0.86	N/S
UK study (Powles et al., 1998)	Family history of breast cancer	2471	Tamoxifen	34	36	0.94	N/S
MORE study (Cummings et al., 1999)	Postmenopausal with osteoporosis	7705	Raloxifene	13	27	0.24	<0.05

MORE, Multiple Outcomes Raloxifene Evaluation; N/S, not stated; RR, relative risk.

communication). The two European studies were smaller in sample size, had major differences in the studied populations and were less well designed than the NSABP-P1 trial.

Risk/benefit assessment of tamoxifen as a preventive agent is a crucial issue (Chlebowski et al., 1999; Fisher, 1999; Gail et al., 1999; Lippman and Brown, 1999). In the NSABP-P1 trial, the administration of tamoxifen was associated with an increased risk of endometrial cancer (RR = 2.5) and thrombo-embolic events (RR for stroke = 1.6; RR for pulmonary embolism = 3; and RR for deep-vein thrombosis = 1.6) (Fisher et al., 1998). These side-effects increased with age. A significant increased rate of thrombo-embolic events was also noted in the Italian Tamoxifen Prevention Study (Veronesi et al., 1998). A woman with a personal or a family history of thrombo-embolic events should be referred to an appropriate clinic to evaluate her haemostatic status before the prescription of tamoxifen. Surprisingly, a recent study revealed that endometrial cancer diagnosed after tamoxifen use could be associated with adverse clinicopathological characteristics and a worse outcome (Bergman et al., 2000). Association of tamoxifen use with poorly differentiated, highly proliferative endometrial cancer with poorer survival is still controversial (Jordan and Assikis, 1995; Barakat, 1998; Lasset et al., 2001; Narod et al., 2001a). Of note, all of the 36 women in the NASBP-P1 study who developed endometrial cancer in the tamoxifen arm had a stage I disease and were alive at the end of the study (Fisher et al., 1998). Interestingly, local administration of progestagens has been suggested to reduce the deleterious effect of tamoxifen on the endometrium (Dickson and Pandiarajan, 2001; Marsh and Mayfield, 2001). Women receiving tamoxifen should have a careful gynaecological history taken and should undergo annual pelvic examination (Chlebowski, 2000). Any abnormal vaginal bleeding or discharge should be strictly evaluated before and during the administration time of tamoxifen by endometrial sampling and transvaginal ultrasound. Outside of clinical trial, routine ultrasonography or endometrial biopsy is not recommended in asymptomatic patients receiving tamoxifen (Barakat, 1999; Suh-Burgmann and Goodman, 1999; Barakat et al., 2000; Gerber et al., 2000; Runowicz, 2000). There was no increased risk of cancer at sites other than the endometrium in any of the three studies.

Treatment with tamoxifen has also been associated with a reduction in breast density in both premenopausal and postmenopausal women (Ursin et al., 1996; Atkinson et al., 1999). Psychological and sexual evaluations were performed among women in tamoxifen-based preventive trials, both in North America and the UK, and no evidence of side-effects associated with tamoxifen was found (Day et al., 1999; Fallowfield et al., 2001).

The efficiency of tamoxifen as a preventive agent of primary breast cancer among *BRCA1/2* mutation carriers has not been extensively studied. The recent data from the P-1 study (see above) is so far all we have, but even this study was not large enough to observe significant effects. To date, a single case-control study evaluating the protection against contralateral breast cancer in *BRCA1/2* mutation carriers has been published (Narod et al., 2000). This matched case-control study compared 209 *BRCA1/2* mutation carriers with bilateral breast cancer with 384 matched controls with unilateral breast cancer. A 75% reduction in risk of contralateral breast cancer was noted among women who used tamoxifen for 2–4 years. According to the authors of this multicentre study, it is reasonable to predict that tamoxifen will also reduce the occurrence of primary cancers in *BRCA1* and *BRCA2* mutation carriers. This postulate is clearly in conflict with that resulting from the mutation results of the P-1 study. It is worth noting that the reduction in new primary cancers noted among women taking tamoxifen in the EBCTCG meta-analysis occurred regardless of whether the initial tumour was ER positive ($30 \pm 6\%$) or 'poor' ($29 \pm 15\%$) (Early Breast Cancer Trialists' Collaborative Group, 1998). Nevertheless, if 80% of *BRCA1*-related breast cancers are ER negative, and the ER status of the first and second cancers are independent, then 64% of *BRCA1* mutation carriers who develop bilateral breast cancer will have two ER-negative tumours, 4% will have two ER-positive cancers, and 32% will have tumours with opposing ER status. It seems implausible that in Narod's study, the entire observed benefit was due to a response in 20% of all mutation carriers (16% who would have had an ER-negative cancer, followed by an ER-positive cancer, and 4% where both the tumours would have been ER positive). Therefore, one question is whether or not tamoxifen can prevent ER-negative second primary breast cancers in *BRCA1* mutation carriers. Narod's analysis has not directly answered this, and it will require documentation of the ER status of all primary and secondary tumours in Narod's series of carriers who did or did not take tamoxifen before tamoxifen will become widely prescribed as a *BRCA1*-related breast cancer preventive drug. Although unlikely, it is possible that in *BRCA1* mutation carriers who have had cancer, tamoxifen is not acting in quite the same way as it is in non-carriers. Certainly, the addition of oophorectomy to tamoxifen had a striking effect on the contralateral breast cancer rate.

Raloxifene – a new selective oestrogen receptor modulator (SERM) – was evaluated in the large, randomized, Multiple Outcomes Raloxifene Evaluation (MORE) study as an agent for the prevention of osteoporosis-related bone fractures in postmenopausal women (Cummings et al., 1999). The major advantage of this SERM should be its absence of oestrogenic-like effects on the endometrial mucosa, associated with a presumably similar protective action to tamoxifen on the mammary gland and blood lipid profile (Love et al., 1994; Chlebowski et al., 1999). In the MORE trial, raloxifene significantly reduced osteoporosis and its complications after a median follow-up of 3.3 years (Cummings et al., 1999). A significant decrease in invasive breast cancer cases was noted in the raloxifene arm (RR = 0.24; 95% CI, 0.13–0.44; $P < 0.001$). Again in this study, the reduction of risk was limited to ER-positive tumours. Thrombo-embolic events were significantly more frequent in women taking raloxifene (RR = 3.1; 95% CI, 1.5–6.2). The breast cancer protective effect associated with raloxifene use has been recently confirmed after 4 years of follow-up (RR = 0.28; 95% CI, 0.17–0.46) (Cauley et al., 2001). The effect of raloxifene in premenopausal women has not been evaluated. According to the recent guidelines elaborated by the American Society of Clinical Oncology, it is premature to prescribe raloxifene to lower the risk of developing breast cancer outside of a clinical trial setting (Chlebowski et al., 1999). The on-going randomized Study of Tamoxifen and Raloxifene (STAR) or the NSABP-P2 trial, initiated in 1999, is assessing the breast cancer risk reduction associated with these two drugs. Eligibility criteria are similar to those used in the NSABP-P1 trial, but currently only postmenopausal women are being enrolled, so this study will not provide information of direct relevance to *BRCA1/2* mutation carriers.

Important issues – such as the optimal dose, length and age to begin chemoprevention, the efficacy of other SERMs (Labrie et al., 1999) and the place of different agents, either alone or in combination with other preventive approaches, such as aromatase inhibitors (Goss and Strasser, 2001), luteinizing hormone-releasing hormone agonists (Spicer and Pike, 2000), retinoids (Lotan, 1996; Lippman et al., 1998; Veronesi et al., 1999) or drugs derived from plants (e.g. isoflavones, indole-3-carbinol) (Osborne, 1999) – are currently being investigated (McCaskill-Stevens et al., 1999; Conley et al., 2000; Cuzick, 2000; Mehta, 2000). For example, the Raloxifene and Zoladex Research Study, a pilot study to assess chemopreventive tolerability and efficiency of raloxifene combined with goserelin in very-high-risk women (presumably *BRCA1/2* mutation carriers) aged 35–45 years, will be launched in the UK and Australia (Eeles and Powles, 2000). All of these chemopreventive strategies are in early stages of development, and drug safety and tolerability are essential issues in chemopreventive treatment dedicated to healthy women.

As most of the *BRCA1*-related breast cancers do not express ER and thus are not expected to respond to anti-oestrogen therapy, the issue of the efficiency of tamoxifen as a preventive drug is important in hereditary cancer. The stage in tumour progression at which hormone independence may arise is not defined. The conjecture that ER expression is absent at the earliest stages of *BRCA1*-related breast cancer carcinogenesis has not been refuted. Indeed, it has been supported by the work of Gusterson and colleagues, who demonstrated that 11 (66%) ductal carcinoma *in situ* lesions associated with 16 *BRCA1/2*-invasive breast cancers were ER negative (Osin et al., 1998).

In summary, the effects of tamoxifen or raloxifene in *BRCA1/2* mutation

Table 15.4. Prophylactic mastectomy and breast cancer prevention

Study	n	Type of mastectomy	Follow-up (yrs)	No. of breast cancers	Risk reduction (%)
Woods, 1983	1400	Subcutaneous	17	3	91
Pennisi and Capozzi, 1989	1500	Subcutaneous	9	6	≥90
Hartmann et al., 1999a	575	Subcutaneous	14	7	≥90
	64	Total	14	0	100
	425 (moderate-risk FH)		14	4	89.5
	214 (high-risk FH)		14	3	94

FH, family history.

carriers is unknown, but some indirect evidence exists that these SERMs effectively reduce breast cancer risk in this particular subgroup. Among some important and currently unresolved issues, we should mention the impact of these drugs in the prevention of *BRCA1* ER-negative breast cancer, the benefit in terms of survival, and the risks/benefits ratio among premenopausal women.

Surgical intervention

The option of prophylactic mastectomy has been a matter of debate (Wapnir et al., 1990; Klijn et al., 1997; Eisen and Weber, 1999). Prophylactic mastectomy has not been rigorously evaluated either among women carrying a genetic predisposition, or in the general population. There are no prospective controlled trials of the reduction of breast cancer risk associated with bilateral prophylactic mastectomy (Hughes et al., 1999). The several published series on prophylactic mastectomy are retrospective and disparate, particularly regarding the eligible criteria for surgery, and none are randomized (Table 15.4). Prophylactic mastectomy has been advocated after multiple previous breast biopsies, unreliable results on physical examination (because of nodular disease), findings of dense breast tissue on mammography or extreme fear of cancer (Hartmann et al., 1999b). Nevertheless, a reduction of breast cancer risk after prophylactic mastectomy was evaluated at 90–100%. In a well-designed retrospective cohort study at the Mayo Clinic between 1960 and 1993, 639 women were classified as having either a moderate or high risk of breast cancer based on their family history (Hartmann et al., 1999a). After a median follow-up of 14 years, a risk reduction of 89.5% ($P < 0.00001$) and 92% was shown in the moderate ($n = 425$) and the high-risk group ($n = 214$), respectively. The reduction in breast cancer mortality has been estimated to be

100% in the moderate-risk group and 81–94% in the high-risk group, depending on the method used to calculate the expected rates (Hartmann et al., 1999a). In the context of *BRCA1* or *BRCA2* mutations, most experts advocate a total mastectomy rather than a subcutaneous procedure, as this latter intervention does not allow an optimal resection of glandular tissue, by preserving the nipple–areolar complex (Hughes et al., 1999; Eisen et al., 2000b). In fact, no comparative studies are available, and cases of breast cancer following either total or subcutaneous pro-phylactic mastectomy have been reported (Eldar et al., 1984; Goodnight et al., 1984; Ziegler and Kroll, 1991). Options of reconstructive surgery, as well as potential surgical complications of this irreversible procedure, should always be discussed with the proband and a plastic surgeon before the intervention.

It has been known for many years that oophorectomy can reduce the incidence of breast cancer (Hirayama and Wynder, 1962; Brinton et al., 1988; Meijer and van Lindert, 1992; Parazzini et al., 1997) and improves survival after breast cancer in an adjuvant setting (Early Breast Cancer Trialists' Collaborative Group, 1996). Recent studies have confirmed the benefit of a prophylactic oophorectomy in women carrying *BRCA1/2* mutations, with a reduction of breast cancer risk of up to 60%, particularly if the oophorectomy was performed before the age of 40 years (Rebbeck et al., 1999; Eisen et al., 2000a; Narod et al., 2000). Interestingly, the lower risk persisted (and is even more marked) after 10 years of follow-up (adjusted hazard ratio (HR) = 0.3; 95% CI, 0.1–0.9) and, perhaps surprisingly, HRT did not seem to significantly reduce the benefits of the procedure (Rebbeck et al., 1999). This latter issue is still controversial, according to the relatively small number of women evaluated in these studies and the previous data concerning HRT and breast cancer risk. Moreover, the effects of oophorectomy and tamoxifen in reducing the risk of contralateral breast cancer among *BRCA1/2* mutation carriers suggested they were independent (Narod et al., 2000). Thus, in *BRCA1/2* mutation carriers, prophylactic oophorectomy at the end of child-bearing years or at age 40 years is often recommended, particularly because no ovarian cancer screening programme has been shown to reduce the mortality from the disease (Rosenthal and Jacobs, 1998). This surgical option is certainly less physically evident than prophylactic mastectomy and is likely to be more popular (Matloff et al., 2000) and may be effective in reducing cancer risks on the two major organs at risk in *BRCA1/2* mutation carriers. A salpingectomy should be associated with the oophorectomy, as rare cases of primary fallopian tube cancer have been described among patients with *BRCA1*, and rarely with *BRCA2* mutations (Delaloge et al., 2000; Zweemer et al., 2000; Aziz et al., 2001; Paley et al., 2001).

Few studies have addressed quality-of-life issues in women who have opted for prophylactic mastectomy or oophorectomy (Eisen et al., 2000b). Five to twenty per cent of women who have undergone prophylactic mastectomy reported at least some dissatisfaction (Borgen et al., 1998; Frost et al., 2000). The potential psychological impact of a prophylactic mastectomy or oophorectomy should always be evaluated and explained to the proband, as well as the current absence of data that demonstrate a benefit in terms of survival gain in the context of *BRCA1/2* mutations (Metcalfe et al., 2000). Interestingly, the first prospective psychosocial study of bilateral prophylactic mastectomy found that 79 English women at high genetic risk of breast cancer who chose to undergo surgery had reduced psychosocial morbidity 6–18 months after surgery (Hatcher et al., 2001). The 64 women who declined surgery showed no such reduction. Neither body image nor sexual functioning significantly changed among women in either group. Cross-cultural and intercultural differences in women's attitudes toward prophylactic surgical procedures, particularly mastectomy, have been discussed (Eisen et al., 2000b; Eisinger et al., 2000). In the Netherlands, among unaffected *BRCA1/2* mutation carriers eligible for prophylactic surgery, the majority of women underwent either bilateral mastectomy (35/68) or oophorectomy (29/45) (Meijers-Heijboer et al., 2000). Most of the surgical procedures were performed in the 12 months following DNA test disclosure.

Some interesting models have been developed to appreciate the potential benefit of various preventive procedures in terms of gain in life expectancy (Schrag et al., 1997, 2000; Grann et al., 1998, 2000). All of these models are based on a series of assumptions (e.g. efficacy of prophylactic interventions, proportion of node-negative breast cancer, similar survival for hereditary breast and ovarian cancer as sporadic cases), which render their estimations of limited value when faced with a real clinical case. Nevertheless, these models can give some insights into the effectiveness of options we regularly discuss with women at risk.

Reducing the risk of second primary breast cancer

Women with a previous diagnosis of breast cancer, particularly if younger than 50 years, may be more likely to opt for prophylactic surgery of the contralateral breast than healthy women (Metcalfe et al., 2000; Wagner et al., 2000). Based on a reduced or delayed incidence of ipsilateral recurrences compared with the high incidence of contralateral breast cancer, a randomized trial of unilateral vs bilateral radiotherapy in *BRCA1/2* mutation carriers who undergo breast-conserving surgery, measuring the incidence of new cancers in the contralateral breast, might be considered (see Chapter 6).

Reducing the risk of ovarian cancer for a woman with no previous cancer
Medical intervention

Oral contraceptives (OC) are known to be associated with a significant reduction of ovarian cancer risk (RR ~ 0.5) (Franceschi et al., 1991; Whittemore et al., 1992).

A similar reduction was reported for *BRCA1* and *BRCA2* mutation carriers that used OC (RR = 0.4; 95% CI, 0.2–0.7) (Narod et al., 1998), and the risk decreased with increasing duration of use. These data have been recently confirmed in an extended and more complete series of women (OR = 0.44; *P* = 0.002) (Narod et al., 2001b). Nevertheless, independent confirmation is required, particularly as the control group in the first study were *BRCA1/2* mutation carriers with intact ovaries, most of whom had had breast cancer. It is indeed problematic to find an adequate control group when cancer risks are so high and mutations are rare.

A meta-analysis of the data from 54 epidemiological studies with 53 297 women with breast cancer and 100 239 women without breast cancer on the relation between OC and breast cancer concluded a slight but significant increase in breast cancer risk (Collaborative Group on Hormonal Factors in Breast Cancer, 1996a). Current users of OC had a higher RR of breast cancer (1.24; 95% CI, 1.15–1.39; *P* < 0.00001) than women who had never used OC. A slightly elevated risk of breast cancer persisted for up to 10 years after cessation of OC. A family history of breast cancer does not modify the effect of OC on risk in general (Collaborative Group on Hormonal Factors in Breast Cancer, 1996b). It is not known if this slight increase in breast cancer risk is similarly present among women carrying *BRCA1/2* mutations. Indeed, one small study of Ashkenazi Jewish women with breast cancer suggested that OC may increase the risk of breast cancer more among *BRCA1/2* mutation carriers than among non-carriers (Ursin et al., 1997). A recent publication showed a worrisome increased risk for breast cancer associated with strong family history of breast cancer and OC use (Grabrick et al., 2000). These authors conducted a large historical cohort and found a significant correlation between ever use of OC and risk of breast cancer in sisters and daughters of 426 consecutively ascertained probands with breast cancer (RR = 3.3; 95% CI, 1.6–6.7). Moreover, the risk to first-degree relatives increased with the number of affected relatives in the family: the RR rose from 4.6 (95% CI, 2.0–10.7) for families with three members with breast/ovarian cancers to 11.4 (95% CI, 2.3–56.4) for families with five or more relatives affected. No data are available regarding the *BRCA1/2* status for these families and the possibility that most of the increased risk is due to formulations of OC with higher levels of oestrogen and progestins has been raised.

In summary, despite a substantial reduction in ovarian cancer risk associated with OC, use of this convenient means of birth control should be carefully discussed with women harbouring *BRCA1/2* mutations, as breast cancer risk may be a real concern (Burke, 2000).

Surgical intervention

Considering the absence of efficient screening programmes, the high mortality rate associated with ovarian cancer and a surgical procedure view as less mutilating than bilateral mastectomy, prophylactic oophorectomy in *BRCA1/2* mutation carriers is regarded as a reasonable option. The optimal type of surgical procedure (laparoscopy vs laparotomy) has not been evaluated, but laparoscopic oophorectomy or adnexectomy has been the option for most women undergoing this preventive surgery (Morice et al., 1999; Eisen et al., 2000b). The risk of ovarian cancer is substantially reduced after oophorectomy, although a precise estimate is not available. In one multicentre retrospective cohort of 248 *BRCA1/2* mutation carriers who underwent prophylactic oophorectomy with a mean follow-up of 9.4 years, Weber et al. (2000) reported a highly significant reduction in ovarian cancer risk with an adjusted hazard ratio (HR) = 0.02 (95% CI, 0.002–0.12). This result needs confirmation in a prospectively designed study. The optimal age to perform the surgery is probably after completion of childbearing or after age 35 years (NIH Consensus Conference, 1995), but probably before 45 years, particularly among *BRCA1* mutation carriers, as an early age at onset of ovarian cancer has been repeatedly observed (Eisen et al., 2000b). Moreover, the induced premature menopause with its potential deleterious consequences (onset of menopausal symptoms, potential risk of accelerated cardiovascular disease or osteoporosis) should also be balanced against the reduction of breast cancer risk, the latter being obvious mainly when the oophorectomy procedure is performed during the premenopausal period. The pathologist should be alerted to the indication for oophorectomy so that a thorough pathological examination can be performed (Salazar et al., 1996). The occurrence of primary serous carcinoma of the peritoneum among *BRCA1/2* carriers, before or after oophorectomy, has been previously discussed (see Chapter 4).

Hysterectomy at the time of prophylactic oophorectomy has been advocated by some experts, as it simplifies the prescription of HRT, the prescription of exogenous progesterone being no longer indicated, and it eliminates the risk of endometrial cancer that is associated with tamoxifen use (Eisen et al., 2000b).

Tubal ligation has been associated with a decreased risk of invasive epithelial ovarian cancer in several case-control and prospective studies (Whittemore et al., 1992; Hankinson et al., 1993; Rosenblatt and Thomas, 1996). The mechanism underlying this effect is not known. The Hereditary Ovarian Cancer Clinical Study Group has conducted a matched case-control study to assess the impact of tubal ligation among 464 women who were found to carry *BRCA1* or *BRCA2* mutations (Narod et al., 2001b). Half of these women had a history of invasive ovarian cancer and were matched for year of birth, country of residence and mutation status with women with both ovaries intact. After adjustment for OC use, parity, breast cancer and ethnic group, the OR for developing ovarian cancer associated with tubal ligation was 0.39 (95% CI, 0.22–0.70; $P = 0.002$) among *BRCA1* mutation carriers. The greatest protection was seen when tubal ligation was performed before age 30 years. No protective effect of tubal ligation was observed among *BRCA2* mutation carriers (OR = 1.19; 95% CI, 0.38–3.68). Interestingly, the combination of tubal ligation and a history of contraceptive use among *BRCA1* mutation carriers was associated with a greater protective effect (OR = 0.28; 95% CI, 0.15–0.52; $P < 0.0001$). Based on these results, the authors concluded that tubal ligation is an attractive option for reducing the risk of ovarian cancer in women with *BRCA1* mutations who had completed childbearing.

Reducing the risk of cancers at other sites
Prostate cancer

Trials are ongoing or will be launched soon to evaluate the effects of finasteride, selenium and vitamin E as chemopreventive agents for prostate cancer in the general population or in men with a higher risk based on their family history of prostate cancer (Costello, 2001; Greenwald, 2001; Nabhan and Bergan, 2001). No particular trial has been designed for male *BRCA1* or *BRCA2* mutation carriers.

Pancreas, head and neck, and stomach cancer

Despite the increased risk associated with *BRCA1/2* germline mutations, the absolute risk for these cancers is still low as they are rare in the general population. No particular approach to prevent these cancer types has been discussed for *BRCA1/2* mutation carriers.

Early detection

The main screening tools that are available and proposed in the hereditary breast/ovarian cancer syndrome are summarized in Table 15.5. All of these measures are based on the same concept, namely that the early detection of a tumour lesion allows the administration of an optimal treatment at a non-advanced stage, which should give the better chance of survival. Whether this concept actually applies equally to *BRCA1/2*-related cancers as it does generally is not known. Indeed, the recommendations proposed for the clinical management of women with an inherited predisposition to breast and ovarian cancer are, in fact, extrapolated from the ones given to the general population (Burke et al., 1997; Eisinger et al., 1998; Vasen et al., 1998). Several variations in these recommendations given by US and French experts have been noted, particularly regarding breast self-examination, lifestyle and prophylactic surgery (Eisinger et al., 1999a). Nevertheless, the uncertainties are similar regarding the incomplete or equivocal scientific evidence on risk reduction for all these areas, and the differences are essentially subtle and may reflect some socio-cultural variations between and within North America and Europe (Julian-Reynier et al., 2001).

Table 15.5. Screening recommendations for women at high risk of breast/ovarian cancer

Measure	Frequency	Age at start (years)
Breast cancer		
Breast self-examination	1 per month	In the early 20s
Clinical breast examination	2–3 per year	25
Mammography	1–2 per year	25–30
Breast ultrasound	Under evaluation	
Breast magnetic resonance imaging (MRI)	Under evaluation	
Ovarian cancer		
Pelvic examination	1 per year	25–35 (regular gynaecological examination)
Transvaginal echography with colour Doppler imaging	1–2 per year	
CA125 level	1–2 per year	

Note: None of these abovementioned measures has formally demonstrated its efficacy in the subgroup of women harbouring germline *BRCA1/2* mutations, particularly in term of breast/ovarian cancer mortality reduction. These recommendations are based on experts' advice, but the type, frequency and the age at which these surveillance methods should start are speculative and not based on data from studies conducted in this particular subgroup. In particular, some authorities have argued that ovarian screening is counterproductive, as it may deter women from considering prophylactic oophorectomy. Variations for some recommendations have been noted between US and French experts (Eisinger et al., 1999b).

As these measures concern a subgroup of women with a particularly high prevalence of the disease, an increase in sensitivity and specificity is expected. Nevertheless, epidemiological data and biological characteristics of hereditary cancers should not be forgotten. Thus, the sensitivity of the mammography in premenopausal women – a subgroup particularly at risk with *BRCA1/2* mutations – may be decreased because of the density of the mammary tissue. Moreover, a high frequency of interval cancers has been reported, probably linked to the characteristics of these lesions, i.e. high grade of malignancy and high proliferative rate. Thus, development and evaluation of new techniques of imaging are eagerly awaited.

The issue of adherence to cancer surveillance guidelines and potential psychological distress are critical in the management of high-risk women (Lerman and Schwartz, 1993; Lynch et al., 1994), as psychological concern may negatively affect the adherence to screening guidelines (Lerman et al., 1993).

Breast cancer

Breast self-examination

A reduction in breast cancer mortality has not been associated with randomized studies that evaluated breast self-examination (Semiglazov et al., 1993; Thomas et al., 1997). Nevertheless, breast self-examination or 'breast awareness' is advocated in women identified as at high risk of developing breast cancer, probably because it is one of the rare proactive measures available (Burke et al., 1997; Møller et al., 1999a; Eisen et al., 2000b). No data are yet available that have assessed the efficacy of this surveillance practice in this particular subgroup.

Clinical examination

Regular clinical breast examination practice in the general population has been reinforced by the provocative conclusion of the second Canadian national breast screening trial (Miller et al., 2000). This study showed that breast examination was as effective (or perhaps, since death rates were not reduced in either arm, as ineffective) as yearly mammography combined with clinical examination in women aged 50–59 years in the reduction of breast cancer mortality after a mean follow-up of 13 years. No study has evaluated the impact of clinical breast examination among *BRCA1/2* mutation carriers. Our clinical impression is that most *BRCA1/2* mutation carriers detect the breast cancers themselves, and that mammography confirms the presence of a probably malignant lesion.

Mammography

Despite a meta-analysis that found a reduction of up to 18% in breast cancer mortality among 40- to 49-year-old women following regular mammographic screening (Hendrick et al., 1997), the effectiveness of this tool for the surveillance of premenopausal women remains debatable (Eckhardt et al., 1994; Kerlikowske et al., 1995; Peer et al., 1996; Gotzsche and Olsen, 2000; Smith, 2000; Ringash, 2001). As mentioned previously, a higher cancer detection rate and a lower false-positive rate are expected in *BRCA1/2* mutation carriers (Gail and Rimer, 1998; Armstrong and Weber, 2001), but some pitfalls should be considered.

Young age and a positive family history of breast cancer have been associated with screening failure (Tabar et al., 1993; Burhenne et al., 1994; Kerlikowske et al., 1996). In the presence of dense breast tissue on mammogram, the absence of detection of suspicious lesion could be misleading, both in young and older women. In a large retrospective study among women aged 40 years or older participating in a mammographic screening programme in western Washington state between 1988 and 1993, mammographic breast density appeared to be a major risk factor for interval cancer, both in women aged less than 50 years and in older women (Mandelson et al., 2000). Preliminary and conflicting data are available regarding the issue of the mammographic features of *BRCA1/2*-associated tumours compared with sporadic tumours, particularly in an age-matched setting (Helvie et al., 1997; Chang et al., 1999; Huo et al., 2000; Kuhl et al., 2000). A nested case-control study of *BRCA1/2* mutation carriers vs non-carriers was performed within a prevalence study of 412 Ashkenazi Jewish women with breast cancer unselected for age or family history and tested for *BRCA1/2* founder mutations (Warner et al., 1999). Forty carriers were age-of-diagnosis-matched with three non-carriers. Tumours among *BRCA1/2* mutation carriers were less frequently visible on the mammogram than among non-carriers (70.6% vs 82.3%; $P = 0.22$, E. Warner, WDF and POC, unpublished data). Interestingly, recent studies that examined the clinicopathological characteristics of interval cancers found that these tumours demonstrated, more frequently than mammographically detected breast cancers, a pattern similar to what is classically seen in *BRCA1*-related breast cancers, i.e. high-grade, ER-negative, p53-positive, highly proliferative tumours (Porter et al., 1999; Gilliland et al., 2000; Narod and Dubé, 2001).

Seven European centres reported preliminary data on the efficacy of surveillance programmes in women with a family history of breast cancer (Møller et al., 1999b). Among women aged less than 50 years at diagnosis, 32% (20 out of 62 prospectively diagnosed breast tumours) were interval cancers and mammography was negative in 23% (14 out of 62). No data regarding the *BRCA1/2* mutation status were available. The first evaluation of a breast cancer surveillance programme among a series of 128 *BRCA1/2* mutation carriers has been recently reported (Brekelmans et al., 2001). The effectiveness of physical examination every 6 months and yearly mammography was evaluated and compared with 449 moderate-risk and 621 high-risk women. Within a median follow-up of 3 years, the highest cancer detection rates and observed/expected ratio were observed among the *BRCA1/2* mutation carriers (nine cases; ratio observed/expected: 23.7), but the cancers were not diagnosed at a particularly early stage (five cases were axillary nodes positive). Five cases were in fact interval cancers, resulting in the worst sensitivity (56%) for screening, being among the *BRCA1/2* mutation carrier subgroup. These preliminary data could be interpreted in favour of mammographic screening at a shorter interval than 1 year or in favour of the development of new approaches, or possibly both. In particular, the effectiveness of magnetic resonance imaging or digital mammography in the early detection of breast cancer in high-risk women could be of great interest (Huo et al., 2000; Kuhl et al., 2000).

Some fears have been reported regarding the potentially hazardous effect of low-dose radiation, which could ultimately be responsible for an increased cancer risk (Den Otter et al., 1996; Gilson, 1997; Vaidya and Baum, 1997; Foray et al., 1999). Despite some *in vitro* evidence of a particular sensitivity of *BRCA1*- or

BRCA2-deficient cells to γ-radiation, no clinical data could support these assumptions (see Chapter 6).

As mammographic screening has become the standard procedure for breast cancer screening, it is particularly important to discuss with high-risk women the obvious limits and potential drawbacks of this screening technique to prevent exaggerated hopes that women might otherwise invest in this technique (Mittra et al., 2000).

Ultrasonography

As a screening tool, ultrasonography has not been shown to be effective in asymptomatic women of the general population (Sickles, 2000). This technique is particularly useful to characterise simple cysts. Several sonographic features have been identified that are sufficiently suggestive of malignancy to perform biopsy, even in the absense of suspicious findings at clinical breast examination or mammography (Sickles, 2000). Ultrasonography has not been rigorously evaluated in women identified as being at high risk of developing breast cancer.

Magnetic resonance imaging

Magnetic resonance imaging (MRI) is a non-ionizing imaging technique that has already been demonstrated to be sensitive for invasive breast cancer. Its sensitivity is less impaired than mammography by dense parenchyma (Weinreb and Newstead, 1995). Preliminary results of a German prospective, non-randomized, pilot project (including 192 asymptomatic women proved or suspected to be *BRCA1/2* mutation carriers) demonstrated that the sensitivity and specificity of breast MRI was superior to conventional mammography and high-frequency breast ultrasound (Kuhl et al., 2000). The triple assessment was performed yearly, plus an additional physical and ultrasound examination every 6 months. Among the nine breast cancers diagnosed (six prevalent, three incident), four were detected and correctly classified by mammography and ultrasound combined. Two other lesions were visible, but were misdiagnosed as fibroadenomas. MRI identified and correctly diagnosed the nine lesions. Of note, the nine cancers were pT1 stage (mean size: 1.05 cm) without axillary node involvement (pN0). The genetic status was not known for all patients, but among the nine women who developed breast cancer, seven had mutations in *BRCA1* ($n = 6$) and *BRCA2* ($n = 1$). Only five false-positive findings were noted with MRI, compared with seven and nineteen with mammography and ultrasound, respectively. Among 105 asymptomatic women with validation of the screening results after the first year, the positive predictive value for mammography, ultrasound and MRI was 30%, 12% and 64% respectively. The cost-effectiveness of screening in this high-risk cohort was not addressed in this study. Preliminary results of this pilot project are encouraging.

Similar prospective evaluations of MRI are ongoing in several centres in North America and Europe.

Other screening techniques

Various approaches have been developed and evaluated for the early detection of breast cancer (Evron et al., 2001), but none has proven its superiority to the existing measures that are currently recommended.

Ovarian cancer

Despite some encouraging reports from studies using established (Jacobs et al., 1999) or new screening methods for early detection of ovarian carcinoma (De-Priest et al., 1997; van Nagell et al., 2000), no statistically significant reductions in ovarian morbidity or mortality have been observed when prospective studies have been carried out in the general population. Limiting ovarian cancer screening programmes to women identified at a significantly increased risk compared with the general population has been proposed as a way of improving the positive predictive value of ovarian screening (Berchuck et al., 1999; Verheijen et al., 1999; Fishman and Cohen, 2000), but the physical location of the ovaries, and possibly the underlying biology of ovarian carcinoma, do not seem to lend themselves to early detection by ultrasound or serum assays, whether the woman is at high or low risk. Improvements in ultrasound technology such as power Doppler and 3-D sonography are currently under investigation in the NCI-supported National Ovarian Cancer Early Detection Program, in a selected population of high-risk women.

Males at risk

Prostate cancer

The increased risk in prostate cancer noted among *BRCA2* mutation carriers (RR = 4.6; 95% CI, 3.5–6.2) is most likely not the result of increased surveillance, as most of the excess risk occurred before screening became widespread (Breast Cancer Linkage Consortium, 1999). The substantially elevated risk of prostate cancer raises the issue of early detection, in that screening by the prostate specific antigen (PSA) test might be justified at a substantially earlier age for mutation carriers (RR for men aged less than 65 years = 7.3; 95% CI, 4.7–11.5) (Breast Cancer Linkage Consortium, 1999). Thus, *BRCA1/2* mutation carriers could also be a particular subgroup for the evaluation of the serum concentration of markers that may improve the sensitivity of the PSA test (Neal et al., 2000; Stephan et al., 2000; Wolk et al., 2000). A note of caution should be struck: no study of unselected males with prostate cancer has ever shown that *BRCA1/2* mutations are over-represented in these men. Thus, the precise risks of prostate cancer for *BRCA1/2* mutation carriers remain uncertain.

Treatment

The issue of the optimal treatment for hereditary breast and ovarian cancer is still largely debatable. Compared with its sporadic counterpart, distinct somatic genetic changes have been reported in hereditary breast cancer (Tirkkonen et al., 1997) and a recent study showed that gene-expression profiles are significantly different between both *BRCA1*- and *BRCA2*-related breast cancers and sporadic cases (Hedenfalk et al., 2001). Pathological features also suggest that there are underlying differences in hereditary breast cancer compared with sporadic cases (see Chapter 7). For example, *BRCA1*-associated tumours are more often poorly differentiated, highly proliferating tumours, with a high frequency of ER negativity, and a higher rate of p53 mutations (Chappuis et al., 2000; Phillips, 2000). Similarly, *BRCA2*-associated tumours exhibit significant differences when compared with age-matched sporadic cases, such as a reduction in tubule formation, a higher proportion of continuous pushing margins and a lower mitotic count (Lakhani et al., 1998).

Breast cancer

Surgery

Currently, the surgical management of breast cancer caused by germline *BRCA1/2* mutations is similar to the sporadic cases, particularly regarding the option of a conservative treatment (lumpectomy or quadrantectomy) associated with radiotherapy. No study that has prospectively evaluated conservative surgery plus radiotherapy versus radical mastectomy among *BRCA1/2* mutation carriers is available. Interestingly, there are currently no definitive data that demonstrate a significant increase in ipsilateral breast tumour recurrence rates among patients with *BRCA1/2* mutations compared with sporadic breast cancer patients (see Chapter 6). When a *BRCA1/2* mutation carrier develops an invasive breast cancer (particularly if this is the result of the failure of preventive strategies), and given the high risk of contralateral breast cancer, the option of bilateral mastectomy with or without reconstruction is a valid option.

Radiotherapy

In vitro, *BRCA1/2*-deficient cells demonstrate an increased sensitivity to radiation (Connor et al., 1997; Sharan et al., 1997; Gowen et al., 1998; Foray et al., 1999), but radiotherapy after breast conservative surgery is not associated with a significant increase of acute or chronic toxicities among *BRCA1/2* mutation carriers (Gaffney et al., 1998; Leong et al., 2000; Pierce et al., 2000). Current results regarding therapeutic radiation in *BRCA1* or *BRCA2* mutation carriers are consistent with the hypothesis that radiotherapy reduces cancer incidence in the treated breast, or significantly delays the appearance of emerging cancers. Radiation scatter has been raised as a contributive factor in the increased incidence of contralateral cancers (Bennett, 1999; Coleman, 1999; Robson et al., 1999), but no clinical data support these hypotheses (discussed in detail in Chapter 6). One test of this hypothesis would be to compare contralateral breast cancer rates in a (historical) cohort of *BRCA1/2* mutation carriers who did or did not receive adjuvant radiotherapy as their only treatment following unilateral breast cancer. If scatter is an important factor, contralateral rates should be higher in the group that received radiotherapy.

Chemotherapy

Indication and types of adjuvant chemo- or hormonotherapy currently in practice with hereditary breast cancer are not different from those proposed for sporadic breast cancers. Some *in vitro* data suggest that cells without functional *BRCA1* or *BRCA2* protein demonstrate a particular sensitivity to several chemotherapeutic drugs. The underlying hypothesis is an increased sensitivity to agents that cause double-strand DNA breaks in *BRCA1*- or *BRCA2*-deficient cells (Biggs and Bradley, 1998; Khanna and Jackson, 2001). This hypersensitivity has been demonstrated for mitoxantrone, amsacrine, etoposide, doxorubicin and cisplatin, with a subsequent increased level of apoptosis (Abbott et al., 1998; Husain et al., 1998; Bhattacharyya et al., 2000; Ren et al., 2001). Of note, in a nude mouse model with *BRCA2*-defective tumour xenograft, tumour growth was very sensitive to mitoxantrone when compared with mice with tumours harbouring *BRCA2*-normal cells (Abbott et al., 1998). A decreased sensitivity to paclitaxel and docetaxel in *BRCA1*-mutated cell-lines has also been observed (Ren et al., 2001). Differences in drug sensitivity might be explained by interaction of *BRCA1* with various pathways that lead to cell death, particularly via a reduction of the anti-apoptotic protein Bcl2 level in cells lacking functional BRCA1 protein (Ren et al., 2001). Interestingly, the higher sensitivity to γ-radiation noted in a *BRCA1*-deficient cell-line was mainly attributed to the mitotic cell death pathway, and not to an increased level of apoptosis (Foray et al., 1999). In one study, initial treatment with chemotherapy reduced the risk of contralateral breast cancer by 60%, and its greatest effect was apparent within 2 years of treatment. At 10 years, the beneficial effect was lost (Narod et al., 2000). It was suggested that chemotherapy eradicates prevalent, sub-clinical cancers. The perspective of specifically designed chemotherapeutic regimens is promising, as the prognosis of hereditary breast cancer may be worse than that of its non-inherited counterpart (Chapter 6).

Ovarian cancer

Several *in vitro* studies showed increased sensitivity of some ovarian cell-lines carrying mutated *BRCA1* alleles to various chemotherapeutic agents (Thangaraju et al., 2000). Supporting these data, the retrospective cohort study by Boyd et al. (2000) demonstrated that ovarian cancer among Ashkenazi Jewish *BRCA1/2* mutation carriers had a better outcome when compared with ovarian cancer in Ashkenazi Jewish non-carriers. Interestingly, although the hereditary and sporadic cancers presented with pathological and treatment (cisplatin-based regimens) characteristics that were remarkably similar, the *BRCA1/2*-associated cancers were more likely to be optimally cytoreduced at primary surgery, and hereditary cases had a significantly longer disease-free interval following primary chemotherapy ($P=0.001$). These data are compatible with the hypothesis of a more favourable response to chemotherapy among hereditary ovarian cancer cases (Boyd et al., 2000). No specific therapeutic approaches of *BRCA1/2*-related ovarian cancer have been proposed.

Perspectives and conclusion

Predictive genetics in oncology opens considerable perspectives in diagnostic and therapeutic approaches of cancer. Multiples issues still exist in the hereditary breast/ovarian cancer syndrome (Kuerer et al., 2000), but the perspective of preventive and screening procedures being potentially effective is very encouraging. Current recommendations for the management of *BRCA1/2* mutation carriers are mostly based on inferences and expert opinions and not on data from randomized controlled trials. Evaluation of the adherent to, or acceptance of, the preventive or surveillance recommendations is an important issue (Lerman et al., 2000). The existing options – both for prevention, early detection and treatment – should be clearly explained in the context of a dedicated counselling process, with the participation of all involved professionals (geneticist, oncologist, surgeon, gynaecologist). Personal characteristics of the proband, such as her experience with cancer within her family, her role within her own nuclear family, and her values and expectations of life, should play a central role in the decision-making process. A concerted multidisciplinary approach, with the application of results from, where possible, prospective studies in well-defined cohorts of *BRCA1* and *BRCA2* carriers, will allow the concerned individuals to fully benefit from this new approach to the medicine.

REFERENCES

Abbott DW, Freeman ML and Holt JT (1998). Double-strand break repair deficiency and radiation sensitivity in BRCA2 mutant cancer cells. *J Natl Cancer Inst* **90**: 978–85.

Armstrong K and Weber BL (2001). Breast cancer screening for high-risk women: too little, too late? *J Clin Oncol* **19**: 919–20.

Armstrong K, Eisen A and Weber B (2000). Assessing the risk of breast cancer. *N Engl J Med* **342**: 564–71.

Atkinson C, Warren R, Bingham SA and Day NE (1999). Mammographic patterns as a predictive biomarker of breast cancer risk: effect of tamoxifen. *Cancer Epidemiol Biomarkers Prev* **8**: 863–6.

Aziz S, Kuperstein G, Rosen B, et al (2001). A genetic epidemiological study of carcinoma of the fallopian tube. *Gynecol Oncol* **80**: 341–5.

Barakat R (1998). Tamoxifen and endometrial cancer: most cancers are early stage and highly curable. *Eur J Cancer* **34** (Suppl.): S49–50.

Barakat RR (1999). Screening for endometrial cancer in the patient receiving tamoxifen for breast cancer. *J Clin Oncol* **17**: 1967–8.

Barakat RR, Gilewski TA, Almadrones L, et al. (2000). Effect of adjuvant tamoxifen on the endometrium in women with breast cancer: a prospective study using office endometrial biopsy. *J Clin Oncol* **18**: 3459–63.

Bennett LM (1999). Breast cancer: genetic predisposition and exposure to radiation. *Mol Carcinog* **26**: 143–9.

Berchuck A, Schildkraut JM, Marks JR and Futreal PA (1999). Managing hereditary ovarian cancer risk. *Cancer* **86**: 1697–704.

Bergman L, Beelen ML, Gallee MP, Hollema H, Benraadt J and van Leeuwen FE (2000). Risk and prognosis of endometrial cancer after tamoxifen for breast cancer. *Lancet* **356**: 881–7.

Bhattacharyya A, Ear US, Koller BH, Weichselbaum RR and Bishop DK (2000). The breast cancer susceptibility gene BRCA1 is required for subnuclear assembly of Rad51 and survival following treatment with the DNA cross-linking agent cisplatin. *J Biol Chem* **275**: 23899–903.

Biggs PJ and Bradley A (1998). A step toward genotype-based therapeutic regimens for breast cancer in patients with BRCA2 mutations? *J Natl Cancer Inst* **90**: 951–3.

Bilimoria MM, Winchester DJ, Sener SF, Motykie G, Sehgal UL and Winchester DP (1999). Estrogen replacement therapy and breast cancer: analysis of age of onset and tumor characteristics. *Ann Surg Oncol* **6**: 200–7.

Blackwood MA and Weber BL (1998). BRCA1 and BRCA2: from molecular genetics to clinical medicine. *J Clin Oncol* **16**: 1969–77.

Borgen PI, Hill AD, Tran KN, et al. (1998). Patient regrets after bilateral prophylactic mastectomy. *Ann Surg Oncol* **5**: 603–6.

Boyd J, Sonoda Y, Federici MG, et al (2000). Clinicopathologic features of BRCA-linked and sporadic ovarian cancer. *J Am Med Assoc* **283**: 2260–5.

Breast Cancer Linkage Consortium (1999). Cancer risks in BRCA2 mutation carriers. *J Natl Cancer Inst* **91**: 1310–6.

Brekelmans CT, Seynaeve C, Bartels CC, et al. (2001). Effectiveness of breast cancer surveillance in BRCA1/2 gene mutation carriers and women with high familial risk. *J Clin Oncol* **19**: 924–30.

Brinton LA, Schairer C, Hoover RN and Fraumeni JF (1988). Menstrual factors and risk of breast cancer. *Cancer Invest* **6**: 245–54.

Brunet JS, Ghadirian P, Rebbeck TR, et al. (1998). Effect of smoking on breast cancer in carriers of mutant BRCA1 or BRCA2 genes. *J Natl Cancer Inst* **90**: 761–6.

Burhenne HJ, Burhenne LW, Goldberg F, et al. (1994). Interval breast cancers in the Screening Mammography Program of British Columbia: analysis and classification. *AJR Am J Roentgenol* **162**: 1067–71.

Burke W (2000). Oral contraceptives and breast cancer: a note of caution for high-risk women. *J Am Med Assoc* **284**: 1837–8.

Burke W, Daly M, Garber J, et al. (1997). Recommendations for follow-up care of individuals with an inherited predisposition to cancer. II. BRCA1 and BRCA2 Cancer Genetics Studies Consortium. *J Am Med Assoc* **277**: 997–1003.

Burstein HJ and Winer EP (2000). Primary care for survivors of breast cancer. *N Engl J Med* **343**: 1086–94.

Cauley JA, Norton L, Lippman ME, et al. (2001). Continued breast cancer risk reduction in postmenopausal women treated with raloxifene: 4-year results from the MORE trial. *Breast Cancer Res Treat* **65**: 125–34.

Chang J, Yang WT and Choo HF (1999). Mammography in Asian patients with BRCA1 mutations. *Lancet* **353**: 2070–1.

Chappuis PO, Nethercot V and Foulkes WD (2000). Clinico-pathological characteristics of BRCA1- and BRCA2-related breast cancer. *Semin Surg Oncol* **18**: 287–95.

Chlebowski RT (2000). Reducing the risk of breast cancer. *N Engl J Med* **343**: 191–8.

Chlebowski RT and McTiernan A (1999). Elements of informed consent for hormone replacement therapy in patients with diagnosed breast cancer. *J Clin Oncol* **17**: 130–42.

Chlebowski RT, Collyar DE, Somerfield MR and Pfister DG (1999). American Society of Clinical Oncology technology assessment on breast cancer risk reduction strategies: tamoxifen and raloxifene. *J Clin Oncol* **17**: 1939–55.

Clemons M and Goss P (2001). Mechanisms of disease: estrogen and the risk of breast cancer. *N Engl J Med* **344**: 276–85.

Cobleigh MA, Norlock FE, Oleske DM and Starr A (1999). Hormone replacement therapy and high S phase in breast cancer. *J Am Med Assoc* **281**: 1528–30.

Col NF, Hirota LK, Orr RK, Erban JK, Wong JB and Lau J (2001). Hormone replacement therapy after breast cancer: a systematic review and quantitative assessment of risk. *J Clin Oncol* **19**: 2357–63.

Colditz GA, Stampfer MJ, Willett WC, Hennekens CH, Rosner B and Speizer FE (1990). Prospective study of estrogen replacement therapy and risk of breast cancer in postmenopausal women. *J Am Med Assoc* **264**: 2648–53.

Coleman CN (1999). Molecular biology in radiation oncology. Radiation oncology perspective of BRCA1 and BRCA2. *Acta Oncol* **38** (Suppl. 13): S55–9.

Collaborative Group on Hormonal Factors in Breast Cancer (1996a). Breast cancer and hormonal contraceptives: collaborative reanalysis of individual data on 53 297 women with breast cancer and 100 239 women without breast cancer from 54 epidemiological studies. *Lancet* **347**: 1713–27.

Collaborative Group on Hormonal Factors in Breast Cancer (1996b). Breast cancer and hormonal contraceptives: further results. *Contraception* **54** (Suppl.): S1–106.

Collaborative Group on Hormonal Factors in Breast Cancer (1997). Breast cancer and hormone replacement therapy: collaborative reanalysis of data from 51 epidemiological studies of 52 705 women with breast cancer and 108 411 women without breast cancer. *Lancet* **350**: 1047–59.

Conley B, O'Shaughnessy J, Prindiville S, et al. (2000). Pilot trial of the safety, tolerability, and retinoid levels of N-(4-hydroxyphenyl) retinamide in combination with tamoxifen in patients at high risk for developing invasive breast cancer. *J Clin Oncol* **18**: 275–83.

Connor F, Bertwistle D, Mee PJ, et al. (1997). Tumorigenesis and a DNA repair defect in mice with a truncating Brca2 mutation. *Nat Genet* **17**: 423–30.

Costello AJ (2001). A randomized, controlled chemoprevention trial of selenium in familial prostate cancer: rationale, recruitment, and design issues. *Urology* **57** (Suppl. 1): S182–4.

Cummings SR, Eckert S, Krueger KA, et al. (1999). The effect of raloxifene on risk of breast cancer in postmenopausal women: results from the MORE randomized trial Multiple Outcomes of Raloxifene Evaluation. *J Am Med Assoc* **281**: 2189–97.

Cuzick J (2000). A brief review of the current breast cancer prevention trials and proposals for future trials. *Eur J Cancer* **36**: 1298–302.

Day R, Ganz PA, Costantino JP, Cronin WM, Wickerham DL and Fisher B (1999). Health-related quality of life and tamoxifen in breast cancer prevention: a report from the National Surgical Adjuvant Breast and Bowel Project P-1 Study. *J Clin Oncol* **17**: 2659–69.

Delaloge S, Morice P, Chompret A and Lhomm C (2000). Prophylactic surgery: oophorectomy or adnexectomy? *J Clin Oncol* **18**: 3454–5.

Den Otter W, Merchant TE, Beijerinck D and Koten JW (1996). Breast cancer induction due to mammographic screening in hereditarily affected women. *Anticancer Res* **16**: 3173–5.

DePriest PD, Gallion HH, Pavlik EJ, Kryscio RJ and Van Nagell JR (1997). Transvaginal sonography as a screening method for the detection of early ovarian cancer. *Gynecol Oncol* **65**: 408–14.

Dickson MJ and Pandiarajan T (2001). Tamoxifen and risk of endometrial cancer. *Lancet* **357** 67–8.

Dunning AM, Healey CS, Pharoah PD, Teare MD, Ponder BA and Easton DF (1999). A systematic review of genetic polymorphisms and breast cancer risk. *Cancer Epidemiol Biomarkers Prev* **8**: 843–54.

Early Breast Cancer Trialists' Collaborative Group (1996). Ovarian ablation in early breast cancer: overview of the randomised trials. *Lancet* **348**: 1189–96.

Early Breast Cancer Trialists' Collaborative Group (1998). Tamoxifen for early breast cancer: an overview of the randomised trials. *Lancet* **351**: 1451–67.

Eckhardt S, Badellino F and Murphy GP (1994). UICC meeting on breast-cancer screening in pre-menopausal women in developed countries. Geneva, 29 September–1 October 1993. *Int J Cancer* **56**: 1–5.

Eeles RA and Powles TJ (2000). Chemoprevention options for BRCA1 and BRCA2 mutation carriers. *J Clin Oncol* **18** (Suppl.): S93–9.

Eisen A and Weber BL (1999). Prophylactic mastectomy: the price of fear. *N Engl J Med* **340**: 137–8.

Eisen A, Rebbeck TR, Lynch HT, et al. (2000a). Reduction in breast cancer risk following bilateral prophylactic oophorectomy in BRCA1 and BRCA2 mutation carriers. *Am J Hum Genet* **67** (Suppl. 2): S58.

Eisen A, Rebbeck TR, Wood WC and Weber BL (2000b). Prophylactic surgery in women with a hereditary predisposition to breast and ovarian cancer. *J Clin Oncol* **18**: 1980–95.

Eisinger F, Alby N, Bremond A, et al. (1998). Recommendations for medical management of hereditary breast and ovarian cancer: the French National Ad Hoc Committee. *Ann Oncol* **9**: 939–50.

Eisinger F, Burke W and Sobol H (1999a). Management of women at high genetic risk of ovarian cancer. *Lancet* **354**: 1648.

Eisinger F, Geller G, Burke W and Holtzman NA (1999b). Cultural basis for differences between US and French clinical recommendations for women at increased risk of breast and ovarian cancer. *Lancet* **353**: 919–20.

Eisinger F, Julian-Reynier C, Sobol H, Stoppa-Lyonnet D, Lasset C and Nogues C (2000). Acceptability of prophylactic mastectomy in cancer-prone women. *J Am Med Assoc* **283**: 202–3.

Eldar S, Meguid MM and Beatty JD (1984). Cancer of the breast after prophylactic subcutaneous mastectomy. *Am J Surg* **148**: 692–3.

Evron E, Dooley WC, Umbricht, et al. (2001). Detection of breast cancer cells in ductal lavage fluid by methylation-specific PCR. *Lancet* **357**: 1335–6.

Fallowfield L, Fleissig A, Edwards R, et al. (2001). Tamoxifen for the prevention of breast cancer: psychosocial impact on women participating in two randomized controlled trials. *J Clin Oncol* **19**: 1885–92.

Fan S, Wang J, Yuan R, et al. (1999). BRCA1 inhibition of estrogen receptor signaling in transfected cells. *Science* **284**: 1354–6.

Fisher B (1999). National Surgical Adjuvant Breast and Bowel Project breast cancer prevention trial: a reflective commentary. *J Clin Oncol* **17**: 1632–9.

Fisher B, Costantino JP, Wickerham DL, et al. (1998). Tamoxifen for prevention of breast cancer: report of the National Surgical Adjuvant Breast and Bowel Project P-1 Study. *J Natl Cancer Inst* **90**: 1371–88.

Fisher B, Powles TJ and Pritchard KJ (2000). Tamoxifen for the prevention of breast cancer. *Eur J Cancer* **36**: 142–50.

Fishman DA and Cohen LS (2000). Is transvaginal ultrasound effective for screening asymptomatic women for the detection of early-stage epithelial ovarian carcinoma? *Gynecol Oncol* 77: 347–9.

Foray N, Randrianarison V, Marot D, Perricaudet M, Lenoir G and Feunteun J (1999). Gamma-rays-induced death of human cells carrying mutations of BRCA1 or BRCA2. *Oncogene* **18**: 7334–42.

Franceschi S, Parazzini F, Negri E, et al. (1991). Pooled analysis of 3 European case-control studies of epithelial ovarian cancer. III. Oral contraceptive use. *Int J Cancer* **49**: 61–5.

Frost MH, Schaid DJ, Sellers TA, et al. (2000). Long-term satisfaction and psychological and social function following bilateral prophylactic mastectomy. *J Am Med Assoc* **284**: 319–24.

Gaffney DK, Brohet RM, Lewis CM, et al. (1998). Response to radiation therapy and prognosis in breast cancer patients with BRCA1 and BRCA2 mutations. *Radiother Oncol* **47**: 129–36.

Gail M and Rimer B (1998). Risk-based recommendations for mammographic screening for women in their forties. *J Clin Oncol* **16**: 3105–14.

Gail MH, Brinton LA, Byar DP, et al. (1989). Projecting individualized probabilities of developing breast cancer for white females who are being examined annually. *J Natl Cancer Inst* **81**: 1879–86.

Gail MH, Costantino JP, Bryant J, et al. (1999). Weighing the risks and benefits of tamoxifen treatment for preventing breast cancer. *J Natl Cancer Inst* **91**: 1829–46.

Gauthier-Villars M, Gad S, Caux V, Pages S, Blandy C and Stoppa-Lyonnet D (1999). Genetic testing for breast cancer predisposition. *Surg Clin North Am* **79**: 1171–87.

Gerber B, Krause A, Muller H, et al. (2000). Effects of adjuvant tamoxifen on the endometrium in postmenopausal women with breast cancer: a prospective long-term study using transvaginal ultrasound. *J Clin Oncol* **18**: 3464–70.

Gilliland FD, Joste N, Stauber PM, et al. (2000). Biologic characteristics of interval and screen-detected breast cancers. *J Natl Cancer Inst* **92**: 743–9.

Gilson E (1997). Benefits and risks of screening mammography in women with BRCA1 and BRCA2 mutations. *J Am Med Assoc* **278**: 289–90.

Goodnight JE, Quagliana JM and Morton DL (1984). Failure of subcutaneous mastectomy to prevent the development of breast cancer. *J Surg Oncol* **26**: 198–201.

Goss PE and Strasser K (2001). Aromatase inhibitors in the treatment and prevention of breast cancer. *J Clin Oncol* **19**: 881–94.

Gotzsche PC and Olsen O (2000). Is screening for breast cancer with mammography justifiable?. *Lancet* **355**: 129–34.

Gowen LC, Avrutskaya AV, Latour AM, Koller BH and Leadon SA (1998). BRCA1 required for transcription-coupled repair of oxidative DNA damage. *Science* **281**: 1009–12.

Grabrick DM, Hartmann LC, Cerhan JR, et al. (2000). Risk of breast cancer with oral contraceptive use in women with a family history of breast cancer. *J Am Med Assoc* **284**: 1791–8.

Grann VR, Panageas KS, Whang W, Antman KH and Neugut AI (1998). Decision analysis of prophylactic mastectomy and oophorectomy in BRCA1-positive or BRCA2-positive patients. *J Clin Oncol* **16**: 979–85.

Grann VR, Sundararajan V, Jacobson JS, et al. (2000). Decision analysis of tamoxifen for the prevention of invasive breast cancer. *Cancer J Sci Am* **6**: 169–78.

Greenwald P (2001). Clinical trials of breast and prostate cancer prevention. *J Nutr* **131** (Suppl.), S176–8.

Gudas JM, Nguyen H, Li T and Cowan KH (1995). Hormone-dependent regulation of BRCA1 in human breast cancer cells. *Cancer Res* **55**: 4561–5.

Hankinson SE, Hunter DJ, Colditz GA, et al. (1993). Tubal ligation, hysterectomy, and risk of ovarian cancer. A prospective study. *J Am Med Assoc* **270**: 2813–8.

Hartmann LC, Schaid DJ, Woods JE, et al. (1999a). Efficacy of bilateral prophylactic mastectomy in women with a family history of breast cancer. *N Engl J Med* **340**: 77–84.

Hartmann LC, Sellers TA, Schaid DJ, et al. (1999b). Clinical options for women at high risk for breast cancer. *Surg Clin North Am* **79**: 1189–206.

Hatcher MB, Fallowfield L and A'Hern R (2001). The psychosocial impact of bilateral prophylactic mastectomy: prospective study using questionnaires and semistructured interviews. *BMJ* **322**: 76–9.

Hedenfalk I, Duggan D, Chen Y, et al. (2001). Gene-expression profiles in hereditary breast cancer. *N Engl J Med* **344**: 539–48.

Helvie MA, Roubidoux MA, Weber BL and Merajver SD (1997). Mammography of breast carcinoma in women who have mutations of the breast cancer gene BRCA1: initial experience. *AJR Am J Roentgenol* **168**: 1599–602.

Hendrick RE, Smith RA, Rutledge JH and Smart CR (1997). Benefit of screening mammography in women aged 40–49: a new meta-analysis of randomized controlled trials. *J Natl Cancer Inst Monogr* **22**: 87–92.

Hilakivi-Clarke L (2000). Estrogens, BRCA1, and breast cancer. *Cancer Res* **60**: 4993–5001.

Hirayama T and Wynder E (1962). Study of epidemiology of cancer of the breast: influence of hysterectomy. *Cancer* **15**: 28–38.

Hughes KS, Papa MZ, Whitney T and McLellan R (1999). Prophylactic mastectomy and inherited predisposition to breast carcinoma. *Cancer* **86**: 2502–16.

Huo Z, Giger ML, Wolverton DE, Zhong W, Cumming S and Olopade OI (2000). Computerized analysis of mammographic parenchymal patterns for breast cancer risk assessment: feature selection. *Med Phys* **27**: 4–12.

Husain A, He G, Venkatraman ES and Spriggs DR (1998). BRCA1 up-regulation is associated with repair-mediated resistance to cis-diaminedichloroplatinum(II). *Cancer Res* **58**: 1120–3.

Jacobs IJ, Skates SJ, MacDonald N, et al (1999). Screening for ovarian cancer: a pilot randomised controlled trial. *Lancet* **353**: 1207–10.

Jernström H, Lerman C, Ghadirian P, et al. (1999). Pregnancy and risk of early breast cancer in carriers of BRCA1 and BRCA2. *Lancet* **54**: 1846–50.

Jordan VC (2000). Tamoxifen: a personal retrospective. *Lancet Oncol* **1**: 43–9.

Jordan VC and Assikis VJ (1995). Endometrial carcinoma and tamoxifen: clearing up a controversy. *Clin Cancer Res* **1**: 467–72.

Julian-Reynier C, Bouchard L, Evans DG, et al. (2001). Women's attitudes towards preventive strategies for hereditary breast/ovarian cancer risk differ from one country to another: differences among English, French and Canadian women. *Cancer* **92**: 959–68.

Karp SE, Tonin PN, Bégin LR, et al. (1997). Influence of BRCA1 mutations on nuclear grade and estrogen receptor status of breast carcinoma in Ashkenazi Jewish women. *Cancer* **80**: 435–41.

Kavanagh AM, Mitchell H and Giles GG (2000). Hormone replacement therapy and accuracy of mammographic screening. *Lancet* **355**: 270–4.

Kerlikowske K, Grady D, Rubin SM, Sandrock C and Ernster VL (1995). Efficacy of screening mammography. A meta-analysis. *J Am Med Assoc* **273**: 149–54.

Kerlikowske K, Grady D, Barclay J, Sickles EA and Ernster V (1996). Effect of age, breast density, and family history on the sensitivity of first screening mammography. *J Am Med Assoc* **276**: 33–8.

Khanna KK and Jackson SP (2001). DNA double-strand breaks: signaling, repair and the cancer connection. *Nat Genet* **27**: 247–54.

King MC, Wieand S, Hale K, et al. (2001). Tamoxifen and breast cancer incidence among women with inherited mutations in BRCA1 and BRCA2: National Surgical Adjuvant Breast and Bowel Project (NSABP-P1) Breast Cancer Prevention Trial. *J Am Med Assoc* **286**: 2251–6.

Klijn JG, Janin N, Cortes-Funes H and Colomer R (1997). Should prophylactic surgery be used in women with a high risk of breast cancer? *Eur J Cancer* **33**: 2149–59.

Kuerer HM, Hwang ES, Anthony JP, et al. (2000). Current national health insurance coverage policies for breast and ovarian cancer prophylactic surgery. *Ann Surg Oncol* **7**: 325–32.

Kuhl CK, Schmutzler RK, Leutner CC, et al. (2000). Breast MR imaging screening in 192 women proved or suspected to be carriers of a breast cancer susceptibility gene: preliminary results. *Radiology* **215**: 267–79.

Labrie F, Labrie C, Belanger A, et al. (1999). EM–652 (SCH 57068), a third generation SERM acting as pure antiestrogen in the mammary gland and endometrium. *J Steroid Biochem Mol Biol* **69**: 51–84.

Lakhani SR, Jacquemier J, Sloane JP, et al. (1998). Multifactorial analysis of differences between sporadic breast cancers and cancers involving BRCA1 and BRCA2 mutations. *J Natl Cancer Inst* **90**: 1138–45.

Lasset C, Bonadona V, Mignotte H and Bremond A (2001). Tamoxifen and risk of endometrial cancer. *Lancet* **357**: 66–7.

Laya MB, Larson EB, Taplin SH and White E (1996). Effect of estrogen replacement therapy on the specificity and sensitivity of screening mammography. *J Natl Cancer Inst* **88**: 643–9.

Leong T, Whitty J, Keilar M, et al. (2000). Mutation analysis of BRCA1 and BRCA2 cancer predisposition genes in radiation hypersensitive cancer patients. *Int J Radiat Oncol Biol Phys* **48**: 959–65.

Lerman C and Schwartz M (1993). Adherence and psychological adjustment among women at high risk for breast cancer. *Breast Cancer Res Treat* **28**: 145–55.

Lerman C, Daly M, Sands C, et al. (1993). Mammography adherence and psychological distress among women at risk for breast cancer. *J Natl Cancer Inst* **85**: 1074–80.

Lerman C, Hughes C, Croyle RT, et al. (2000). Prophylactic surgery decisions and surveillance practices one year following BRCA1/2 testing. *Prev Med* **31**: 75–80.

Lesko SM, Rosenberg L, Kaufman DW, et al. (1985). Cigarette smoking and the risk of endometrial cancer. *N Engl J Med* **313**: 593–96.

Lippman SM and Brown PH (1999). Tamoxifen prevention of breast cancer: an instance of the fingerpost. *J Natl Cancer Inst* **91**: 1809–19.

Lippman SM, Lee JJ and Sabichi AL (1998). Cancer chemoprevention: progress and promise. *J Natl Cancer Inst* **90**: 1514–28.

Lotan R (1996). Retinoids in cancer chemoprevention. *FASEB J* **10**: 1031–9.

Love RR, Wiebe DA, Feyzi JM, Newcomb PA and Chappell RJ (1994). Effects of tamoxifen on cardiovascular risk factors in postmenopausal women after 5 years of treatment. *J Natl Cancer Inst* **86**: 1534–9.

Lynch HT, Lynch J, Conway T and Severin M (1994). Psychological aspects of monitoring high risk women for breast cancer. *Cancer* **74**: 1184–92.

Mamounas EP (2000). Breast cancer chemoprevention. *Hematol Oncol Clin North Am* **14**: 727–38.

Mandelson MT, Oestreicher N, Porter PL, et al. (2000). Breast density as a predictor of mammographic detection: comparison of interval- and screen-detected cancers. *J Natl Cancer Inst* **92**: 1081–7.

Marks JR, Huper G, Vaughn JP, et al. (1997). BRCA1 expression is not directly responsive to estrogen. *Oncogene* **14**: 115–21.

Marquis ST, Rajan JV, Wynshaw-Boris A, et al. (1995). The developmental pattern of Brca 1 expression implies a role in differentiation of the breast and other tissues. *Nat Genet* **11**: 17–26.

Marsh F and Mayfield M (2001). Tamoxifen and risk of endometrial cancer. *Lancet* **357**: 68.

Matloff ET, Shappell H, Brierley K, Bernhardt BA, McKinnon W and Peshkin BN (2000). What would you do? Specialists' perspectives on cancer genetic testing, prophylactic surgery, and insurance discrimination. *J Clin Oncol* **18**: 2484–92.

McCaskill-Stevens W, Hawk ET, Flynn PJ and Lippman SM (1999). National Cancer Institute-supported cancer chemoprevention research: coming of age. *J Clin Oncol* **17**: 53–62.

Mehta RG (2000). Experimental basis for the prevention of breast cancer. *Eur J Cancer* **36**: 1275–82.

Meijer WJ and van Lindert AC (1992). Prophylactic oophorectomy. *Eur J Obstet Gynecol Reprod Biol* **47**: 59–65.

Meijers-Heijboer EJ, Verhoog LC, Brekelmans CT, et al. (2000). Presymptomatic DNA testing and prophylactic surgery in families with a BRCA1 or BRCA2 mutation. *Lancet* **355**: 2015–20.

Metcalfe KA, Liede A, Hoodfar E, Scott A, Foulkes WD and Narod SA (2000). An evaluation of needs of female BRCA1 and BRCA2 carriers undergoing genetic counselling. *J Med Genet* **37**: 866–74.

Miller AB, To T, Baines CJ and Wall C (2000). Canadian National Breast Screening Study-2, 13-year results of a randomized trial in women aged 50–59 years. *J Natl Cancer Inst* **92**: 1490–9.

Mittra I, Baum M, Thornton H and Houghton J (2000). Is clinical breast examination an acceptable alternative to mammographic screening? *BMJ* **321**: 1071–3.

Møller P, Evans G, Haites N, et al. (1999a). Guidelines for follow-up of women at high risk for inherited breast cancer: consensus statement from the Biomed 2 Demonstration Programme on Inherited Breast Cancer. *Dis Markers* **15**: 207–11.

Møller P, Reis MM, Evans G, et al. (1999b). Efficacy of early diagnosis and treatment in women with a family history of breast cancer European Familial Breast Cancer Collaborative Group. *Dis Markers* **15**: 179–86.

Morice P, Pautier P, Mercier S, et al. (1999). Laparoscopic prophylactic oophorectomy in women with inherited risk of ovarian cancer. *Eur J Gynaecol Oncol* **20**: 202–4.

Nabhan C and Bergan R (2001). Chemoprevention in prostate cancer. *Cancer Treat Res* **106**: 103–36.

Narod SA (1998). Host susceptibility to cancer progression. *Am J Hum Genet* **63**: 1–5.

Narod SA and Dubé MP (2001). Biologic characteristics of interval and screen-detected breast cancers. *J Natl Cancer Inst* **93**: 151.

Narod SA, Goldgar D, Cannon-Albright L, et al. (1995). Risk modifiers in carriers of BRCA1 mutations. *Int J Cancer* **64**: 394–8.

Narod SA, Risch H, Moslehi R, et al. (1998). Oral contraceptives and the risk of hereditary ovarian cancer. Hereditary Ovarian Cancer Clinical Study Group. *New Engl J Med* **339**: 424–8.

Narod SA, Brunet JS, Ghadirian P, et al. (2000). Tamoxifen and risk of contralateral breast cancer in BRCA1 and BRCA2 mutation carriers: a case-control study. *Lancet* **356**: 1876–81.

Narod SA, Pal Y, Graham T, Mitchell M and Fyles A (2001a). Tamoxifen and risk of endometrial cancer. *Lancet* **357**: 65–6.

Narod SA, Sun P, Ghadirian P, et al. (2001b). Tubal ligation and the risk of ovarian cancer in carriers of BRCA1 or BRCA2 mutations. *Lancet* **357**: 1467–70.

Nathanson KN, Wooster R and Weber BL (2001). Breast cancer genetics: what we know and what we need. *Nat Med* **7**: 552–6.

Neal DE, Leung HY, Powell PH, Hamdy FC and Donovan JL (2000). Unanswered questions in screening for prostate cancer. *Eur J Cancer* **36**: 1316–21.

NIH Consensus Conference (1995). Ovarian cancer. Screening, treatment, and follow-up. NIH Consensus Development Panel on Ovarian Cancer. *J Am Med Assoc* **273**: 491–7.

Osborne MP (1999). Chemoprevention of breast cancer. *Surg Clin North Am* **79**: 1207–21.

Osin P, Crook T, Powles T, Peto J and Gusterson B (1998). Hormone status of in-situ cancer in BRCA1 and BRCA2 mutation carriers. *Lancet* **351**: 1487.

Paley PJ, Swisher EM, Garcia RL, et al. (2001). Occult cancer of the fallopian tube in BRCA-1 germline mutation carriers at prophylactic oophorectomy: a case for recommending hysterectomy at surgical prophylaxis. *Gynecol Oncol* **80**: 176–80.

Parazzini F, Braga C, La Vecchia C, Negri E, Acerboni S and Franceschi S (1997). Hysterectomy, oophorectomy in premenopause, and risk of breast cancer *Obstet Gynecol* **90**: 453–6.

Peer PG, Verbeek AL, Straatman H, Hendriks JH and Holland R (1996). Age-specific sensitivities of mammographic screening for breast cancer. *Breast Cancer Res Treat* **38**: 153–60.

Pennisi VR and Capozzi A (1989). Subcutaneous mastectomy data: a final statistical analysis of 1500 patients. *Aesthetic Plast Surg* **13**: 15–21.

Phillips KA (2000). Immunophenotypic and pathologic differences between BRCA1 and BRCA2 hereditary breast cancers. *J Clin Oncol* **18** (Suppl.): S107–12.

Pierce LJ, Strawderman M, Narod SA, et al. (2000). Effect of radiotherapy after breast-conserving treatment in women with breast cancer and germline BRCA1/2 mutations. *J Clin Oncol* **18**: 3360–9.

Porter PL, El-Bastawissi AY, Mandelson MT, et al. (1999). Breast tumor characteristics as predictors of mammographic detection: comparison of interval- and screen-detected cancers. *J Natl Cancer Inst* **91**: 2020–8.

Powles T, Eeles R, Ashley S, et al. (1998). Interim analysis of the incidence of breast cancer in the Royal Marsden Hospital tamoxifen randomised chemoprevention trial. *Lancet* **352**: 98–101.

Rahman N and Stratton MR (1998). The genetics of breast cancer susceptibility. *Annu Rev Genet* **32**: 95–121.

Rajan JV, Marquis ST, Gardner HP and Chodosh LA (1997). Developmental expression of Brca2 colocalizes with Brca1 and is associated with proliferation and differentiation in multiple tissues. *Dev Biol* **184**: 385–401.

Rebbeck TR (2000). Prophylactic oophorectomy in BRCA1 and BRCA2 mutation carriers. *J Clin Oncol* **18** (Suppl): S100–3.

Rebbeck TR, Levin AM, Eisen A, et al. (1999). Breast cancer risk after bilateral prophylactic oophorectomy in BRCA1 mutation carriers. *J Natl Cancer Inst* **91**: 1475–9.

Ren Q, Potoczek MB, Krajewski S, et al. (2001). Transcriptional regulation of the Bcl-2 gene by wild type BRCA1 is important in regulating response to DNA damage-induced apoptosis. *Proc Am Assoc Cancer Res* **42**: 2991 (abstr.).

Ringash J (2001). Preventive health care, 2001 update: screening mammography among women aged 40–49 years at average risk of breast cancer. *CMAJ* **164**: 469–76.

Risch HA, McLaughlin JR, Cole DE, et al. (2001). Prevalence and penetrance of germline BRCA1 and BRCA2 mutations in a population series of 649 women with ovarian cancer. *Am J Hum Genet* **68**: 700–10.

Robson M, Levin D, Federici M, et al. (1999). Breast conservation therapy for invasive breast cancer in Ashkenazi women with BRCA gene founder mutations. *J Natl Cancer Inst* **91**: 2112–17.

Rosenblatt KA and Thomas DB (1996). Reduced risk of ovarian cancer in women with a tubal ligation or hysterectomy. The World Health Organization Collaborative Study of Neoplasia and Steroid Contraceptives. *Cancer Epidemiol Biomarkers Prev* **5**: 933–5.

Rosenthal A and Jacobs I (1998). Ovarian cancer screening. *Semin Oncol* **25**: 315–25.

Rossing MA, Cushing KL, Voigt LF, Wicklund KG and Daling JR (2000). Risk of papillary thyroid cancer in women in relationship to smoking and alcohol consumption. *Epidemiology* **11**: 49–54.

Runowicz CD (2000). Gynecologic surveillance of women on tamoxifen: first do no harm. *J Clin Oncol* **18**: 3457–8.

Salazar H, Godwin AK, Daly MB, et al. (1996). Microscopic benign and invasive malignant neoplasms and a cancer-prone phenotype in prophylactic oophorectomies. *J Natl Cancer Inst* **88**: 1810–20.

Schairer C, Lubin J, Troisi R, Sturgeon S, Brinton L and Hoover R (2000). Menopausal estrogen and estrogen–progestin replacement therapy and breast cancer risk. *J Am Med Assoc* **283**: 485–91.

Schrag D, Kuntz KM, Garber JE and Weeks JC (1997). Decision analysis: effects of prophylactic mastectomy and oophorectomy on life expectancy among women with BRCA1 or BRCA2 mutations. *N Engl J Med* **336**: 1465–71.

Schrag D, Kuntz KM, Garber JE and Weeks JC (2000). Life expectancy gains from cancer prevention strategies for women with breast cancer and BRCA1 or BRCA2 mutations. *J Am Med Assoc* **283**: 617–24.

Schuurman AG, van den Brandt PA and Goldbohm RA (1995). Exogenous hormone use and the risk of postmenopausal breast cancer: results from The Netherlands Cohort Study. *Cancer Causes Control* **6**: 416–24.

Semiglazov VF, Sagaidak VN, Moiseyenko VM and Mikhailov EA (1993). Study of the role of breast self-examination in the reduction of mortality from breast cancer. The Russian Federation/World Health Organization Study. *Eur J Cancer* **29A**: 2039–46.

Sharan SK, Morimatsu M, Albrecht U, et al. (1997). Embryonic lethality and radiation hypersensitivity mediated by Rad51 in mice lacking Brca2. *Nature* **386**: 804–10.

Sickles EA (2000). Breast imaging: from 1965 to the present. *Radiology* **215**: 1–16.

Smith RA (2000). Breast cancer screening among women younger than age 50: a current assessment of the issues. *CA Cancer J Clin* **50**: 312–36.

Spicer DV and Pike MC (2000). Future possibilities in the prevention of breast cancer: luteinizing hormone-releasing hormone agonists. *Breast Cancer Res* **2**: 264–7.

Stephan C, Jung K, Lein M, Sinha P, Schnorr D and Loening SA (2000). Molecular forms of prostate-specific antigen and human kallikrein 2 as promising tools for early diagnosis of prostate cancer. *Cancer Epidemiol Biomarkers Prev* **9**: 1133–47.

Suh-Burgmann EJ and Goodman A (1999). Surveillance for endometrial cancer in women receiving tamoxifen. *Ann Intern Med* **131**: 127–35.

Tabar L, Duffy SW and Burhenne LW (1993). New Swedish breast cancer detection results for women aged 40–49. *Cancer* **72**: 1437–48.

Thangaraju M, Kaufmann SH and Couch FJ (2000). BRCA1 facilitates stress-induced apoptosis in breast and ovarian cancer cell lines. *J Biol Chem* **275**: 33487–96.

Thomas DB, Gao DL, Self SG, et al. (1997). Randomized trial of breast self-examination in Shanghai: methodology and preliminary results. *J Natl Cancer Inst.* **89**: 355–65.

Thompson D and Easton D (2001). Variation in cancer risks, by mutation position, in BRCA2 mutation carriers. *Am J Hum Genet* **68**: 410–9.

Tirkkonen M, Johannsson O, Agnarsson BA, et al. (1997). Distinct somatic genetic changes associated with tumor progression in carriers of BRCA1 and BRCA2 germ-line mutations. *Cancer Res* **57**: 1222–7.

Ursin G, Pike MC, Spicer DV, Porrath SA and Reitherman RW (1996). Can mammographic densities predict effects of tamoxifen on the breast? *J Natl Cancer Inst* **88**: 128–9.

Ursin G, Henderson BE, Haile RW, et al. (1997). Does oral contraceptive use increase the risk of breast cancer in women with BRCA1/BRCA2 mutations more than in other women? *Cancer Res* **57**: 3678–81.

Ursin G, Astrahan MA, Salane M, et al. (1998). The detection of changes in mammographic densities. *Cancer Epidemiol Biomarkers Prev* **7**: 43–7.

Vaidya JS and Baum M (1997). Benefits and risks of screening mammography in women with BRCA1 and BRCA2 mutations. *J Am Med Assoc* **278**: 290.

van Nagell J, DePriest PD, Reedy MB, et al. (2000). The efficacy of transvaginal sonographic screening in asymptomatic women at risk for ovarian cancer. *Gynecol Oncol* **77**: 350–6.

Vasen HF, Haites NE, Evans DG, et al. (1998). Current policies for surveillance and management in women at risk of breast and ovarian cancer: a survey among 16 European family cancer clinics. European Familial Breast Cancer Collaborative Group. *Eur J Cancer* **34**: 1922–6.

Verheijen RH, von Mensdorff-Pouilly S, van Kamp GJ and Kenemans P (1999). CA 125: fundamental and clinical aspects. *Semin Cancer Biol* **9**: 117–24.

Verheul HA, Coelingh-Bennink HJ, Kenemans P, et al. (2000). Effects of estrogens and hormone replacement therapy on breast cancer risk and on efficacy of breast cancer therapies. *Maturitas* **36**: 1–17.

Veronesi U, Maisonneuve P, Costa A, et al. (1998). Prevention of breast cancer with tamoxifen: preliminary findings from the Italian randomised trial among hysterectomised women. Italian Tamoxifen Prevention Study. *Lancet* **352**: 93–7.

Veronesi U, De Palo G, Marubini E, et al. (1999). Randomized trial of fenretinide to prevent second breast malignancy in women with early breast cancer. *J Natl Cancer Inst* **91**: 1847–56.

Vogel VG (2000). Breast cancer prevention: a review of current evidence. *CA Cancer J Clin* **50**: 156–70.

Wagner TM, Moslinger R, Langbauer G, et al. (2000). Attitude towards prophylactic surgery and effects of genetic counselling in families with BRCA mutations. Austrian Hereditary Breast and Ovarian Cancer Group. *Br J Cancer* **82**: 1249–53.

Wapnir IL, Rabinowitz B and Greco RS (1990). A reappraisal of prophylactic mastectomy. *Surg Gynecol Obstet* **171**: 171–84.

Warner E, Foulkes W, Goodwin P, et al. (1999). Prevalence and penetrance of BRCA1 and BRCA2 gene mutations in unselected Ashkenazi Jewish women with breast cancer. *J Natl Cancer Inst* **91**: 1241–7.

Weber BL, Punzalan C, Eisen A, et al. (2000). Ovarian cancer risk reduction after bilateral prophylactic oophorectomy (BPO) in BRCA1 and BRCA2 mutation carriers. *Am J Hum Genet* **67** (Suppl. 2): S59.

Weinreb JC and Newstead G (1995). MR imaging of the breast. *Radiology* **196**: 593–610.

Welcsh PL, Schubert EL and King MC (1998). Inherited breast cancer: an emerging picture. *Clin Genet* **54**: 447–58.

Whittemore AS, Harris R and Itnyre J (1992). Characteristics relating to ovarian cancer risk: collaborative analysis of 12 US case-control studies. II. Invasive epithelial ovarian cancers in white women Collaborative Ovarian Cancer Group. *Am J Epidemiol* **136**: 1184–203.

Willett WC, Colditz G and Stampfer M (2000). Postmenopausal estrogens: opposed, unopposed, or none of the above. *J Am Med Assoc* **283**: 534–5.

Willis DB, Calle EE, Miracle-McMahill HL and Heath CW (1996). Estrogen replacement therapy and risk of fatal breast cancer in a prospective cohort of postmenopausal women in the United States. *Cancer Causes Control* **7**: 449–57.

Wolk A, Andersson SO, Mantzoros CS, Trichopoulos D and Adami HO (2000). Can measurements of IGF-1 and IGFBP-3 improve the sensitivity of prostate-cancer screening? *Lancet* **356**: 1902–3.

Woods JE (1983). Subcutaneous mastectomy: current state of the art. *Ann Plast Surg* **11**: 541–50.

Ziegler LD and Kroll SS (1991). Primary breast cancer after prophylactic mastectomy. *Am J Clin Oncol* **14**: 451–4.

Zweemer RP, van Diest PJ, Verheijen RH, et al. (2000). Molecular evidence linking primary cancer of the fallopian tube to BRCA1 germline mutations. *Gynecol Oncol* **76**: 45–50.

16

Management of familial ovarian cancer

Dirk Brinkmann and Ian Jacobs

St Bartholomew's and The Royal London School of Medicine & Dentistry, London, UK

Should the management of familial ovarian cancer differ from that of sporadic ovarian cancer?

The management of familial ovarian cancer (FOC) is currently essentially the same as for sporadic ovarian cancer, but is FOC biologically different from sporadic ovarian cancer and should we be managing it differently? There is some conflicting evidence. Greggi examined eight families with two or more first-degree relatives affected with epithelial ovarian cancer (EOC) among a series of 138 consecutive ovarian cancer patients. No significant difference was detected in clinical and pathological features between sporadic and familial cases. Papillary serous adenocarcinoma was the predominant histological type. However, in three high-risk families, EOC tended to develop at a younger age compared with other familial cases and with sporadic cancers, and nulliparity was less frequent in the familial group (Greggi et al., 1990). Similarly, Bewtra identified 37 FOC patients from FOC syndrome kindreds with documented cancers of the ovary, breast, colon or endometrium in two or more first-degree relatives. The age and clinical stage at diagnosis and overall 5-year survival of FOC patients were compared with those of sporadic EOC patients. The mean age of FOC patients at diagnosis was significantly lower (50.2 years) than that of the unselected control population (59 years) ($P < 0.001$). Histologically, all (100%) FOC tumours were EOC, with a predominance of serous papillary type, moderate to high grade (89 vs 71% in control; $P = 0.07$). No other pathological features appeared to be significant (Bewtra et al., 1992). Chang described the characteristics of patients with FOC and their response rates to chemotherapy and 5-year survival, and compared them with matched controls with sporadic ovarian cancer. There were 28 cases of FOC presenting to the Royal Marsden Hospital, London, from January 1983 to September 1993. The incidence of FOC over this time-period was 2.2% (28/1268). There was a statistically significant difference in histological subtype: 83% of patients with FOC had serous cystadenocarcinoma compared with 49% in the matched control group ($P = 0.0025$). However, there were no differences in median age or FIGO (Federation of Gynaecology and Obstetrics) stage between patients with FOC and the sporadic cases and no difference in overall response to chemotherapy or 5-year survival (Chang et al., 1995). Rubin, however, found improved survival in FOC patients. He identified 53 patients with germline mutations of *BRCA1*. The average age at diagnosis was 48 years (range 28–78). Histologically, 43 out of the 53 patients showed serous adenocarcinoma. They included three tumours of low malignant potential (borderline). With a median follow-up among survivors of 71 months from diagnosis, 20 patients had died of ovarian cancer, 27 had no evidence of the disease, 4 were alive with the disease, and 2 had died of other diseases. Actuarial median survival for the 43 patients with advanced-stage disease was 77 months, compared with 29 months for the matched controls ($P < 0.001$) (Rubin et al., 1996). Zweemer compared 42 confirmed cases of EOC with 84 matched controls. The median survival in the familial cases was 10 months longer than in the matched controls (Zweemer et al., 1999). Boyd found that the hereditary group had a longer disease-free interval following primary chemotherapy in comparison with the non-hereditary group, with a median time to recurrence of 14 months and 7 months, respectively ($P < 0.001$). Those with hereditary cancers had improved survival compared with the non-hereditary group ($P = 0.004$). For stage III cancers, *BRCA* mutation status was an independent prognostic variable ($P = 0.03$). They concluded that, although *BRCA*-associated hereditary ovarian cancers have surgical and pathological characteristics similar to those of sporadic cancers, advanced-stage hereditary cancer patients survive for longer than non-hereditary cancer patients (Boyd et al., 2000).

Presentation

A patient with FOC may present in a number of ways. The peak incidence of sporadic ovarian cancer is 40–60 years of age. Familial ovarian cancer has an earlier average age of onset, but cancers under 40 years of age are still uncommon (Bewtra et al., 1992; Boyd et al., 2000). Ovarian tumours rarely give rise to specific symptoms at an early stage, the commonest being vague gastrointestinal disturbance such as dyspepsia or increased abdominal girth. A result of this is that the majority of patients still present as stage III disease with spread to the abdominal cavity. It is the aim of screening to be able to identify the disease before it has spread from its primary site of origin, i.e. stage 1A, as one is then able to cure the majority of patients. More and more patients with FOC are presenting via some sort of screening programme.

Special investigations

- Ultrasound
- Tumour markers
- Cross-sectional imaging: magnetic resonance imaging (MRI), CT scan

Transvaginal ultrasound has a high sensitivity for detecting adnexal pathology. The main features that would raise one's index of suspicion for cancer are: complexity of the mass, solid components, papillary protrusions into cysts, fixity, increased blood flow on Doppler imaging – particularly if intratumoural – bilaterality and the presence of ascites or metastatic deposits. Ultrasound also has a high specificity. The results of an ultrasound scan are usually combined with a CA125 level to give a composite score or weighting. In a general population, with an overall low incidence of ovarian cancer and a relatively high incidence of benign adnexal pathology, the positive predictive value of a 'positive' scan is relatively low at about 20%. Stated another way, one is subjecting about five women to surgery for every cancer detected (Jacobs et al., 1999; Aslam et al., 2000). In an FOC population where the ratio of benign to malignant tumours would be expected to be higher, one would expect the screening tests to perform better. Good data on screening in an FOC population don't exist. A randomized screening trial would be unethical in such a high-risk population. The results of a prospective trial – the UK Familial Ovarian Cancer Screening Study – will be eagerly awaited. This aims to recruit 5000 volunteers with a family history of ovarian cancer and offer them screening in the form of transvaginal ultrasound scanning and a CA125 test.

Cross-sectional imaging in the form of CT scanning or MRI can provide valuable additional information, particularly as regards preoperative staging. Ovarian cancer staging is primarily a surgical one. However, if the preoperative imaging were to suggest intra-parenchymal liver or pulmonary metastases, this might alter the decision as to whether or not to operate.

Management

Management is broadly divided into:

1 Surgery
2 Chemotherapy
3 Neoadjuvant chemotherapy with interval debulking
4 Palliative care

Surgery

Prophylactic surgery will be dealt with later. The aim of surgery is to remove as much of the disease as possible and stage it completely. The standard operation for this is a laparotomy via a subumbilical midline incision and a total abdominal hysterectomy, bilateral salpingo-oophorectomy, infra-colic omentectomy, washings and selected biopsies. In cases where there is extensive peritoneal spread of disease, surgically removing the majority bulk of the disease appears to provide some benefits to the patient as regards response to subsequent chemotherapy and possibly a small survival benefit (Griffiths, 1975; Griffiths et al., 1979; Hacker et al., 1983; Goodman et al., 1992; Hoskins et al., 1992; Hunter et al., 1992; Curtin et al., 1997). During the past two decades, maximum cytoreductive surgery (also called debulking surgery) has been the recommended surgical approach for advanced stages of ovarian carcinoma. The residual tumour volume after surgery is one of the strongest prognostic factors, and only patients who undergo complete or optimal surgery are likely to be long-term survivors (Allen et al., 1995; Munkarah et al., 1997). A well-trained surgeon in the field of gynaecological oncology can achieve an optimal tumour reduction in up to 75% of patients with advanced-stage ovarian cancer.

In a small subset of patients, particularly the younger patients with apparent stage Ia disease, it may be possible to perform a unilateral salpingo-oophorectomy with appropriate staging in an attempt to preserve subsequent fertility. In FOC, this conservative approach would be counter-intuitive as one would not be able to fully stage the patient and there would be an 'at-risk' ovary left behind.

Chemotherapy

- Platinum-based chemotherapy
- Taxanes
- Combination chemotherapy

In advanced-stage ovarian cancer, long-term survival is unusual. However, many patients achieve a significant response to chemotherapy with a significant disease-free interval.

Until the mid-1970s, standard therapy for ovarian carcinoma was a single alkylating agent, typically melphelan. Subsequently, combination chemotherapy was shown to be superior to such therapy. During the 1980s, cisplatin-based combination chemotherapy became the standard chemotherapy regimen for advanced ovarian cancer; however, other classes of agents with documented activity against ovarian tumours appeared to be cross-resistant with platinum (Vogl et al., 1979). The introduction of paclitaxel in the early 1990s, with its apparent lack of cross-resistance with platinum compounds, was a notable advance in ovarian cancer management. During the 1990s, the combination of platinum (cisplatin or carboplatin) plus paclitaxel rapidly evolved into front-line chemotherapy for advanced ovarian cancer. The series of randomized phase III studies that have compared the activity of platinum/paclitaxel with alternative regimens supports the combination of platinum/paclitaxel as the current standard chemotherapy for advanced ovarian cancer. Outstanding issues that stem from this phase III experience include the impact of non-protocol salvage regimens on survival and the potential benefits of sequential single-agent regimens (Advanced Ovarian Cancer Trialists' Group, 2000).

Neoadjuvant chemotherapy with interval debulking

This involves establishing the diagnosis via a biopsy. This is then followed by between three and six cycles of chemotherapy, followed by an interval debulking operation as for primary surgery. Retrospective analyses suggest that a subgroup of patients with stage III and IV ovarian carcinoma can be managed in this way. The indications for neoadjuvant chemotherapy appear to be stage IV disease or extensive stage III disease where optimal debulking appears unlikely (Lawton et al., 1989; Jacob et al., 1991; Schwartz et al., 1994; Onnis et al., 1996; Vergote et al., 1998; Eisenkop et al., 1999; Vergote et al., 2000). Interval debulking surgery in patients with suboptimal primary debulking surgery has been proven effective in increasing overall survival and progression-free survival in a large, prospective, randomized trial of the European Organization for Research and Treatment of Cancer (van der Burg et al., 1995). The same group is assessing the strategy of neoadjuvant chemotherapy, followed by interval debulking surgery, in a prospective randomized trial.

Another trial, OVO6, assesses the role of interval debulking surgery in newly diagnosed ovarian cancer patients with residual macroscopic disease after surgery. Many patients are left with residual disease after surgery. Despite advances in chemotherapy, the prognosis for these patients is poor and a new surgical strategy for improving survival rates would be an important contribution.

Palliative care

As most patients present with advanced disease, and long-term survival in this group is unusual, palliative care is assuming a growing role. A full discussion is beyond the scope of this chapter. Two specific problems should be mentioned: abdominal distention due to ascites, which may require repeated ascitic taps, and bowel obstruction, which not infrequently requires defunctioning bowel surgery.

Prevention

The combined oral contraceptive pill (COCP) has a protective effect against ovarian cancer when used for 5 years, with a 50% reduction in risk. Narod enrolled 207 women with hereditary ovarian cancer and 161 of their sisters as controls in a case-control study. All of the patients carried a pathogenic mutation in either

BRCA1 (179 women) or *BRCA2* (28 women). Lifetime histories of oral-contraceptive use were obtained by interview or by written questionnaire and were compared between patients and control women, after adjustment for year of birth and parity. The adjusted odds ratio (OR) for ovarian cancer associated with any past use of oral contraceptives was 0.5 (95% CI, 0.3–0.8). The risk decreased with increasing duration of use ($P > 0.001$); use for 6 or more years was associated with a 60% reduction in risk. Oral-contraceptive use protected against ovarian cancer both for carriers of the *BRCA1* mutation (OR 0.5; 95% CI, 0.3–0.9) and for carriers of the *BRCA2* mutation (OR 0.4; 95% CI, 0.2–1.1) (Narod et al., 1998). There is some evidence to suggest that use of the COCP may slightly increase the risk of breast cancer. Although this is a small effect, it may be more significant in breast/ovarian cancer families. Tamoxifen, which is used for primary chemoprophylaxis against breast cancer, and to reduce recurrence, has no overall effect on the incidence or behaviour of ovarian cancer. However, its use is associated with an increased risk of endometrial cancer. Other agents currently undergoing evaluation are the retinoids and progestins (levonorgestrel).

Prophylaxis

Some patients with familial ovarian cancer syndromes have a lifetime cumulative risk of developing ovarian cancer of 60–70%. In these situations, a prophylactic bilateral oophorectomy is warranted. Prophylactic oophorectomy is divided into primary prophylactic surgery, where apparently normal ovaries are removed, and secondary prophylactic surgery, where ovaries are removed at surgery for a benign condition. The main dilemma lies in the correct timing of the procedure, how the procedure is performed and whether a concomitant hysterectomy should be performed.

One needs to weigh up the balance of waiting, and thereby possibly risking the development of cancer, versus performing an early oophorectomy and leaving the patient prematurely hypo-oestrogenic. One would then need to address the issue of hormone replacement therapy (HRT). There is some evidence to suggest that the prolonged use of HRT is associated with an increased risk of breast cancer. In an extended follow-up of the participants in the Nurses' Health Study, Colditz found that the risk of breast cancer was significantly increased among women who were currently using oestrogen alone (relative risk (RR), 1.32; 95% CI, 1.14–1.54) or oestrogen plus progestins (RR, 1.41; 95% CI, 1.15–1.74) when compared with postmenopausal women who had never used hormones. Women currently taking hormones, who had used such therapy for 5–9 years, had an adjusted relative risk of breast cancer of 1.46 (95% CI, 1.22–1.74). Those currently using hormones, who had done so for a total of 10 or more years, had a relative risk of 1.46 (95% CI,

1.20–1.76). The increased risk of breast cancer associated with 5 or more years of postmenopausal hormone therapy was greater among older women (RR for women aged 60–64 years, 1.71; 95% CI, 1.34–2.18). The RR of death due to breast cancer was 1.45 (95% CI, 1.01–2.09) among women who had taken oestrogen for 5 or more years (Colditz et al., 1995). We believe that women who undergo prophylactic oophorectomy and are rendered prematurely hypo-oestrogenic are at increased risk of cardiovascular disease and osteoporosis. We feel that giving HRT until the age of the natural menopause does not increase their risk of breast cancer and protects them from the adverse effects of being hypo-oestrogenic.

In a special report, Schrag et al. (1997) calculated that, on average, 30-year-old women who carry *BRCA1* or *BRCA2* mutations gain 2.9–5.3 years of life expectancy from prophylactic mastectomy and 0.3–1.7 years of life expectancy from prophylactic oophorectomy, depending on their cumulative risk of cancer. Gains in life expectancy declined with age at the time of prophylactic surgery and were minimal for 60-year-old women. Among 30-year-old women, oophorectomy could be delayed for 10 years with little loss of life expectancy. On the basis of a range of estimates of cancer incidence, prognosis, and efficacy of prophylactic surgery, this model suggests that prophylactic mastectomy provides substantial gains in life expectancy, and prophylactic oophorectomy more limited gains, for young women with *BRCA1* or *BRCA2* mutations.

The preferred surgical procedure in our unit is a laparoscopic bilateral salpingo-oophorectomy without a concomitant hysterectomy. We believe that the fallopian tubes have an 'at-risk' epithelium and should be removed. A concomitant hysterectomy increases the operating time, increases the short-term morbidity of the operation and, we believe, adversely affects bowel and bladder function. The laparoscope also allows an adequate assessment of the overall peritoneal surface.

The age at which we would recommend oophorectomy depends on the overall lifetime risk of developing cancer. Virtually all studies show that the incidence of ovarian cancer increases strikingly only after age 40 years. Mutations in *BRCA2* may confer a lower risk of ovarian cancer than mutations in *BRCA1* (Ford et al., 1994; Goldberg et al., 1997; Boyd et al., 2000).

Tobacman initially raised the question of primary peritoneal carcinoma. Prophylactic oophorectomy was performed in 28 female members of 16 families at high risk of ovarian carcinoma. Of these women, three subsequently developed disseminated intra-abdominal malignancy where there was uncertainty about the primary site, despite extensive investigation. These tumours were indistinguishable histopathologically from ovarian carcinoma. It would seem that, in cancer-prone families, the susceptible tissue is not limited to the ovary, but includes other derivatives of the coelomic epithelium, from which primary peritoneal adenocarcinomas may arise (Tobacman et al., 1982). The records from the Gilda

Radner Familial Ovarian Cancer Registry were reviewed for instances of prophylactic oophorectomy and cases of primary peritoneal carcinoma occurring after prophylactic oophorectomy. As a preventive measure against the subsequent development of ovarian cancer, 324 women in 931 families underwent prophylactic oophorectomy. Primary peritoneal carcinoma, indistinguishable histologically from primary ovarian adenocarcinoma, developed in six of these women 1–27 years after prophylactic oophorectomy (Piver et al., 1993).

In families where a mutation in *BRCA1/2* was demonstrated, Berchuck would recommend prophylactic oophorectomy in mutation carriers. In addition, he recommended that oophorectomy should also be considered in women aged over 35 years with germline mutations in DNA-repaired genes (hereditary non-polyposis colon cancer) undergoing laparotomy for colonic resection or other indications (Berchuck et al., 1999a). Berchuck questioned the value of oophorectomy in mutation carriers. It was at first thought that the lifetime risk of ovarian cancer in *BRCA* carriers was as high as 60%. More recent studies have suggested risks in the range of 15–30%. In addition, peritoneal papillary serous carcinoma that is indistinguishable from ovarian cancer occurs in some women after oophorectomy. He felt that, in view of the uncertainty regarding the efficacy of prophylactic oophorectomy, chemopreventive and early detection approaches also deserved consideration as strategies for decreasing ovarian cancer mortality in women who carry mutations in ovarian cancer susceptibility genes (Berchuck et al., 1999b).

Removed normal ovaries need to undergo careful histopathological analysis by an experienced pathologist who is interested in gynaecological pathology (Werness et al., 2000).

Counselling

Heritable cancer risk assessment is an increasingly common method of deriving valuable information relevant to deciding on appropriate screening regimens and preventive treatments. Assessments of heritable risk typically include familial–genetic evaluation, where analyses relate family pedigree to cancer risk, and DNA testing, where analyses indicate genetic mutations associated with cancer risk (e.g. *BRCA1/BRCA2* mutations) or their absence.

The first step in appropriate counselling is establishing risk. This involves taking a detailed family history to include three generations, with diagnosis, age of onset and, ideally, confirmation in the form of a death certificate or histology report. The probability that a patient carries an autosomal dominant germline mutation depends on this pedigree. If she has two affected first-degree relatives then they have a 66% risk of carrying the mutation. She will have a 50% risk of inheriting the gene if present, i.e. a 33% risk of carrying the gene. The lifetime risk of developing ovarian cancer in a carrier is 45%. Her risk is therefore 45% × 33% = 15%. If she were to have a live affected relative, then this would raise the possibility of genetic testing for *BRCA1/2* germline mutations. The first step is to identify a live affected relative and test for a mutation. If this is informative, one can then search for the mutation in the unaffected relative who is seeking counselling.

There is much talk about the psychological impact of counselling. In a paper reporting on the psychological responses of women given familial–genetic evaluations of ovarian cancer risk, sizeable differences were found in the prevalence of clinically significant depression (Ritvo et al., 2000). In a review, none of the 15 papers reviewed reported increased distress (general and situational distress, anxiety and depression) in carriers or non-carriers of heritable disease. Both carriers and non-carriers showed decreased distress after testing; this was greater and more rapid amongst non-carriers. The studies reviewed suggest that those undergoing predictive genetic testing do not experience adverse psychological consequences. However, most of the papers involved screening for Huntington's chorea and not FOC (Broadstock et al., 2000).

Conclusion

Patients who come from FOC families who have established ovarian cancer should be managed in the same way as those from sporadic ovarian cancer families. It may be that, with time, subtle biological differences will emerge. For the asymptomatic patient there are some very difficult decisions to make, particularly as regards genetic testing and prophylactic oophorectomy. The results of screening trials will hopefully go some way to help in making these decisions informed decisions.

REFERENCES

Advanced Ovarian Cancer Trialists' Group (2000). Chemotherapy for advanced ovarian cancer. *Cochrane Database Syst Rev* **2000**(2): CD001418.

Allen DG, Heintz AP and Touw FW (1995). A meta-analysis of residual disease and survival in stage III and IV carcinoma of the ovary. *Eur J Gynaecol Oncol* **16**(5): 349–56.

Aslam N, Banerjee S, Carr JV, et al. (2000). Prospective evaluation of logistic regression models for the diagnosis of ovarian cancer. *Obstet Gynecol* **96**(1): 75–80.

Berchuck A, Schildkraut JM, Marks JR, et al. (1999a). Managing hereditary ovarian cancer risk. *Cancer* **86** (11 Suppl.): 2517–24.

Berchuck A, Carney ME and Futreal PA (1999b). Genetic susceptibility testing and prophylactic oophorectomy. *Eur J Obstet Gynecol Reprod Biol* **82**(2): 159–64.

Bewtra C, Watson P, Conway T, et al. (1992). Hereditary ovarian cancer: a clinicopathological study. *Int J Gynecol Pathol* **11**(3): 180–7.

Boyd J, Sonoda Y, Federici MG, et al. (2000). Clinicopathologic features of BRCA-linked and sporadic ovarian cancer. *JAMA* **283**(17): 2260–5.

Broadstock M, Michie S and Marteau TM (2000). Psychological consequences of predictive genetic testing: a systematic review. *Eur J Hum Genet* **8**(10): 731–8.

Chang J, Fryatt I, Ponder B, et al. (1995). A matched control study of familial epithelial ovarian cancer: patient characteristics, response to chemotherapy and outcome. *Ann Oncol* **6**(1): 80–2.

Colditz GA, Hankinson SE, Hunter DJ, et al. (1995). The use of estrogens and progestins and the risk of breast cancer in postmenopausal women. *N Engl J Med* **332**(24): 1589–93.

Curtin JP, Malik R, Venkatraman ES, et al. (1997). Stage IV ovarian cancer: impact of surgical debulking. *Gynecol Oncol* **64**(1): 9–12.

Eisenkop SM, Spirtos NM and Friedman RL (1999). Neoadjuvant chemotherapy for advanced ovarian cancer. *Gynecol Oncol* **74**(2): 311–12.

Ford D, Easton DF, Bishop DT, et al. (1994). Risks of cancer in BRCA1-mutation carriers. Breast Cancer Linkage Consortium. *Lancet* **343**(8899): 692–5.

Goldberg JM, Piver MS, Jishi MF, et al. (1997). Age at onset of ovarian cancer in women with a strong family history of ovarian cancer. *Gynecol Oncol* **66**(1): 3–9.

Goodman HM, Harlow BL, Sheets EE, et al. (1992). The role of cytoreductive surgery in the management of stage IV epithelial ovarian carcinoma. *Gynecol Oncol* **46**(3): 367–71.

Greggi S, Genuardi M, Benedetti-Panici P, et al. (1990). Analysis of 138 consecutive ovarian cancer patients: incidence and characteristics of familial cases. *Gynecol Oncol* **39**(3): 300–4.

Griffiths CT (1975). Surgical resection of tumor bulk in the primary treatment of ovarian carcinoma. *Natl Cancer Inst Monogr* **42**: 101–4.

Griffiths CT, Parker LM and Fuller AF (1979). Role of cytoreductive surgical treatment in the management of advanced ovarian cancer. *Cancer Treat Rep* **63**(2): 235–40.

Hacker NF, Berek JS, Lagasse LD, et al. (1983). Primary cytoreductive surgery for epithelial ovarian cancer. *Obstet Gynecol* **61**(4): 413–20.

Hoskins WJ, Bundy BN, Thigpen JT, et al. (1992). The influence of cytoreductive surgery on recurrence-free interval and survival in small-volume stage III epithelial ovarian cancer: a Gynecologic Oncology Group study. *Gynecol Oncol* **47**(2): 159–66.

Hunter RW, Alexander ND and Soutter WP (1992). Meta-analysis of surgery in advanced ovarian carcinoma: is maximum cytoreductive surgery an independent determinant of prognosis? *Am J Obstet Gynecol* **166**(2): 504–11.

Jacob JH, Gershenson DM, Morris M, et al. (1991). Neoadjuvant chemotherapy and interval debulking for advanced epithelial ovarian cancer. *Gynecol Oncol* **42**(2): 146–50.

Jacobs IJ, Skates SJ, MacDonald N, et al. (1999). Screening for ovarian cancer: a pilot randomised controlled trial. *Lancet* **353**(9160): 1207–10.

Lawton FG, Redman CW, Luesley DM, et al. (1989). Neoadjuvant (cytoreductive) chemotherapy combined with intervention debulking surgery in advanced, unresected epithelial ovarian cancer. *Obstet Gynecol* **73**(1): 61–5.

Munkarah AR, Hallum AV, Morris M, et al. (1997). Prognostic significance of residual disease in patients with stage IV epithelial ovarian cancer. *Gynecol Oncol* **64**(1): 13–17.

Narod SA, Risch H, Moslehi R, et al. (1998). Oral contraceptives and the risk of hereditary ovarian cancer. Hereditary Ovarian Cancer Clinical Study Group. *N Engl J Med* **339**(7): 424–8.

Onnis A, Marchetti M, Padovan P, et al. (1996). Neoadjuvant chemotherapy in advanced ovarian cancer. *Eur J Gynaecol Oncol* **17**(5): 393–6.

Piver MS, Jishi MF, Tsukada Y, et al. (1993). Primary peritoneal carcinoma after prophylactic oophorectomy in women with a family history of ovarian cancer. A report of the Gilda Radner Familial Ovarian Cancer Registry. *Cancer* **71**(9): 2751–5.

Ritvo P, Robinson G, Irvine J, et al. (2000). Psychological adjustment to familial genetic risk assessment: differences in two longitudinal samples. *Patient Educ Couns* **40**(2): 163–72.

Rubin SC, Benjamin I, Behbakht K, et al. (1996). Clinical and pathological features of ovarian cancer in women with germ-line mutations of BRCA1. *N Engl J Med* **335**(19): 1413–16.

Schrag D, et al. (1997). Decision analysis – effects of prophylactic mastectomy and oophorectomy on life expectancy among women with BRCA1 or BRCA2 mutations. *N Engl Med* **336**(20): 1465–71.

Schwartz PE, Chambers JT and Makuch R (1994). Neoadjuvant chemotherapy for advanced ovarian cancer. *Gynecol Oncol* **53**(1): 33–7.

Tobacman JK, Greene MH, Tucker MA, et al. (1982). Intra-abdominal carcinomatosis after prophylactic oophorectomy in ovarian-cancer-prone families. *Lancet* **2**(8302): 795–7.

van der Burg ME, van Lent M, Buyse M, et al. (1995). The effect of debulking surgery after induction chemotherapy on the prognosis in advanced epithelial ovarian cancer. Gynecological Cancer Cooperative Group of the European Organization for Research and Treatment of Cancer. *N Engl J Med* **332**(10): 629–34.

Vergote I, De Wever I, Tjalma W, et al. (1998). Neoadjuvant chemotherapy or primary debulking surgery in advanced ovarian carcinoma: a retrospective analysis of 285 patients. *Gynecol Oncol* **71**(3): 431–6.

Vergote IB, De Wever I, Decloedt J, et al. (2000). Neoadjuvant chemotherapy versus primary debulking surgery in advanced ovarian cancer. *Semin Oncol* **27** (3 Suppl. 7): 31–6.

Vogl SE, Greenwald E, Kaplan BH, et al. (1979). Ovarian cancer. Effective treatment after alkylating-agent failure. *JAMA* **241**(18): 1908–11.

Werness BA, Ramus SJ, Whittemore AS, et al. (2000). Histopathology of familial ovarian tumors in women from families with and without germline BRCA1 mutations. *Hum Pathol* **31**(11): 1420–4.

Zweemer RP, Verheijen RH, Menko FH, et al. (1999). Differences between hereditary and sporadic ovarian cancer. *Eur J Obstet Gynecol Reprod Biol* **82**(2): 151–3.

17

Prophylactic mastectomy in mutation carriers

D. G. R. Evans[1], F. I. Lalloo[1] and A. D. Baildam[2]

[1]St Mary's Hospital, Manchester, UK
[2]Withington Hospital, Manchester, UK

Introduction

Management options available for women at high lifetime risk of breast cancer due to their family history, or carriage of a mutation in *BRCA1/2* (which confer a lifetime risk of breast cancer of 85% (Ford et al., 1994; Wooster et al., 1994) are limited. Screening with mammography or even magnetic resonance imaging (MRI) is one option, and this can be combined with entering trials of chemo-prevention. However, many women are now seriously considering or undertaking prophylactic mastectomy if found to be mutation carriers for *BRCA1* or *BRCA2*. The efficacy of surgical procedures to reduce the risk of breast cancer is controversial (Goodnight et al., 1984; Zeigler and Kroll, 1991), although it would appear that the residual risk of breast cancer is dependent upon the amount of remaining breast tissue following the surgical procedure. Recent work suggests that more women than previously are considering prophylactic mastectomy (JW et al., 1996; Lynch et al., 1997) and that protocols should be in place to deal with these requests. It has been suggested that surgery will increase life expectancy in *BRCA1* or *BRCA2* mutation carriers (Schrag et al., 1997). A recent study by Hartmann et al. (1999) has demonstrated that women with a high risk of breast cancer can significantly reduce the incidence of the disease with prophylactic surgery. However, the level of reduction in those at highest risk (*BRCA1/BRCA2* carriers) is still unclear.

Genetic counselling and the family history clinic

Breast cancer family history clinics started to be established in the UK in 1987 (Evans et al., 1996a,b) and these have burgeoned across Europe and North America. They are generally administered by consultants in medical oncology, clinical genetics and breast surgery, often with a multidisciplinary approach, with close involvement of radiologists, and a psychiatrist/psychologist. At these clinics, unaffected women at increased risk of breast cancer are assessed for their lifetime and shorter-term risks of breast cancer. In most family history clinics, the Cancer and Steroid Hormone study risk estimation is used (Claus et al., 1994) and can be supplemented with information about risks for relatives in *BRCA1* or *BRCA2* families (Ford et al., 1994, 1998). After assessing risks, women are presented with a number of choices, including regular surveillance usually with a combination of mammography and clinical examination, which could commence at 30–40 years depending on the age of cancers in the family and the overall risk (Evans et al., 1994; Eccles et al., 2000). Women are, in general, now split into three risk groups: average, moderate and high risk. It is only really in the high-risk group that prophylactic surgery would be considered. This usually equates to a lifetime risk of 1 in 4 (25%) or greater. As a rough guide, this equates to having a heterozygote risk of 1 in 4 with two relatives, including one first degree diagnosed with an average age of less than 50 years, or with three relatives aged less than 60 years. All affected relatives should be first-degree relatives or related through a male.

In a recent survey of 10 European centres (Evans et al., 1999), only three (Manchester, Edinburgh, Heidelberg/Dusseldorf) routinely mention the possibility of prophylactic mastectomy to those women with a lifetime risk of 1 in 4 or greater. This is often done with a single sentence or a statement of the availability of the procedure as an option for the prevention of breast cancer. This then allows women to extend the discussion if they wish to do so, or to state that they are not interested in surgery. However, many centres would only mention prophylactic surgery to potential mutation carriers who are undertaking a genetic test. Indeed, there appears to be a cultural shift across Europe from North to South where prophylactic mastectomy becomes less acceptable to both physician and patient (Julian-Reynier et al., 2000, 2001). In the US it is interesting that, where mastectomies were commonplace in the 1970s and 1980s (Hartmann et al., 1999), there appears to be less enthusiasm for this now, even amongst gene mutation carriers. What is absolutely clear is that adequate preparation of a woman for risk-reducing mastectomy is essential.

The prophylactic mastectomy protocol

If women wish to discuss the procedure in greater detail, most centres in our European survey offered a further appointment at least 1 month later. This gives women time to consider the procedure more fully and to discuss it with appropriate members of the family. Involvement of the partners is important and they can be invited to attend each appointment. At the second appointment, with the geneticist or oncologist, a basic description of the surgery is given, including the potential residual risk of various procedures. It is emphasized that the residual risk and complication rate may be higher if the surgery preserves the nipple/areolar complex. It is also usually made clear that these procedures are largely unproven (Goodnight et al., 1984; Zeigler and Kroll, 1991) as regards their efficacy in reducing the risk of breast cancer. The patient is also challenged to consider the complications, which may result in a potentially poor cosmetic result, as well as the possible impact upon her personal life and family dynamics.

The possibility of genetic testing is also discussed in terms of the availability of a living affected member of the family and the basic underlying structure of the family (Eeles, 1996). If possible, a time-scale for genetic testing is discussed, and the woman is asked to consider the potential impact of having proceeded with surgery, if she then undergoes genetic testing that shows that she does not carry the causative mutation. Centres also emphasize that the genetic risk of breast cancer decreases with age and that the remaining risk of breast cancer if the woman is older (over 40 years) is lower than the lifetime risk (Claus et al., 1994; Evans et al., 1994). If a woman wishes to proceed, a psychological assessment is arranged. At this stage, most centres proactively seek confirmation of the breast cancers in the family if they have not already done so. This ensures that the risk assessment is as accurate as possible. We have previously reported the presence of factitious histories within some families where women fabricate their family history in order to obtain surgery or are innocently implicated as being at risk by another family member (Evans et al., 1996a).

After a psychological assessment, a more detailed surgical consultation is arranged to discuss the type of procedure best suited to the woman and whether a one- or two-stage procedure is preferable. This would usually involve discussion of three basic options: (1) total bilateral mastectomy, (2) bilateral mastectomy with reconstruction, either with implants or tissue flaps, and (3) bilateral subcutaneous mastectomy that retains the overlying skin and nipple/areolar complex. The potential complications are also discussed together with the expected cosmetic result. Surgeons will usually have photographs available for women to view if they wish.

The whole process of consultations through to surgical procedure usually takes 6–12 months. This time delay is deliberate in most centres, with the greatest delay at the beginning of the protocol in order to allow women time for the decision-making process. If the protocol is run concurrently with a decision for predictive genetic testing, then the wait would generally be shorter. The number of women who are known to have undergone prophylactic surgery in each centre is shown in Table 17.1. The full protocol of two sessions at the family history clinic, a session with a psychiatrist and sessions with the surgeons was established in 1993 in Manchester. While only two other centres have a similar written protocol, the

Table 17.1. Number and type of prophylactic mastectomies carried out by centres

Centre	No.	Age (years)	Mean	SM	MM	Bilateral	Contralateral	BRCA1/2 cases
Manchester	116	21–60	40	25	91	100	16	19
Edinburgh	47	32–60	43	3	44	17	30	2
Aberdeen	22	34–58	43.5	6	16	20	2	4
Leiden	15	20–37	36.5	8	7	15	0	?
Dusseldorf	8	29–46	38	3	5	8	0	1
Oslo	12	27–51	39.5	6	6	11	1	0
Southampton	9	32–57	43.5	6	3	5	3	3
Belfast	11	32–57	40	11	0	5	6	1

MM, modified mastectomy; SM, simple mastectomy.

remaining clinics adhere to the basic principles in most instances. The major difference is that several centres are mainly reactive. Thus, prophylactic surgery would usually only be formally discussed in women proven to be *BRCA1/2* mutation carriers. No centre recommends the procedure, even in the latter category.

There was also no clear pattern in terms of the surgical procedure recommended in women who had decided on surgery. While some units were cautious about offering skin/nipple-preserving mastectomies, these options were generally available in every case.

Surgical technique

Women with *BRCA1/2* mutations carry that genotype in all cells, but those who develop cancer of the breast seldom develop multicentric disease. Like most women with sporadic breast cancer, they are more likely to have a unifocal breast cancer, but are at a much higher risk of bilateral cancers. The objective of surgery is to reduce the incidence of, and mortality from, breast cancer in women at high risk, and to do so in a way that is most consistent with quality of life and aesthetic concerns. Breast restorative procedures for women who undergo mastectomy for breast cancer have progressed rapidly, with significantly improved aesthetic results compared with those possible a decade ago. The use of skin-sparing mastectomy with immediate submuscular expander/implant or myocutaneous flap volume replacement is one such advance. Risk-reducing mastectomy has been developed using the techniques of skin-sparing surgery and volume replacement.

At all stages of operative planning, the patient must be involved in the decisions that are made. Women must be told that no operation will remove all risk, but risk reduction may be of the order of over 80%. Whether or not to conserve the nipple is controversial. Breast tissue immediately deep to the nipple/areolar complex (NAC) is uncommonly a site of primary breast cancer, but retention of this tissue must theoretically carry a slight diminution in risk reduction. With awareness of this, most women who undergo risk-reducing mastectomy with immediate reconstruction do request NAC preservation, but are warned that NAC sensory loss is likely and NAC ischaemic loss possible.

The operation described is the procedure developed and now most commonly requested by women from the Manchester Family Clinic. It comprises a skin-sparing mastectomy with NAC conservation when requested, and immediate breast volume replacement by means of submuscular tissue expansion.

At a second procedure some months later after tissue expansion in the clinic, the infra-mammary fold is recreated on each breast and the tissue expander replaced with permanent implants. This second procedure affords the best chance to adjust the aesthetic quality of the breast reconstructions such that, ideally, the woman will look as near-normal as possible, not only when wearing a bra but also when undressed. Pre- and postoperative photographs are mandatory.

Operative sequence

1 Positioning of the patient. The patient lies supine with both hands under her waist and with the shoulder and elbow slightly flexed.
2 Mastopexy-type skin incisions. These are made transversely across the outer half of the breast towards the axillary tail and extended around the areola and, depending on the size of the breast, medially for 11 cm. Otherwise, lower pole skin dropout looks unsightly and is difficult to correct.
3 Marking the incision. With removal of the skin in the mastopexy shape, a paper template can be made to orientate and mark the incision on the contralateral breast. De-epithelialized skin bridges are left in place around the upper half of the NAC, to preserve the subdermal vascular plexus. Transverse scars are used to enable direct access to all quadrants of the breast, including the peripheral upper outer quadrant and axillary tail.
4 Breast parenchyma removal. The breast is removed en bloc with the axillary tail, but the axillary lymph nodes as far as possible are left *in situ*. The breast is removed laterally at the lateral border of latissimus dorsi. The breast is weighed.
5 Submuscular expander. Once the submuscular pocket has been developed as far as possible the tissue expander is selected for size and shape to make the nearest

possible match with the removed breast. Its handling involves utmost precaution to prevent infection.

6 Outpatient care. Following discharge, the woman is seen in the outpatient clinic and the tissue expanders expanded with injected normal saline using a butterfly needle 23 gauge and a sterile technique. Up to 100 ml may be installed at any time, depending upon the tension in the overlying muscle and skin. For most women two expansions are sufficient, but occasionally more are needed. Following optimum expansion, the patient waits for three months so that maximum ptosis can develop.

7 The second procedure. The tissue expander is aspirated and removed. Where necessary to achieve better shape, an inferior and medial capsulotomy can be performed using bipolar scissors. The definitive prosthesis is selected and inserted. If the NAC has not been conserved, the NAC reconstruction followed by NAC tattoo is performed later under local anaesthetic.

Outcomes

The concept of a single operation to include mastectomy and reconstruction is an attractive ideal but seldom gives good cosmesis. This new technique allows development of the medial and inferior poles of the reconstructed breasts, together with the opportunity for accurate nipple placement. The aesthetic results of the two-stage process for most women are a significant improvement over a one-stage operation. The procedure has evolved by attention to detail to correct possible cosmetic inadequacies.

The cosmetic key is the match of the skin envelope surface area to that achievable by the expanded muscle pocket that constitutes the neo-breast mound. In any breast with natural, minor or moderate ptosis, a good match can be achieved if breast volume is not much larger than approximately 500 cm^3. If there is major ptosis, then infra-mammary fold de-epithelialization and shortening is essential if the nipple position is to be accurate whilst at the same time avoiding redundant inferior pole skin.

In a natural breast of greater than 700 cm^3 in size or with gross ptosis, nipple elevation using a mastopexy technique is not possible, and in these cases the nipple should be removed and reconstructed at a later date.

Complications were uncommon in this series. One patient underwent ischaemic NAC loss followed by infection of both tissue expanders. These were removed, but delayed reconstruction was successful 6 months later. In two cases, partial depigmentation of the natural NAC was corrected by tattoo.

This series has but short follow-up. Nevertheless, there have been no women so far diagnosed with any breast disease following surgery. There are potential psychosocial morbidities associated with this procedure, and those are the subject of an ongoing multicentre study in the UK to which many of these women have contributed.

Follow-up

Follow-up of women who have undergone surgery is considered to be an important part of the protocol. In Manchester, women who have undergone prophylactic mastectomy are followed up annually at a multidisciplinary day. As well as discussion of problems/issues with all the relevant clinicians (geneticist/oncologist/psychiatrist/surgeons), each patient is examined. Clinical examination by palpation of the breasts is felt to be adequate as remaining breast tissue is very superficial in all types of surgical procedure. No cancers occurred prospectively in the 174 women who had undergone surgery in the European group (Evans et al., 1999). Using data from Claus et al. (1994) and the International Linkage Consortium (Ford et al., 1994), it is possible to calculate annual age-dependent expected incidence rates for breast cancer in women who have not undergone surgery. The mean expected rate for our cohort of women was 1% annually, reflecting a lifetime risk that ranged from 25% to 80%. Even though this cohort already had a follow-up in excess of 400 woman years, only four cancers would have been expected. Follow-up of an extended cohort for more than 5 years will be necessary to address the issue of risk reduction. If this is to be analysed by type of surgery or by confining to known *BRCA1/2* mutation carriers only (17/174), even longer follow-up will be necessary.

Uptake

Our own data from Manchester have shown that 8–10% of women at 1 in 4 lifetime risk or above have sought further advice about risk-reducing mastectomy and 6% have proceeded, rising to 11% in those at 40% lifetime risk. Of those proven unaffected mutation carriers aged less than 60 years, 17 out of 35 (48%) have now opted for risk-reducing surgery (Lalloo et al., 2000). Results from the Netherlands show a similarly high uptake (52%) (Meijers-Heijboer et al., 2000). Thus far, two patients in our series and several in the Dutch series that initially opted not to have surgery have developed breast cancer, contrasting with none of the operated cases (Meijers-Heijboer et al., 2000).

REFERENCES

Claus EB, Risch N and Thompson WD (1994). Autosomal dominant inheritance of early-onset breast cancer; implications for risk prediction. *Cancer* **73**: 643–51.

Eccles DM, Evans DGR and Mackay J (2000). Guidelines for a genetic risk based approach to advising women with a family history of breast cancer. *J Med Genet* **37**: 203–9.

Eeles R 1996. Testing for the breast cancer predisposition gene, BRCA1. *Br Med J* **313**: 572–3.

Evans DGR, Fentiman IS, McPherson K, Asbury D, Ponder BAJ and Howell A (1994). Familial breast cancer. *Br Med J* **308**: 183–7.

Evans DGR, Cuzick J and Howell A (1996a). Cancer Genetics Clinics. *Eur J Cancer* **32**: 391–2.

Evans DGR, Kerr B, Cade D, Hoare E and Hopwood P (1996b). Fictitious breast cancer family history. *Lancet* **348**: 1034.

Evans DGR, Anderson E, Lalloo F, et al. (1999). Utilisation of preventative mastectomy in 10 European centres. *Disease Markers* **15**: 148–51.

Ford D, Easton DF, Bishop DT, Narod SA and Goldgar DE (1994). Risks of cancer in BRCA1-mutation carriers. *Lancet* **343**: 692–5.

Ford D, Easton M, Stratton S, et al. (1998). Genetic heterogeneity and penetrance analysis of the BRCA1 and BRCA2 genes in breast cancer families. *Am J Hum Genet* **62**: 676–89.

Goodnight JE, Quagliana JM and Morton DL (1984). Failure of subcutaneous mastectomy to prevent the development of breast cancer. *J Surg Oncol* **26**: 198–201.

Hartmann LC, Schiad DJ, Woods JE, et al. (1999). Efficacy of bilateral prophylactic mastectomy in women with a family history of breast cancer. *N Engl J Med* **340**: 77–84.

Julian-Reynier C, Eisinger F, Moatti J-P and Sobol H (2000). Physician's attitudes towards mammography and prophylactic surgery for hereditary breast/ovarian cancer risk and subsequently published guidelines. *Eur J Hum Genet* **8**: 204–8.

Julian-Reynier C, Bouchard L, Evans G, et al. (2001). Women's attitudes toward preventive strategies for hereditary breast/ovarian cancer risk differ from one country to another: differences between Manchester (UK), Marseilles (F) and Montreal (Ca). *Cancer* **92**: 959–68.

JW, Eeles R, Cole T, Taylor R, Lunt P and Baum M (1996). Prophylactic mastectomy for genetic predisposition to breast cancer: the proband's story. *Clin Oncol* **8**: 222–5.

Lalloo F, Baildam A, Brain A, Hopwood P, Howell A and Evans DGR (2000). Preventative mastectomy for women at high risk of breast cancer. *Eur J Surg Oncol* **26**: 711–13.

Lynch HT, Lemon SJ, Durham C, et al. (1997). A descriptive study of BRCA1 testing and reactions to disclosure of test results. *Cancer* **79**: 2219–28.

Meijers-Heijboer EJ, Verhoog LC, Brekelmans CTM, et al. (2000). Presymptomatic DNA testing and prophylactic surgery in families with a BRCA1 or BRCA2 mutation. *Lancet* **355**: 2015–20.

Schrag D, Kuntz KM, Garbor JE and Weeks JC (1997). Decision analysis – effects of prophylactic mastectomy and oophorectomy on life expectancy among women with BRCA1 or BRCA2 mutations. *N Engl J Med* **336**: 1465–71.

Wooster R, Neuhausen SL, Mangion J, et al. (1994). Localization of a breast cancer susceptibility gene, BRCA2, to chromosome 13q12–13. *Science* **265**: 2088–90.

Zeigler LD and Kroll SS (1991). Primary breast cancer after prophylactic mastectomy. *Am J Clin Oncol* **14**: 451–4.

18

Psychosocial aspects of genetic counselling for breast and ovarian cancer

Alison Bish[1] and Steven Sutton[2]

[1]Cancer Research UK, London
[2]Institute of Public Health, University of Cambridge, UK

Introduction

The population risk of developing breast cancer in the UK is 1 in 12 and the risk of ovarian cancer is 1 in 100. A small proportion (approximately 5–10%) of women who develop breast and ovarian cancers have an inherited genetic susceptibility to these cancers (Easton and Peto, 1990; Claus et al., 1991). To date, two breast and ovarian cancer predisposing genes have been identified: *BRCA1* (Miki et al., 1994; Easton et al., 1995; Narod et al., 1995) and *BRCA2* (Wooster et al., 1995). Women who have inherited a mutation in the *BRCA1* or *BRCA2* gene have approximately an 80% risk of developing breast cancer over their lifetime, particularly at a young age, and a 40%–60% lifetime risk of developing ovarian cancer (Easton et al., 1995).

Widespread publicity about the possible genetic basis of some breast and ovarian cancers has led to an increase in concern amongst women with a family history of these cancers. Increasing numbers of women are attending clinics in hospitals in the UK for genetic counselling about their family history of breast or ovarian cancer, where most will want information about their future risk of developing cancer (Brain et al., 2000a) and about what steps they can take to minimize this risk. A further motivation for attending for genetic counselling is to undergo genetic testing. Both risk counselling and genetic testing have psychosocial effects. An overview of these will be covered in this chapter, including the psychological impact of risk counselling and risk perceptions, and changes in these following counselling, attitudes towards genetic testing, and impact of test results on psychological state and behaviour.

Psychological distress associated with genetic counselling for breast/ovarian cancer

Relevant psychological issues have been raised and discussed regarding hereditary breast cancer (Lerman and Croyle, 1994). A point to note is that much of the current research work in this area is theoretical, and a variety of measures and inclusion criteria are used that make comparison between studies difficult. As studies have used different assessment tools for measuring psychological distress, apparent prevalence rates for distress vary (Hopwood et al., 1998), which has implications for clinicians who provide genetic counselling. A variety of measures are used. Some are specific to anxiety or depression (e.g. Hospital Anxiety and Depression Scale – Zigmond and Snaith, 1983; Beck Depression Inventory – Beck and Steer, 1987; State-Trait Anxiety Inventory – Spielberger et al., 1983), others assess more general psychiatric distress (e.g. General Health Questionnaire – Goldberg and Williams, 1988), and others are cancer specific, or can be adapted to be so (Cancer Worry Scale – Lerman et al., 1991; Impact of Events Scale – Horowitz et al., 1979).

What seems to be clear from the research is that women at risk of hereditary breast/ovarian cancer do suffer some level of psychological distress. Research in the USA has found that relatives of breast cancer patients, who are therefore at increased risk themselves, may suffer psychological distress (Wellisch et al., 1991; Kash et al., 1992). Twenty-seven per cent of the women in the study carried out by Kash et al. were suffering psychological distress that warranted psychological counselling. Some studies in the UK and USA have found that levels of anxiety and general distress among women at risk who are attending for genetic counselling are higher than those found in the general population (e.g. Lerman et al., 1994; Valdimarsdottir et al., 1995; Cull et al., 1999).

Some research has used standard measures, which give an indication of the proportion of women who can be classified as clinical cases in terms of their levels of anxiety, depression and general psychological distress, and has found fairly high proportions of individuals to be under stress. In a recent study it was found that 41% of the women had a possible anxiety disorder, as measured by the Hospital Anxiety and Depression Scale, and 11% had a possible depression disorder, prior to attending for genetic counselling (Bish et al., 2002). These proportions are comparable to those found in other studies of women undergoing genetic counselling for breast/ovarian cancer risk (e.g. Dudokdewit et al., 1998; Lodder et al., 1999; Kent et al., 2000). Other studies (e.g. Cull et al., 1999; Watson et al., 1999) have found approximately 30% of their sample of women undergoing genetic counselling to be classifiable as 'cases' on a psychiatric measure (General Health Questionnaire).

There is also growing research evidence that a substantial minority of women attending for genetic counselling suffer from specific worries about developing cancer (e.g. Brain et al., 1999; Bish et al., 2002). For example, in the study by Bish et al. (2002), 34% of women reported that they worry often or almost all the time about developing breast cancer. Worry about developing ovarian cancer amongst women attending for genetic counselling is rarely assessed, despite the fact that if women have a *BRCA1* or *BRCA2* mutation they are at a greatly increased lifetime risk of developing ovarian cancer. Worry about developing ovarian cancer tends to be found to be lower in studies where this has been assessed (e.g. Bish et al., 2002), probably due to the fact that it receives less media coverage than breast cancer and is less common.

Aside from the negative psychological impact of distress, raised levels of distress can have detrimental behavioural effects. Women who are distressed may fail to take in the information they have been given during counselling about risk and surveillance behaviours (Hopwood et al., 1998; Cull et al., 1999) and act on this information appropriately (Lerman et al., 1995). In addition, anxiety may diminish women's willingness to participate in screening and surveillance (Kash et al., 1992; Lerman et al., 1993) or may lead to excessive self-examination (Brain et al., 1999).

Genetic counselling may have positive effects on pre-existing levels of distress. Some of the few prospective studies that have examined how genetic counselling may influence levels of distress have found that general distress (Cull et al., 1999; Brain et al., 2000b) and cancer-specific worry (Bish et al., 2002; Brain et al., 2000b; Kent et al., 2000) reduce following counselling, although other research has found no change (Watson et al., 1999). However, the group in the study by Watson et al. was not split on the basis of their actual risk of developing cancer, which may be likely to influence level of worry, with those individuals at the most risk being least reassured by counselling.

A point to note is that much research is neither prospective nor includes a long-term follow-up. The advantage of prospective studies is that they enable the effect of counselling on pre-existing baseline anxiety, depression and specific worry to be examined. Longitudinal studies with a long-term follow-up enable an examination of whether any observed changes in distress are sustained in the long-term. Such information is obviously important for organizing clinical services and providing the care to individuals at the most appropriate time.

Psychological distress amongst previously affected women

Women who have already had and been treated for breast or ovarian cancer ('affected' women) make up a significant proportion of those being counselled in genetic centres. Evaluation of the psychological effects of genetic counselling among such affected women has been relatively neglected in the literature on psychological distress. The assumption seems to be that these women will be less distressed and worried in the face of being at increased risk as they have already had cancer and therefore received the 'worst possible news'. However, some research has found that in fact such women are more worried, particularly about developing ovarian cancer, and show raised perceptions of risk in comparison with unaffected women (Bish et al., 2002). Such findings indicate the need for sensitive counselling of these women.

Perceptions of risk

Most women with a family history of breast or ovarian cancer seem to have an unrealistic view of their risk of developing such cancers; whether this is pessimistic or optimistic varies from study to study. The variation seems to be due to the type of measures used. Some studies use comparative measures where women are asked to compare themselves with other women, while other studies use ratios where women are asked to select the ratio (e.g. 1 in 2, 1 in 100) that they believe corresponds with their risk. There is some evidence that women attending for genetic counselling over-estimate their risk before their consultation (Lerman et al., 1995). Lerman studied first-degree relatives of breast cancer patients (often the type of woman attending for genetic counselling) and found that 21% thought they were at a much higher risk of developing breast cancer than the average woman; 57% thought they were at higher risk and only 21% thought their risk was the same or less than the average woman. In a recent UK study (Bish et al., 2002) it was found that 47% of women attending for genetic counselling felt that their risk was slightly higher than other women, and a further 36% felt that it was much higher. Perceptions of the likelihood of carrying a genetic mutation were also elevated, with 43% of the women feeling that this was fairly likely and 20% extremely likely. Other research has found that women with a family history of breast cancer are as likely to under-estimate as over-estimate their risk (Evans et al., 1993) or indeed be more likely to under-estimate their risk (Cull et al., 1999). These studies used the same measure, which was selection of a ratio to assess perceived risk.

The aim of genetic counselling is to impart a realistic perception of risk so that women are able to make informed decisions about health management strategies, such as screening and surveillance. There is some evidence that genetic counselling can increase accuracy in perceptions of risk (e.g. Evans et al., 1994; Cull et al., 1999; Watson et al., 1999). Evans et al. (1994) found that improvements in accuracy were more common amongst those women who had previously over-estimated their risk. Watson et al. (1999) reported that, whilst there were initially good improvements in accuracy, at 1-year follow-up substantially fewer women were accurate. This is important to note as it may be that information is not retained for long enough to influence behaviour and screening intentions.

Genetic testing

Mutation searches and predictive testing

Before an individual who has not had cancer can be tested to determine whether or not they have inherited a susceptibility to breast or ovarian cancer, it is first necessary to undertake a germline mutation test. This involves taking a blood sample from a member of the family who has had breast or ovarian cancer and where there is a high chance of a genetic mutation. The *BRCA1* and *BRCA2* genes are then analysed to determine whether a mutation exists. If a mutation is found, a 'predictive test' will then be available for individuals in the family who have not had these types of cancer.

Genetic testing for the presence of mutations in *BRCA1* or *BRCA2* is still relatively new, and individuals undergoing genetic testing carry a substantial stress burden. If the results of the test are positive they cannot, of course, indicate when the disease will develop, or indeed whether it will, as the genes do not have full penetrance. Also, sporadic breast cancer risk factors are still present for these women (e.g. age of menarche, menopause, pregnancy and age).

Genetic testing also has implications for an individual's family, whose personal risk estimates will change as a result of a family member's test. In the case of predictive testing, children of an affected parent are at increased risk of having inherited the genetic mutation. Negative results may not provide relief if other family members have positive results, and guilt may be associated with worry about passing a gene on to children. Mutation searching also has implications for family members. Positive results will mean that close relatives' personal risk estimates change, whereas inconclusive results mean that no further testing can be carried out in the family. Research evidence for the psychological impact of test results is outlined below.

Attitudes towards testing

Reported intention to undergo genetic testing is high (e.g. Lerman et al., 1994; Lerman et al., 1995; Struewing et al., 1995; Meiser et al., 2000; Sutton et al., submitted for publication), with most research finding percentages over 75% saying that they would be tested (usually the questions are posited for hypothetical testing rather than in advance of an actual test, which may influence results). Some research has examined actual uptake of testing and shows that uptake is also high –

in most cases over 50% (Lynch et al., 1993; Valdimarsdottir et al., 1995; Watson et al., 1996; Dudokdewit et al., 1997). Such findings are in contrast to Huntington's disease, where reported interest in testing was found not to be matched by actual uptake. This discrepancy may be because of the lack of treatment for Huntington's disease and also its inevitability, as this gene has full penetrance. As uptake seems to be high for *BRCA1/2* testing, this has implications for support services. A variety of individuals may undergo testing and a greater proportion may have difficulty in adjusting to a bad news result. It may be the case that only those who felt able to cope with bad news underwent testing for Huntington's disease and that this is why the predicted catastrophic reactions to the results have not been borne out by research evidence.

A number of studies have examined motivations to undergo testing. The strongest motivations seem to be desire for certainty in order to plan for the future and to make informed decisions about screening and preventive options (e.g. Tessaro et al., 1997). A recent longitudinal UK study has examined factors that affect intentions to have a test (Sutton et al., submitted). Sutton et al. found that the strongest-held beliefs among women at risk of developing breast and ovarian cancer were that a test would make them aware of problems with their breasts before a cancer developed and that a test would give them certainty about whether or not they would develop cancer in the future. This latter belief was strongly associated with a high intention to have a test. In addition, the study also found that in deciding whether or not to have a genetic test, women would take into account what they thought their family would want them to do.

Brief note about gender differences

Most research focuses almost exclusively on women, as women make up the vast majority of those individuals seeking genetic counselling or being referred to such services. In addition, the cancers involved are more likely to affect women, in the case of breast cancer, and to exclusively affect women, in the case of ovarian cancer. Some research has also included men (e.g. Struewing et al., 1995) and has found that men tend to be more reluctant to undergo genetic testing. However, a point to note is that if potential male carriers are not tested, then the risk to their daughters could remain hidden. In addition, some research has found that women with sons do not see genetic testing as being advantageous for their children (Meiser et al., 2000).

Inconclusive results

Reduction of uncertainty is thought to be one of the major psychological benefits of genetic testing[1] (Dudokdewit et al., 1997). However, the results from a

---

[1] Uncertainty about developing breast cancer cannot be eliminated even with predictive testing as population risk remains and the gene does not have 100% penetrance.

mutation search can be far from conclusive. Whilst a positive finding is conclusive, if no mutation is found this does not indicate that there is no mutation in the family, as an as yet unidentified genetic mutation may be causing the cancer. This type of result is complex and may be difficult for patients to understand. Some research suggests that psychological distress is caused by 'not knowing', and that any result at all is beneficial. For example, Lerman et al. (1998) found that: (1) women who declined testing who had a high level of baseline distress were more distressed 1 month later; (2) there was no change in carriers; and (3) in non-carriers distress reduced. In the case of Huntington's disease, Wiggins et al. (1992) found that individuals who were tested for this disease who could not be given a result (or who declined to go ahead with the testing) scored higher on depression at 12 months in comparison with their baseline than those who were carriers or non-carriers.

Psychological impact of results

Studying the impact of receiving predictive test results for *BRCA1/2* is in its infancy. Research has tended to show that pre-existing mood is the best predictor of impact of *BRCA1/2* results rather than the result itself (Dudokdewit et al., 1998). It is therefore important to carry out prospective research in order to take into account pre-existing psychological state. Some studies have not found serious short-term psychological effects after undergoing *BRCA1/2* predictive testing (Lynch et al., 1993; Lerman et al., 1996). Lerman et al. (1996) found that non-carriers had a reduction in depression in comparison with carriers and non-tested individuals, but that carriers did not show any increase in distress at 1-month follow-up. Some research has found that the order of testing can be important. For example, Smith et al. (1999) found that women undergoing predictive *BRCA1* testing who were first in the family had the greatest adverse psychological conse-quences to the test result. In fact they found that levels of distress amongst carriers were higher than levels found amongst cancer patients shortly after diagnosis. Another important factor can be personal experience of cancer. Croyle et al. (1997) found that carriers had more cancer-related worries than non-carriers, the highest levels being amongst those carriers who had had no cancer themselves. General distress reduced after testing for both carriers and non-carriers, showing the clinical importance of using specific measures to examine levels of psychologi-cal distress as general assessments may fail to identify those in need of assistance. It is possible that, in the longer term, differences will not show. For example, Wiggins et al. (1992) found that carriers and non-carriers of the Huntington's gene differed immediately after receiving their result, differed less at 6 months and did not differ at all at 12 months.

Effect of results on behaviour

It is important to assess how the recipients perceive results as the result can have an impact on an individual's future behaviour. It is possible that the inconclusive result given for germline mutations for *BRCA1/2* may in fact be seen as a true negative result. Some preliminary research examining the psychological impact of an inconclusive result suggests that this may be the case (Bish et al., submitted for publication). There is a risk that if people test negative (or perhaps perceive that they have done so), then intentions to attend for screening may reduce (Bish et al., 2002) or they may fail to attend for surveillance and be breast aware (Lerman et al., 1996). Indeed, evidence from the USA would support this. Lerman et al. (2000) found that a year after receiving their test result large numbers of carriers were not attending for recommended breast and ovarian screening.

Conclusions

Individuals undergoing genetic counselling for breast and ovarian cancer may suffer psychological distress in terms of raised levels of anxiety and depression and specific worries about developing cancers. In addition, risk perceptions are likely to be inaccurate. Genetic counselling can help both to alleviate levels of distress and also to increase accuracy of risk perceptions. Interest in, and uptake of, genetic testing is high but preliminary research findings suggest that there is no serious psychological effect of testing. However, test results may have an impact on an individual's future willingness to participate in screening and surveillance. In view of the fact that this area is relatively new, further well-designed rigorous research is required to build on the findings available so far, in particular to explore the long-term psychological and behavioural effects of genetic testing on individuals and on their families.

REFERENCES

Beck A and Steer R (1987). *The Beck Depression Inventory Manual.* San Antonio, Texas: Psychological Corporation.

Bish A, Sutton S, Jacobs C, Levene S, Ramirez A and Hodgson S (2002). Changes in psychological distress after cancer genetic counselling: a comparison of affected and unaffected women. *Br J Canc* (in press).

Brain K, Norman P, Gray J and Mansel R (1999). Anxiety and adherence to breast self-examination in women with a family history of breast cancer. *Psychosom Med* **61**: 181–7.

Brain K, Gray J, Norman P, et al. (2000a). Why do women attend familial breast cancer clinics? *J Med Genet* **37**: 197–202.

Brain K, Gray J, Norman P, et al. (2000b). A randomised trial of a specialist genetic assessment service for familial breast cancer. *J Natl Cancer Inst* **92**(16): 1345–51.

Claus EB, Risch N and Thompson WD (1991). Genetic analysis of breast cancer in the cancer and steroid hormone study. *Am J Hum Genet* **48**(2): 232–42.

Croyle RT, Smith KR, Botkin JR, Baty B and Nash J (1997). Psychological responses to BRCA1 mutation testing: preliminary findings. *Health Psychol* **16**(1): 633–72.

Cull A, Anderson EDC, Campbell S, Mackay J, Smyth E and Steel M (1999). The impact of genetic counselling about breast cancer risk on women's risk perceptions and levels of distress. *Br J Cancer* **79**(3/4): 501–8.

Dudokdewit AC, Tibben A, Dujvenvoorden HJ, et al., Niermeijer MF, Passchier J and other members of the Rotterdam/Leiden Genetics Workgroup (1997). Psychological distress in applicants for predictive DNA testing for autosomal dominant, heritable, late onset disorders. *J Med Genet* **34**: 382–90.

Dudokdewit AC, Tibben A, Duivenvoorden HJ, Niermeijer MF, Passchier J and the other members of the Rotterdam/Leiden Genetics Workgroup (1998). Predicting adaption to pre-symptomatic DNA testing for late onset disorders: who will experience distress? *J Med Genet* **35**: 745–54.

Easton D and Peto J (1990). The contribution of inherited predisposition to cancer incidence. *Cancer Surv* **9**(3): 395–416.

Easton DF, Ford D, Bishop DT and the Breast Cancer Linkage Consortium (1995). Breast and ovarian cancer incidence in BRCA1 mutation carriers. *Am J Hum Genet* **56**: 265–71.

Evans DGR, Burnell LD, Hopwood P and Howell A (1993). Perception of risk in women with a family history of breast cancer. *Br J Cancer* **67**: 612–14.

Evans DGR, Blair V, Greenhalgh R, Hopwood P and Howell A (1994). The impact of genetic counselling on risk perception in women with a family history of breast cancer. *Br J Cancer* **70**: 934–8.

Goldberg D and Williams P (1988). *A User's Guide to the General Health Questionnaire*. Windsor, UK: NFER-Nelson.

Hopwood P, Keeling F, Long A, Pool C, Evans G and Howell A (1998). Psychological support needs for women at high genetic risk of breast cancer: some preliminary indicators. *Psycho-oncology* **7**: 402–12.

Horowitz M, Wilner N and Alvarez W (1979). Impact of event scale: a measure of subjective stress. *Psychosom Med* **41**(3): 209–18.

Kash KM, Holland JC, Halper MS and Miller DG (1992). Psychological distress and surveillance behaviors of women with a family history of breast cancer. *J Natl Cancer Inst* **84**(1): 24–30.

Kent G, Howie H, Fletcher M, Newbury-Ecob R and Hosie K (2000). The relationship between perceived risk, thought intrusiveness and emotional well-being in women receiving counselling for breast cancer risk in a family history clinic. *Br J Health Psychol* **5**(1): 15–26.

Lerman C and Croyle R (1994). Psychological issues in genetic testing for breast cancer susceptibility. *Arch Intern Med* **154**: 609–16.

Lerman C, Trock B, Rimer BK, Jepson C, Brody D and Boyce A (1991). Psychological side effects of breast cancer screening. *Health Psychol* **10**: 259–67.

Lerman C, Daly M, Sands C, et al. (1993). Mammography adherence and psychological distress among women at risk for breast cancer. *J Natl Cancer Inst* **85**(13): 1074–80.

Lerman C, Kash K and Stefanek M (1994). Younger women at increased risk for breast cancer: perceived risk, psychological well-being, and surveillance behavior. *J Natl Cancer Inst Monogr* **16**: 171–6.

Lerman C, Lustbader E, Rimer B, et al. (1995). Effects of individualized breast cancer risk counseling: a randomized trial. *J Natl Cancer Inst* **87**(4): 286–92.

Lerman C, Narod S, Schulman K, et al. (1996). BRCA1 testing in families with hereditary breast–ovarian cancer. *JAMA* **275**(24): 1885–92.

Lerman C, Hughes C, Lemon SJ, et al. (1998). What you don't know can hurt you: adverse psychological effects in members of BRCA1-linked and BRCA2-linked families who decline genetic testing. *J Clin Oncol* **16**(5): 1650–4.

Lerman C, Hughes C., Croyle RT, et al. (2000). Prophylactic surgery decisions and surveillance practices one year following BRCA1/2 testing. *Prev Med* **31**(1): 75–80.

Lodder LN, Frets PG, Trijsburg RW, et al. (1999). Presymptomatic testing for BRCA1 and BRCA2: how distressing are the pre-test weeks? *J Med Genet* **36**: 906–13.

Lynch HT, Watson P, Conway TA, et al. (1993). DNA screening for breast/ovarian cancer susceptibility based on linked markers. *Arch Intern Med* **153**: 1979–87.

Meiser B, Butow P, Barratt A, et al. (2000). Attitudes to genetic testing for breast cancer susceptibility in women at increased risk of developing hereditary breast cancer. *J Med Genet* **37**: 472–6.

Miki Y, Swensen J, Shattuck-Eidens D, et al. (1994). A strong candidate for the breast and ovarian cancer susceptibility gene BRCA1. *Science* **266**(5182): 66–71.

Narod SA, Ford D, Devilee P, et al. (1995). An evaluation of genetic heterogeneity in 145 breast–ovarian cancer families. Breast Cancer Linkage Consortium. *Am J Hum Genet* **56**(1): 254–64.

Smith KR, West JA, Croyle RT and Botkin JR (1999). Familial context of genetic testing for cancer susceptibility: moderating effect of siblings' test results on psychological distress one to two weeks after BRCA1 mutation testing. *Cancer Epidemiol Biomarkers Prev* **8**: 385–92.

Spielberger C, Gorsuch R, Lushene R, Vagg P and Jacobs G (1983). *The Handbook of the State-Trait Anxiety Inventory*. Palo Alto, CA: Consulting Psychologists Press.

Struewing JP, Lerman C, Kase RG, Giambarresi TR and Tucker MA (1995). Anticipated uptake and impact of genetic testing in hereditary breast and ovarian cancer families. *Cancer Epidemiol Biomarkers Prev* **4**: 169–73.

Tessaro I, Borstelmann N, Regan K, Rimer BK and Winer E (1997). Genetic testing for susceptibility to breast cancer: findings from women's focus groups. *J Womens Health* **6**(3): 317–27.

Valdimarsdottir HB, Bovbjerg DH, Kash KM, Holland JC, Osborne MP and Miller DG (1995).

Psychological distress in women with a familial risk of breast cancer. *Psychooncology* **4**: 133–41.

Watson M, Lloyd SM, Eeles R, et al. (1996). Psychological impact of testing (by linkage) for the BRCA1 breast cancer gene: an investigation of two families in the research centre. *Psychooncology* **5**: 233–9.

Watson M, Lloyd S, Davidson J, et al. (1999). The impact of genetic counselling on risk perception and mental health in women with a family history of breast cancer. *Br J Cancer* **79**(5/6): 868–74.

Wellisch DK, Gritz ER, Schain W, Wang HJ and Siau J (1991). Psychological functioning of daughters of breast cancer patients. Part II. Characterising the distressed daughters of the breast cancer patient. *Psychosomatics* **33**(3): 171–9.

Wiggins S, Whyte P, Huggins M, et al. (1992). The psychological consequences of predictive testing for Huntington's disease. *N Engl J Med* **327**: 1401–5.

Wooster R, Bignell G, Lancaster J, et al. (1995). Identification of the breast cancer susceptibility gene BRCA2. *Nature* **378**(6559): 789–92.

Zigmond AS and Snaith RP (1983). The Hospital Anxiety and Depression Scale. *Acta Psychiatr Scand* **67**: 361–70.

19

BRCA1/2 testing: uptake and its measurement

Lucy Brooks, Andrew Shenton, F. I. Lalloo and D. G. R. Evans

St Mary's Hospital, Manchester, UK

Introduction

From the time that a family is informed of the identification of a *BRCA1/2* mutation, every individual in that bloodline has, in theory, the opportunity to have a genetic test. Each person has the option to have counselling and can choose to have the test, to postpone the decision, or to take no action. The issues that affect this decision and the potential personal sequelae are discussed elsewhere, and are different for men and women.

In the simplest terms, the level of uptake of a test is the number of family members who opt for testing divided by the number of people in the bloodline. The ideal measurement of uptake would involve contacting all family members, and offering counselling and testing. However, in routine clinical practice, family members unknown to clinic are not informed out of the blue about their risk or invited to attend.

This practice respects the confidentiality of patients, and avoids the potential for unexpected anxiety, but anecdotal accounts from the Huntington's disease experience suggest that neither the direct approach nor a non-interventionist course is appropriate for everyone. This also leaves questions about the group of family members not known to clinicians. These are the hardest to quantify because it is impossible to know whether they know about the test and have made an informed decision not to attend clinic, or whether they are unaware of either their family history or the availability of a predictive test.

Studies of families used in research contexts have demonstrated variable uptake, but the protocols for testing have varied between studies. In some protocols, an affected proband is the only person to be informed when a mutation is found. In studies with unaffected proband(s), if a mutation is subsequently found in a sample obtained with permission from an affected relative, several people may be informed of the result.

These different approaches, and the usual range of family communication and dynamics, may affect the numbers of persons attending for counselling, and therefore the size of the 'unknown' group. Whilst it is important to know what proportion of clinic attendees will have testing, the 'unknowns' must also be considered, as these are potential future patients.

Within publicly funded health systems, it is useful for service providers and budget holders to have an estimate of the likely level of uptake. The following sections will be discussed in more depth: (1) the experience from other genetic tests, (2) expectations of levels of test utilization, and (3) the theoretical measurement of uptake and how this compares with research on actual uptake.

The experience from other genetic tests

Late-onset disorders are unique in that the implications for the individual usually have priority over reproductive decisions. As a result, protocols for testing for late-onset disorders have been developed using Huntington's disease (HD) as a model. The anticipated rate of utilization of a predictive test for HD was high (70%+) (Schoenfeld et al., 1984) when the question was hypothetical, but actual uptake is 10–15% (Craufurd et al., 1989; Tibben et al., 1992; Quaid and Morris, 1993). This may be due to the lack of a cure or any preventive measures as well as to the inevitability of developing the degenerative disorder.

The word 'predictive' is less appropriate than 'pre-symptomatic' when discussing testing for cancer predisposing genes. A mutation-positive result does not always mean that the patient will develop cancer, and effective screening may reduce the mortality rate. The option of prophylaxis (often surgery) is available in some cases and so a bad-news result is not a death sentence. This does not negate the 'worry of waiting for cancer' that such a result can cause, but the rate of uptake of testing for cancer predisposing genes was anticipated to be higher, after counselling, than for HD.

A Finnish study of uptake of predictive testing for hereditary non-polyposis colorectal cancer (HNPCC) showed a rate of 88% of the study sample, qualified as 75% of the whole sample (including non-responders), and redefined as 96% of those who attended for the first counselling session (Aktan-Collan et al., 2000). This involved one-to-one counselling, as opposed to the family group counselling offered in the Lerman et al. (1999) study, which reported a 43% test uptake for HNPCC.

Evans et al. (1997) discussed von Hippel–Lindau disease, familial adenomatous polyposis and neurofibromatosis type 2, and found that the rate of uptake of testing was high, with combined figures of 95% for those aged under 16 years, 77% for adult males and 93% for adult females. This was a register-based study of three different conditions where there is some advantage to be conferred from early screening. This means that childhood testing is offered (unlike HNPCC or BRCA1/2), and the high rates in under-16s may be due to parental influence.

The exception here is Li–Fraumeni or Li–Fraumeni-like syndrome, where there is no clear screening protocol due mostly to the characteristics of these syndromes. This has led to a lower rate of uptake, at about 25% (Schneider et al., 1995; Evans et al., 1997), which is in line with the HD rate.

In general, for late-onset conditions, it can be said that experience of pre-symptomatic genetic testing suggests that the better the prognosis and preventive measures, the higher the rate of uptake. However, where there is no screening or preventive steps that can be taken, careful non-directive counselling often results in fewer family members taking the test.

Anticipated rates for BRCA1/2

As breast cancer is the most common form of cancer in women, with a population rate of 1 in 12 in the UK and 1 in 9–10 in the USA, most women know of someone affected by the disease. In addition, there have been many public health campaigns aiming to raise women's awareness of the need for screening.

In general, the population rate of ovarian cancer of 1 in 70 is less well known, and there is less general awareness of the disease.

Women are usually better both at reporting health concerns and utilizing healthcare services than men. Thus, the hypothetical offer of a genetic test for two 'women's cancers' may be expected to elicit a high positive response rate. A negative result would reduce potential worry about these cancers, and for women without a family history of breast/ovarian cancer, this may be seen as another way of looking after their general health.

Research into the potential uptake of BRCA1/2 testing

Hypothetical studies of various groups of subjects have been carried out regarding their intentions and attitudes towards genetic tests. These include: general population samples, groups of first-degree relatives of affected individuals, patients with cancer, women and men with and without a defined family history of hereditary breast/ovarian cancer, those of Ashkenazi Jewish descent, and other social groups. The methods and results are summarized in Table 19.1 and discussed below.

Many of these studies were undertaken prior to the cloning of BRCA1 and BRCA2. Mutations are spread throughout both BRCA genes. However, founder mutations in up to 2% of Ashkenazi Jews mean that a meaningful test can be offered without a mutation search or a strong family history (Lalloo et al., 1998).

For most other families in Britain, finding the gene fault can take some time. This is confounded by the potential for mutations to be in uncharacterized genes (*BRCA3/4*), and has led to recent psychosocial studies into the effects of a long wait for a definite result (Broadstock et al., 2000). Early papers reported on linkage studies prior to cloning of the genes, and in some families, despite full sequencing, mutations have not been found.

As can be seen in Table 19.1, there are a variety of methods used for the studies undertaken prior to cloning. These all have the potential to alter the result of any uptake measurement (actual or hypothetical) and are discussed on p. 319 of this chapter. It is important at this stage to encourage the reader to consider the study methodology in context with the predicted rate of test utilization.

The general population

The main difference between hypothetical and retrospective studies is that the 'general population' can be offered a 'gene test for breast cancer', as opposed to a test for a faulty family gene. This expression was used by Ulrich et al. (1998), who also offered men 'a gene test for prostate cancer', in a random telephone poll in Washington State, USA, in 1995–96. They found that 76% of women and 83% of men said that they would definitely or probably take this test, for which no fee was mentioned. The sample included 6.9% of participants who had a personal history of (non-specific) cancer, and no assessment was made of the family history reported by 5% of men and 9% of women. It was noted that the very-well-educated women showed less interest in this hypothetical test than those who were less educated.

Hereditary breast/ovarian cancer families

Prior to the detailed characterization of *BRCA1* (and the discovery of *BRCA2*), a number of studies focused on individuals with a proven family history of breast and ovarian cancer, two reported rates of interest (definite or probable) in a genetic test being approximately 95% (Lerman et al., 1994; Struewing et al., 1995). A third study (Julian-Reynier et al., 1996) found a similar rate amongst unaffected women with at least one first-degree relative (FDR) affected, but a lower rate of interest (76%) in affected women. Struewing et al. (1995) added a note regarding the fact that their sample was made up of people involved in linkage studies (some having given blood), and that this was possibly a factor in the high rate. Lerman et al. (1994) suggested that the request rate for tests among low-risk women would be high, based on a telephone poll of FDRs of women with ovarian cancer.

Lerman et al. (1995), in a similar study that examined the FDRs of breast cancer

Table 19.1. Estimates in advance

Author	Lerman et al.	Lerman et al.	Struewing et al.	Julian-Reynier et al.	Tambor et al.	Ulrich et al.	Cappelli et al.	Meiser et al.
Title	Attitudes about genetic testing for breast–ovarian cancer susceptibility	Interest in genetic testing among FDRs of breast cancer patients	Anticipated uptake and impact of genetic testing in hereditary breast and ovarian cancer families	Attitudes towards cancer predictive testing and transmission of information to the family	Genetic testing for breast cancer susceptibility: awareness and interest among women in the general population	Genetic testing for cancer risk: a population survey on attitudes and intention	Psychological and social determinants of women's decisions to undergo genetic counselling and testing for breast cancer	Attitudes to genetic testing for breast cancer susceptibility in women at increased risk of developing hereditary breast cancer
Year	1994	1995	1995	1996	1997	1998	1999	2000
Source	J Clin Oncol	Am J Med Genet	Cancer Epidemiol Biomarkers Prev	J Med Genet	Am J Med Genet	Community Genet	Clin Genet	J Med Genet
Volume and page nos	12(4): 843–50	57: 385–92	4: 169–73	33: 731–6	68: 43–9	1: 213–22	55: 419–30	37: 472–6
Country	USA	USA	USA	France	USA	USA	Canada	Australia
Description of paper	Telephone interview of relatives of Ov Ca patients' relatives	Telephone interview of relatives of Br Ca patients' relatives	Interview of NCI study family members about testing and anticipated impact	Questionnaire to unaffected patients at cancer genetics clinic about testing	Telephone questionnaire to HMO 50 yrs+ mammography adherers and non-adherers	Random phone survey asking about gene testing without any fine detail	Questionnaire comparison between general population and affecteds	Questionnaire to high-risk women about reasons for and against testing
Family mutation already identified? Risk status of sample population	None – FDRs, with 39% having 2+ FDRs or SDRs with breast or ovarian cancer	None – FDRs, but 86% had risk estimate of less than 15%	None – consistent with linkage to BRCA1	None – in 78% of the cases studied, a genetic risk of cancer was likely to run in the families	None – 2% considered at increased risk from family history	No – theoretical test for breast cancer for women, prostate cancer for men	BRCA1/2 or none – control group	None – history consistent with a dominantly inherited predisposition (80%) or at moderately increased risk

Individual level of risk	FDRs only	FDRs only	Affected and FDRs, SDRs or TDRs	Affected and first-degree relatives	10% had an affected FDR	Variable	Affected and general population	80% at 1 in 2 to 1 in 4; 20% at 1 in 8 to 1 in 4
Type of clinic	Cancer	Cancer	Registry families	Cancer genetics	Mammography clinic	N/A Phone poll	Cancer	Familial cancer
Response rate	91%	78%	98%	84%	53%	64%	67%	89%
Reported level of interest in test	95% (75% 'definitely' + 20% 'probably' interested)	91%	95% ('definitely' + 16% 'probably')	76.2% (affecteds), 95.8% (FDRs)	69%	76% of women, 83% of men	60% (72% affecteds; 46% unaffecteds)	92% (70% 'definitely' and 22% 'probably' interested)
Quotations/notes from the text	Unlike HD, high rates of interest in genetic testing for *BRCA1* are likely to translate into widespread utilization. Carriers of *BRCA1* will have options for possible prevention, early detection and treatment.	Given the greater potential for early detection and treatment of Br Ca (compared with Ov Ca) one would expect demand for genetic testing to be greater among relatives of Br Ca patients than among Ov Ca patients. Observed interest may be (partly due) to an inflated sense of personal risk – common (in) FDRs of Br Ca patients.	Not unexpectedly, we found a high level of interest in genetic testing among this group of highly educated subjects who were participating in a genetic linkage study.	96.6% assumed that health surveillance would improve from BNR. 15.5% would want active dissemination. More women in favour of the test may have participated in the survey.	This population was less interested. This may be because our study consisted only of women aged 50 years+. Older women were less likely than younger women to be interested.	Well-educated women expressed less intent. Respondents were concerned about the potential misuses and confidentiality of the genetic tests results, and a large majority supported laws.	Women with Br Ca were almost six times more likely to want the test than the general population of women. However, of the Br Ca participants who intended to have the test, only 49% had actually sought advice about testing 3–15 months later.	Understanding what steps to take to reduce one's cancer risk was endorsed by 87% of women. In contrast, surveys of attitudes to HD testing identified wanting 'to be certain' as the most commonly reported reason.

BNR, bad news result; FDR, first-degree relative; HMO, Health Management Organization; SDR, second-degree relative; TDR, third-degree relative.

patients, found a 91% interest in genetic testing, despite 83% and 80% of subjects anticipating that a mutation-positive result would cause anxiety and depression respectively. In this group, only 10% had more than one FDR with breast cancer, and 14% had a risk of breast cancer that was greater than 15%, as reported by the researchers.

Calculating uptake

Mathematically speaking, the definition of uptake is the number of people tested divided by the number of people who could potentially be tested, or $U = n/N$, where U is uptake, n is the number of people who have had a test, and N is the maximum number of people who could be tested.

The most simply categorized term refers to the people who have had a test. It can be easily stated that in clinical studies and situations, any person who gives blood but then declines to receive their result has in effect *not* been tested. This reflects the patient's experience and confidentiality, as even if the clinician is aware of the patient's mutation status, they are unable to act upon it.

What kind of test?

The first expression to be defined must be 'test'. Does this refer to predictive/pre-symptomatic tests only, to tests on people with and without a diagnosis of cancer, or to mutation searches carried out on samples from affected individuals? If it is to include mutation searches, then the status of the sample donor must be given – are they alive or deceased? – and there must be guides as to when an inconclusive result (no mutation found) counts as a gene test. Is linkage included? What is the status of a test for a founder mutation (especially Ashkenazi Jewish) in a woman without a strong family history of breast or ovarian cancer? Currently, it is realistic to define a test as being for a known family mutation (previously detected in the affected proband) or for a relevant founder mutation.

What is the study population?

Whose uptake is being measured? Is it the rate for the family (U_f), or the rate for those seen at a particular clinic (U_c)? In situations where a test is only offered as part of a study protocol, and an active approach is made to recruit family members to the study, these can be seen as one and the same. However, in routine practice, this cannot be controlled, as mutations are found one by one, and information allowed to naturally disseminate through the family. Many kindreds are spread across regions, and unless active recruitment takes place or information is cross-checked between centres, it is possible that the information recorded on a family in one centre is at best out of date, with the potential to be very inaccurate. In this situation, U_c becomes more important.

Changes over time

It is very important to put a time component into the equation, as every family's situation can change, until every member has had a test. Until an individual has received their test result, they have the option to move from the 'untested' group to the 'tested' group. This is a weakness in research counselling/testing protocols where a test is offered at a particular time, as other life factors such as deaths or marriages may have priority for the participants at that point in time. Also, an individual who has initially declined testing may be triggered to reconsider their decision by an outside event. It may be more revealing to consider the rate of uptake within each family, where $\Delta U_f = \Delta n/N \times \Delta \text{time}$, and how this changes.

The way in which information is passed around the family now becomes relevant, as the starting point ($t=0$) must be defined. A precise measure of the rate of uptake would be from the time that each individual became aware of the availability of a genetic test to the time when they made a decision to take the test. This shows the advantage of studies using the proactive approach, as this point can be defined, and the time taken to testing by each individual can be measured accurately.

The difficulties involved in measuring time delays without interfering in or prompting family communication routes make calculation of an exact figure for the time from being informed to having a test difficult. For example, it would be unlikely that patients could accurately recall when each and every family member was informed of the availability of a test. Without very specific records, it is impossible to establish whether significant delays in attending for testing are due to periods of reflection, or cancellations, or natural delays in referrals and clinic waiting times.

Defining $t=0$ as the date on which the first individual(s) in the family was informed that a mutation had been identified (the affected proband and/or previously known at-risk relatives) gives the most realistic starting point for a retrospective study or audit. However, it may be possible to record the time taken from the commencement of counselling at clinic for each individual.

Attendance for education and counselling

Only when an individual attends clinic is it possible to be sure that they are aware of their family history and the implications it may have for them. It may be preferable to measure uptake as a proportion of those who have attended clinic, rather than of the whole family. This would change the equation to: $U_i = n/C$, where U_i is the uptake amongst people known to have received counselling about testing, and C is the total number who have had counselling. If this were the calculation used, then the relationship between N and C must be stated, so that it can be seen how many at-risk family members have attended clinic ($A = C/N$, where A is attendance at clinic).

The proportion of family members (A) who have attended clinic (and their whereabouts on the pedigree) gives some indication as to the spread of information around the family. The 'unknowns' are those who have not come forward to clinic, and therefore might not know about the availability of testing. These are potential future patients (F), and cannot be discounted unless they have actively declined counselling and testing. It is questionable as to whether non-response to an invitation to participate in an education/testing research programme counts as informed non-utilization. 'A' cannot be measured in studies involving active recruitment to a research testing protocol, and U_i has less meaning in these studies, as it only shows the participation level in the study, unless testing in that area is available solely as part of a research protocol.

Eligibility

Who is eligible for pre-symptomatic testing? The definition of the denominator includes more clauses and sub-clauses than any other part of the equation. It may be simplest to count everybody in the bloodline of the family. However, it is not usual practice to test those under the age of 18 years, or those unable to give informed consent due to mental health or learning problems. In a National Health System setting, when calculating the uptake amongst patients of one particular clinic (U_c), the family members resident in another region or country become ineligible for testing by that clinic.

It is unnecessary to test the children (and grandchildren) of anybody found to be a non-carrier. This reinforces the importance of including a time component in the calculation, as the number of people in the denominator is dynamic and may be reduced or increased by mutation-negative or mutation-positive results respectively.

Some descendants of a mutation-negative individual may have been counselled by a clinic prior to reduction of their risk. They must therefore be removed from the updated calculation of uptake with respect to counselling (C). Conversely, it is not usual to test children without having already tested the parent. Therefore, theoretically, until the parent has had a test, the children are 'ineligible'. If this is formally phrased, it could be said that only those at 50% risk of having inherited the mutation were 'eligible' for inclusion in the denominator, at any point in time.

This definition is too narrow because there may be an intervening relative who is unavailable for testing (probably deceased). As mutations in the *BRCA1/2* genes are not fully penetrant, the children of an unaffected woman are still at risk of having inherited the faulty gene copy. So, the group of people who could be tested includes those in each vertical bloodline at most risk of inheriting the mutation, i.e. those at 50% risk, or those at 25% (or 12.5%) risk where the intervening generation is unavailable for testing.

And finally, any obligate carriers (usually alive and well parents of the affected proband in whom the mutation was found) could be said to be ineligible for inclusion in the denominator of an uptake calculation, as their status is known by default.

Pedigree studies

Who is included in audit-based research, using the family trees held in patients' notes? Broadly speaking, this comprises those local, unaffected family members made up of the siblings, sons and daughters of affected women and men, or the nieces, nephews, granddaughters and grandsons, where their bloodline parent has died (Figure 19.1).

If the information recorded on a pedigree has been provided by a patient and not been exhaustively researched, it is likely to contain inaccuracies. This is unavoidable, as the patient(s) may not have been in touch with his/her relatives for years. In large extended families, it is unlikely that the different branches will even know of each other, however geographically proximate they are. Therefore, if the denominator in a calculation of uptake includes only those at 50% risk, and contact has been lost, the patients at one regional clinic may not be aware of all diagnostic and clinical activity in the family. As Figure 19.2 shows, the whole picture may be quite different, and the level of attendance and testing measured by one centre may be inaccurate.

Research contexts

Calculating the level of uptake from information ordinarily recorded in clinic can be seen to be fraught with potential mistakes and problems. Audit-style research based on clinical notes can only reflect the general trend, but it is difficult to see how a research study could be designed such that accurate data collection could be ensured without interfering in routine clinical practice. One possibility is through a national register, or a similar system where information from a number of sources is collated and compared.

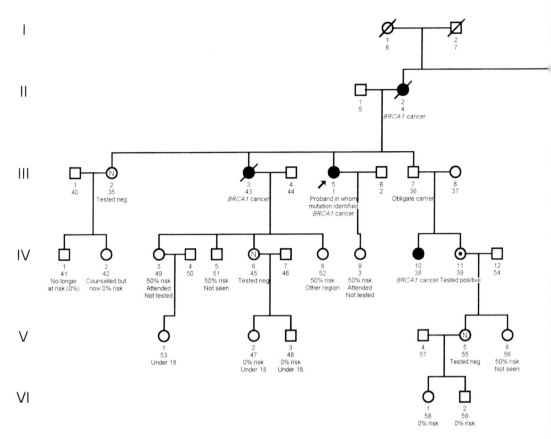

Figure 19.1 Fictitious pedigree, recorded from one branch of the family. Based on this information, the uptake (U_f) in this kindred is 31%, the uptake amongst clinic attenders (U_i) is 67% with an attendance rate of 46% (those at 50% risk only) (RTA, road traffic accident).

Most investigations into the level of uptake of *BRCA1/2* tests have been in the context of other research protocols, usually psychosocial questionnaires and sociodemographic measures. The advantages and disadvantages of studies based on the proactive recruitment of patients have been mentioned, but other differences between approaches and clinic structures also warrant discussion. Table 19.2 shows a summary of these reports, and the papers are discussed in more detail in the next section.

Summarizing the theoretical arguments given above, the equations for U_f, ΔU_f, U_i, U_c and U_s must now have the following definitions and include the following terms:

$$U_f = n/N \text{ at } t = \text{'}X\text{'}$$
$$\Delta U_f = \Delta n/N \times \Delta t$$

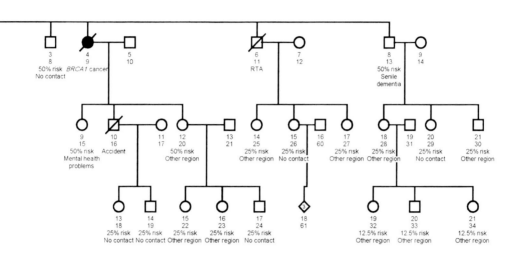

$U_i = n/C$ at $t = `X`$, where $A = `Y`$

$U_c = n/N_a$ at $t_{ave} = `X`$

$A = C/N$

$F = N - A$

U_f	= the level of uptake in a family, wherever its members are
ΔU_f	= the change in uptake in a family (see below)
U_i	= the level of uptake amongst informed patients
U_c	= the combined uptake for all the families seen at a clinic
A	= the proportion of eligible family members who have attended for counselling
F	= the group who have not voluntarily come forward to clinic and whose level of awareness is unknown; potential future patients
n	= the number of people who have received the results of a genetic test for a known familial *BRCA1/2*-disease-causing mutation
N	= the number of people in the bloodline who could be tested. This excludes those under the age of 18 years, obligate carriers and those with mental health or learning difficulties. The level of risk must also be defined to reflect clinical practice, so that only those in each vertical bloodline at greatest risk (apart from healthy obligate carriers) are included
$t = X$	= the time after the family has been informed of the identification of a mutation in *BRCA1/2*

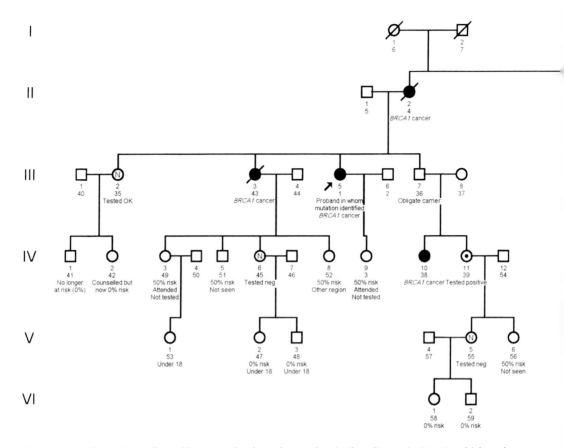

Figure 19.2. Information collected from another branch reveals a further diagnosis (III:18), which makes II:8 an obligate carrier, and raises his descendants' risks. Now $U_f = 26\%$, while U_i remains similar at 71%, and attendance is 37%. However, without tracing II:3, and checking directly with the descendants of II:4 and II:6, can we be sure that the pedigree is complete, or that all testing activity has been recorded?

C = the number of people eligible for testing under the criteria listed for N who have attended clinic for counselling about the issues involved in testing

N.B. The total number of people who have attended for counselling would be $U_i + P$, where P is any known patients whose risk has been reduced to that of the general population by a mutation-negative result in a parent

N_a = the number of people eligible for testing under the criteria above who are resident in the area covered by that specific regional centre

t_{ave} = the average time since the families were informed of their various mutations

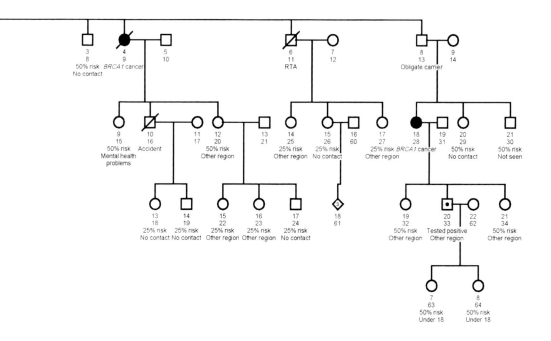

Review of the literature to date

Having outlined the theoretical measurement and methods of uptake in the previous section, Table 19.3 examines the context in which a number of studies have been carried out to date. It can be seen that the eight reports that specifically deal with the rate of utilization of *BRCA1/2* testing have arrived at a number of different figures, the lowest and highest quoted being 27% and 84% respectively. The fact that both of these figures are from Julian-Reynier et al. (2000a) illustrates that these 'headline rates of uptake' can be very different, depending on the population included, and the study protocol.

Where the focus of the study has been on psychological or other measures, in order to obtain the maximum number of responses active recruitment methods have been used, such as by Lerman et al. (1996) and Bowles Biesecker et al. (2000). Other research has concentrated on particular families (Watson et al., 1995; Smith et al., 1999), again using proactive recruitment, whereas Reichelt et al. (1999) and Julian-Reynier et al. (2000a,b) have reported on national rates. Finally, Hagoel et al. (2000) provide data on the utilization of counselling rather than testing in a national study, and Meijers-Heijboer et al. (2000) report on consecutive families

Table 19.2. Investigations into the level of uptake of *BRCA1/2* tests

	Watson et al.	Lerman et al.	Reichelt et al.	Smith et al.	Bowles Biesecker et al.	Hagoel et al.	Julian-Reynier et al.	Meijers-Heijboer et al.
Author	Watson et al.	Lerman et al.	Reichelt et al.	Smith et al.	Bowles Biesecker et al.	Hagoel et al.	Julian-Reynier et al.	Meijers-Heijboer et al.
Title	Genetic testing in breast/ovarian cancer (BRCA1) families	BRCA1 testing in families with hereditary breast–ovarian cancer. A prospective study of patient decision making and outcomes	Uptake of genetic testing and pre-test levels of mental distress in Norwegian families with known BRCA1 mutations	Familial context of genetic testing for cancer susceptibility: moderating effect of siblings' test results on psychological distress one to two weeks after BRCA1 mutation testing	Psychosocial factors predicting BRCA1/BRCA2 testing decisions in members of hereditary breast and ovarian families	Proband family uptake of familial genetic counselling	Uptake of hereditary breast ovarian cancer genetic testing in a French national sample of BRCA1 families	Presymptomatic DNA testing and prophylactic surgery in families with a BRCA1 or BRCA2 mutation
Year	1995	1996	1999	1999	2000	2000	2000a	2000
Source	*Lancet*	*JAMA*	*Dis Markers*	*Cancer Epidemiol Biomarkers Prev*	*Am J Med Genet*	*Psychooncology*	*Psychooncology*	*Lancet*
Volume and page nos	**346**: 583	**275**: 1885–92	**15**: 139–43	**8**: 385–92	**93**: 257–63	**9**: 522–7	**9**: 504–10	**355**: 2015–20
Country	UK	USA	Norway	USA	USA	Israel	France	Netherlands
Description of paper	Early account of take-up in two linkage families	Prospective cohort study; results offered after education; interviews with concerned predictor variables	Prospective questionnaire to patients attending clinic	Interviews measuring distress in large kindred members	Prospective sociodemographic, personality and family functioning measures taken	Retrospective pedigree audit to assess attendance on invitation to counselling	Survey of clinicians' experience of families	Audit of individuals and families attending clinic and their actions
Family mutation	*BRCA1* 95+% probability of linkage	*BRCA1*	*BRCA1*	*BRCA1*	*BRCA1* and *BRCA2*	*BRCA1* (3 AJ and *BRCA2* mutations)	*BRCA1*	*BRCA1* and *BRCA2*

Cancer status of patients	Unaffected	Unaffected and affected	Unaffected and affected	Unaffected and affected	Unaffected and affected	Unaffected and affected	Unaffected and affected	Unaffected
Who pays?	Not discussed – free	Research	Public health care	Research	Research pays?	Not discussed	Public health system?	Public and private health insurance
Research protocol/routine practice	Research	Research	Routine	Research	Research	Routine	Routine	Routine
Active dissemination/cascade (by clinic or family)	Families involved in Br/Ov cancer consortium study	Families previously enrolled for genetics study	Not clear	Active, family involved in other research	Families previously enrolled for genetics study	Through proband but encouraged by clinic	Cascade only by law	Cascade
Individual's level of risk	Not stated	Family members	Family members	Not stated	Affected (8%) and 'at risk'	Affected, first-degree relatives (at 50% risk)	First- and second-degree relatives	50% and 25%
Type of clinic	Cancer genetics	Hereditary cancer institute	Cancer	University of Utah	Cancer	Familial cancer	Cancer genetics	Family cancer clinic
Checking of information	From clinic records	Personal: questionnaire 69% response	Personal: questionnaire 89% response (Founder effect)	Personal, and through family members	Personal: questionnaire 70% response	Proband made all contacts	From family files	Unsure
Who was told of mutation	Families involved in Br/Ov cancer consortium study	Families previously enrolled for genetics study	Known mutations	Family previously in other studies (+ unknown members)	Families previously enrolled for NCI study	Proband only	Affected only	All known patients

Table 19.3. Results of studies in the context of the definitions they have used

Author	Watson et al.		Lerman et al.		Reichelt et al.		Smith et al.	
Year	1995		1996		1999		1999	
Title	Genetic testing in breast/ovarian cancer (BRCA1) families		BRCA1 testing in families with hereditary breast–ovarian cancer. A prospective study of patient decision making and outcomes		Uptake of genetic testing and pre-test levels of mental distress in Norwegian families with known BRCA1 mutations		Familial context of genetic testing for cancer susceptibility: moderating effect of siblings' test results on psychological distress 1–2 weeks after BRCA1 mutation testing	
Headline rate quoted	41%		60% or 43% interviewees vs sample		78%		54%	
	Definitions	Results	Definitions	Results	Definitions	Results	Definitions	Results
U_f at $t=X$ or U_c at t_{ave}	Uptake of linkage test, prior to cloning of the gene	41%	Uptake in registry families	43%	Uptake among persons already counselled and offered testing when it became available	All = 78% UF = 76%	Uptake in one large kindred	54% of SPs (92% of final analysis group) (= 35%* of EFMs)
No. of families		2 families		13 families		27 families		1 family
Year		1995		1996		1/5/99		1999
$\Delta U_f \times \Delta t$	n/a	(Two persons awaiting an appointment)	n/a	n/a		(6% undecided)	Offer of free testing restricted to study period	Not discussed
Time to report after offer of test		Unclear		Up to 17 months		Unclear		Unclear
U_i	Uptake amongst clinic attendees at time of report	13/15 = 87% Or 93%* after death	Uptake among attendees of pre-test education in the study / Uptake in EFMs	99%* (SPs)	Uptake in this sample	78%	Uptake among those who attended for counselling in the study	91%

	Study 1	Study 2	Study 3	Study 4
Attendance level	47% – see below (One died suddenly before testing)	60% (SPs)	100% of sample	59.2% of SPs had counselling
Quote in the discussion	These highly selected individuals may not be representative of the whole population of BRCA1 families		We found an uptake of testing much higher than in any previous report and this may be an effect of self-referral to our health-service	
A	Proportion of individuals entered into programme to have attended for pre-test counselling — 47% (or 52%* after those living out of area removed from calculation)	SPs who attended for pre-test education — 60% (SPs)	Had earlier attended counselling sessions – offered testing when it became available — 100%	Proportion attending for counselling — 59.2% of SPs (= 39% of EFMs)
Sample	Families at 95% probability of linkage — Two families	Members of BRCA1 families on registry, already in genetics studies — 13 families	Members of BRCA1 families — 27 families	Members of kindred: 2082 — One family
Further criteria	In breast/ovarian cancer consortium study — 32 individuals entered programme (How many didn't?)	Participated in research interview, or just had decision re-testing recorded — 279 (192 interviewed, 87 declined interview)	Had earlier attended counselling sessions – offered testing when it became available — 232 (How many other family members had not attended for counselling?)	Participants in ongoing longitudinal psychosocial study — 759 individuals (500 fully informed about study; 124 refused to participate; 135 not contacted)
n	Number tested — 13 (41%)	Number requesting BRCA result — 121 EFMs = 43% 115 SPs = 60%	Received the results of genetic testing — 180 (78%)	Had test — 269
No. tested; breakdown by gender	Females 10 (59%*); Males 3 (20%*)	Females SPs = 85 (66%*); Males SPs = 30 (48%*)	Females UF = 120 (76%); Males No further data given	Females 125; Males (in final analysis) 87; No data on SPs in final analysis

Table 19.3. (cont.)

	Watson et al. Definitions	Watson et al. Results	Lerman et al. Definitions	Lerman et al. Results	Reichelt et al. Definitions	Reichelt et al. Results	Smith et al. Definitions	Smith et al. Results
N	Age not specified	32 females = 17 (53%) males = 15 (47%)	EFMs 18+ (SPs)	279 EFMs (192 SPs females = 129 (67%) males = 63 (31%))	Age not specified	232 females = 186 (80%) males = 46 (20%)	EFMs 18+	759 EFMs (500 SPs, but only 212 used in final analysis females = 125 (59% males = 87 (41%))
Individual's risk status/ relationship to AP/other affected individual(s) (quote from paper)	In linkage family		Members of extended hereditary Br/Ov cancer families with and without cancer	38 (14%*) affected with cancer (various)	Members of families with demonstrated *BRCA1* mutations		Recruitment strategy designed so that at-risk parents tested before their children – staged	Eligible family members included affected individuals
Note on this	Individuals risk not specified – short letter		Precise risk for family members not given – 50%? Or 25% or less?	Categories split into 2(+) affected FDRs and 0–1 affected FDRs – difficult to estimate risk status	Exact risk for unaffecteds not given		Non-participants more likely to have a parent who had already tested negative – ?eligible?	Proportion of affecteds not discussed, or the uptake in this group
Cancer status	Unaffected only		Unaffected and affected (some sporadic Br/Ov or other sites)	38 (14%*) affected with cancer	Unaffected and affected	AF = 30 (13%) UM = 0 (0%) UF = 156 (67%) UM = 46 (20%)	Unaffected and affected	No breakdown given
No. tested, breakdown by cancer status	Unaffected only	13 (41%)	Unaffected Affected	87 (56%) 28 (74%)	Unaffected	UF = 120 (76%) No other data given	Unaffected Affected	No breakdown given

t	Not discussed	Not discussed	n/a – active approach with test offer	n/a	Not discussed	Not discussed	Not discussed	n/a – active offer in study context
C	Number to have attended pre-test counselling	15 (47%)	Number of SPs who attended for pre-test education	116 (60% of SPs)	Had earlier attended counselling sessions	232 (100%)	Number of SPs to have completed first genetic counselling session	296/500 SPs (59%) (296/759 EFMs – 39%)
N_a	Number close enough to travel to clinic	29 (91%)	n/a (research centre)	n/a	n/a (national study)	n/a	N/a – one family actively recruited	n/a
Other		No reply 5 Declined entering programme 2 Did not proceed with testing 9 Did not attend 2 Out of area 3 Awaiting appointment 2						Family part of a religious minority (Mormons)

Table 19.3. (cont.)

	Bowles Biesecker et al.		Hagoel et al.		Julian-Reynier et al.		Meijers-Heijboer et al.	
Author	Bowles Biesecker et al.		Hagoel et al.		Julian-Reynier et al.		Meijers-Heijboer et al.	
Year	2000		2000		2000a		2000	
Title	Psychosocial factors predicting BRCA1/BRCA2 testing decisions in members of hereditary breast and ovarian families		Proband family uptake of familial genetic counselling		Uptake of hereditary breast/ovarian cancer genetic testing in a French national sample of BRCA1 families		Presymptomatic DNA testing and prophylactic surgery in families with a BRCA1 or BRCA2 mutation	
Headline rate quoted	55% and 78% EFMs vs SPs		34% had counselling		26.7% and 84.2% F/SDRs vs attendees		38%	
	Definitions	Results	Definitions	Results	Definitions	Results	Definitions	Results
U_f at $t = X$ or U_c at t_{ave}	Uptake in NCI study families	EFMs = 55% SPs = 78%	n/a Focus of paper is on uptake of counselling, not of testing	n/a (34% had counselling)	Uptake in families with ≥1 FDR or SDR: information from 36 clinics and checked with other clinics	0 in 14.7% of families AF = 69% UF = 31% UM = 13% (56%: 23%: 7%) Total = 27% (19%)	Uptake in family members at 50% risk: series of consecutive families attending Rotterdam clinic	EFMs = 38% UF = 57% (at 50% risk) UM = 22% (at 50% risk)
No. of families Year	11 families 2000		67 families 2000		37 families 8+ months after family informed		53 families 24 months after mutation found	
$\Delta U_t \times \Delta t$	Not discussed	Not discussed	n/a	n/a (change in attendance rate over time not discussed)	Data include those still in the process of testing	Data broken down – above (Is assumption safe that all will receive a result?)	Graph used to show proportion that did not have DNA test vs time since genetic diagnosis (9, 12, 24 months)	UF (9:12:24/12) = 51%: 54%: 58% UM (9:12:24/12) = 19%: 19%: 24%

Time to report after offer of test			Up to 35 months		Mean follow-up = 26 months (range: 16–62 months)
U_i	Uptake amongst education and counselling attendees — 78%	n/a — Focus of paper is on uptake of counselling, not of testing	Uptake amongst attendees, including those still in the process — 84% (59% had actually had a result*)	Not discussed	Not discussed
Attendance level	70.5%*	34%	32%		
Quote in the discussion	Before testing was possible, Struewing et al. (1995) reported that 79% of participants in the same population would definitely want to be tested and that 16% would probably want to be tested	Study service providers consider that the participation of invited individuals in genetic counselling has potential benefits for each family member	From these data, we can say that, on average for every BRCA1 mutation detected, we have two 'at risk' female FDRs that can be tested, and that 50% of them will ask for testing	The time-dependent rates suggest that most individuals interested in DNA testing had already come forward during the period of our study. Therefore, it is unlikely that uptake of DNA testing will significantly increase over time	Not discussed
A	Proportion participating in education and counselling sessions — 70.5%	Proportion of those at-risk family members to attend clinic on invitation from the AP — 34% (Only 1 EFM in 27 families gave possible attendance of 0% or 100%)	Proportion of FDRs and SDRs attending clinic after the AP had received her result — FDR AF: UF: UM = 96%: 60%: 25%; total = 34%; SDR AF: UF: UM = 58%: 21%: 10%; total = 18%; All total = 32%	Not discussed	
Sample	Families with known BRCA1/2 mutations — 11 families	Families with at least one AJ founder mutation — 67 families	First three families known to clinicians — 15% of French families; 34 families	Mutation identified between 1/1/94 and 1/1/98	53 families

Table 19.3. (cont.)

	Bowles Biesecker et al.		Hagoel et al.		Julian-Reynier et al.		Meijers-Heijboer et al.	
	Definitions	Results	Definitions	Results	Definitions	Results	Definitions	Results
Further criteria	Previously enrolled in NCI familial cancer study	38% of protocol participants had never taken part in other research studies	Excluding (2) families with no residents in Israel	First to be tested must be affected	Excluding (3) families with no FDRs or SDRs. AP had result for minimum of 8 months	(12 families excluded where *t* < 8 months)		
n	Number tested	135 (55%)	Number of individuals to have had counselling (decision to have testing not recorded)	(34% had counselling)	Data include numbers tested as well as those in the process of testing	79 (19%) had test 33 (8%) in the process of testing	DNA testing utilization	257 (38%)
No. tested; breakdown by gender	Females Males	87 (66%*) females = 132 (54%) 48 (43%*) males = 112 (46%)	Females Males	(no breakdown given)	Females Males (tested + in process)	67 + 23 (37% total) 12 + 10 (13% total)	Females Males	198 (48%) 59 (22%)
N	Aged ≥18	244 females = 244 (66.1%) (actually it's 65.8%!) males = 127 (34.2%)	Aged ≥22	371 EFMs females = 244 (66.1%) (actually it's 65.8%!) males = 127 (34.2%)	Aged 18+	419 females = 244 (58.2%) males = 175 (41.8%)	Aged 20+	682 females = 411 (60.2%) males = 271 (39.7%)

	Study 1		Study 2		Study 3		Study 4	
Individual's risk status / relationship to AP/other affected individual(s) (quote from paper)	In extended families, affected or unaffected	Affected = 8% At least one affected FDR = 41%	Blood relatives on side of family where mutation found	Affected = 54 (15%) FDR with cancer = 260 (70%)	FDR or SDR of the AP	FDR = 173 (41.3%) SDR = 246 (58.7%)	50% risk of inheriting the mutation and 25% (daughters of untested men) AF excluded	50% risk UF = 275 (40%) 50% risk UM = 271 (40%) 25% risk UF = 136 (20%)
Note on this			At-risk status redefined step-by-step after every test result		SDRs said to be 'at risk' but not clear if status redefined after (FDRs) test result		Not stated if this was redefined after each new result	
Cancer status	Unaffected and affected	Affected = 14 (8%)	Unaffected and affected	Affected (Br/Ov ca) = 54 (14.5%) Affected (other ca) = 14 (3.8%) No cancer = 303 (81.7%)	Unaffected and affected (affected men excluded)	AF = 36 (8.6%) UF = 208 (49.6%) UM = 175 (41.8%)	Unaffected only	Unaffected only
No. tested, breakdown by cancer status	Unaffected Affected % Breakdown by risk status	UF SPs = 76 (79%) AF SPs = 11 (79%) Not possible to analyse by risk status	Unaffected Affected % Breakdown by risk status (counselled)	(76 (25%) counselled) (49 (72%) counselled) FDR of cancer patient = 40% Not FDR of a cancer patient = 21%	Unaffected (tested + in process) Affected % Breakdown by risk status	59 + 28 (23% total) 20 + 5 (69% total) FDRs = 36% (= 51% UF, 18% UM) SDRs = 14% (= 18% UF, 9% UM)	Unaffected only % Breakdown by risk status	UF 50% risk = 158 (57%) UF 25% risk = 40 (29%) UM = 59 (22%) Total = 38% Total at 50% risk = 36% UF at 25% risk = 29%

Table 19.3. (*cont.*)

	Bowles Biesecker et al.		Hagoel et al.		Julian-Reynier et al.		Meijers-Heijboer et al.	
	Definitions	Results	Definitions	Results	Definitions	Results	Definitions	Results
t	Not discussed	Not discussed	Not discussed	Not discussed	Time from AP being informed of mutation detection to first result in relation	In 24 families: Mean = 6.5 m Median = 4 m Range = 0–35 months Subsequent cut-off at 75th centile = 8 months	Time from mutation identification	9, 12 and 24 months
C	Number to have attended pre-test education and counselling	172 (70.5%)	Number to have accepted invitation to participate in counselling	(34%)	n/a (national study)	All total = 133 (32%)	Not discussed	Not discussed
N_a	Not discussed	Travelling may have deterred those who were ambivalent about testing	Two families with no EFMs in Israel excluded	n/a	n/a (national study)	n/a	Not discussed (national study?)	Not discussed

AF, affected female; AM, affected male; AP, affected proband in whom mutation identified; EFM, eligible family member; FDR, first-degree relative; SDR, second-degree relative; SP, study participant (where uptake measured in a wider, e.g. psychosocial, study); UF, unaffected female; UM, unaffected male.

*Some figures calculated from data given for this table, not supplied in the original paper.

attending one particular clinic. To make the quoted results of these different and equally valid works more directly comparable, Table 19.3 includes a thorough break-down of how these figures were calculated, extracted from the papers.

To facilitate ease of reading, the following discussion refers to the above studies by the initials of the first author, for example Julian-Reynier et al. (2000) becomes 'J-R'; BB, Bowles Biesecker et al. (2000); H, Hagoel et al. (2000); L, Lerman et al. (1996); M-H, Meijers-Heijboer et al. (2000); R, Reichelt et al. (1999); S, Smith et al. (1999); W, Watson et al. (1995).

Cultural differences between the populations in the different studies may have influenced the decisions made by family members. However, the cost of the test was not a consideration.

Attendance

When considering the numbers of eligible family members in each study, there are difficulties in making comparisons. R, whose study population was composed of family members who had previously attended for counselling and who were offered a test when it became available, reports the highest rate. Therefore an attendance rate of 100% was quoted. In contrast, L only supplies information about study participants, and M-H doesn't mention attendance. The lowest rate is 32% (J-R), but this is without active recruitment. In the case of the Norwegian study (R), it is unclear whether there were family members who had declined counselling at any time, and in the Watson paper (1995), it is unclear how many individuals declined entry into the programme.

Where there has been active recruitment, it is easier to be sure that every eligible family member is aware of their risk and of the availability of a test. In these studies, the range of attendance is 39% (S) (one family) to 70% (BB). This may be as high as 100% (R) as the recruitment method is unclear in two reports. In the studies of families where fewer informative interventions have been recorded, there is much greater agreement, with 32% attendance in France (J-R) and 34% in Israel (H).

Making a broad generalization from these reports, it could be suggested that one-third of family members attend for counselling spontaneously, and perhaps two-thirds of family members have been definitely informed of their potential to be tested. This raises the issue of whether it is the clinician's responsibility to ensure that every family member is aware of their risk status; this is a moral and legal question that deserves wider debate than could be given here.

Uptake amongst attendees

Once an individual has come forward for counselling, they are much more likely to have testing than to decline the offer. Across the six reports that discussed this, there was broad agreement that 78–99% of those attending clinic or research education sessions will proceed to testing. The method of initiating attendance appears not to impact on the rate of test utilization. However, it must be remembered that those unwilling to undergo testing are more likely to refuse to participate in research or to not make contact spontaneously, and so will not attend.

Participation in ongoing research

It might be expected that participation in research for up to 20–25 years (BB) may affect individual's attitudes to, and reasons for, having testing. Thirty-eight per cent of this sample were new to research, and comparisons showed no effect. However, their very involvement may undermine this calculation, as they have become 'study participators'. Other authors generally acknowledge that the well-researched families may not be typical.

There are privacy and confidentiality issues connected to the use of pedigree information provided by one family member in genetic studies, and its trans-mission to others. For example, Benkendorf et al. (1997) report that 56–57% of first-degree relatives of cancer patients felt that written consent should be gained before a member of the immediate family was informed of a genetic test result. These and other workers (Powers, 1993; Winter et al., 1996; Julian-Reynier et al., 2000b) remind us of the care that must be taken in using such information.

'Time since genetic diagnosis' as a selection criterion

Only two papers (J-R and M-H) refer directly to the time when the family's mutation was found. J-R used a cut-off point based on the 75th centile of elapsed time in the initial sample, and excluded any families who had had less than 8 months to attend for counselling, while M-H used a date cut-off. Where testing was offered as part of a specific research programme, this limitation may have affected results. M-H showed that the rate of uptake had stabilized by 24 months, but most of the finite offer periods are likely to have been shorter than this, and this is often unclear. J-R includes those 'in the process of testing' in the headline rate of uptake, therefore assuming that they will go ahead with testing. Anecdotal evidence shows that some individuals will postpone testing for considerable periods, or decline to receive their results after blood has been drawn, making this assumption unsafe.

Cancer and risk status

Up to 18% of the family members offered testing were affected with cancer (B), with two papers (W and M-H) concentrating only on pre-symptomatic testing, and one further work (S) not specifying what proportion of individuals contacted had a diagnosis of cancer. In most cases, the uptake amongst affecteds and unaffecteds is either directly reported or deducible from the data provided. Unsurprisingly perhaps, every paper that provided complete data on cancer status showed a higher rate of utilization of counselling (H) or testing in affecteds than in unaffecteds, except where data were only available for study participants (BB), where a rate of 79% was reported for both groups. J-R reports the lowest figures in each group, while L consistently reports the highest (23% vs 56% and 69 vs 74%: unaffecteds and affecteds respectively). This may once more reflect differences in recruitment methodology.

Eligibility criteria definitions given ranged from being the first- or second-degree relative (J-R) of the affected proband (i.e. having a risk of inheriting the mutation of 50% or 25%, M-H) to a much looser given definition such as 'being a member of the extended family' (W, L, R, BB). S and BB can both be criticized for offering testing to, or contacting, the children of untested parents. The former stated that: 'non-participants were more likely to have a parent who had already tested negative', which would make them ineligible for testing under the usual clinical criteria. Later in the text it is stated that the recruitment strategy was designed so that at-risk parents were tested before their children, which further confuses the analysis. In the latter, this was justified as allowing independent decision-making, but negated by the fact that up to five family members were present at each education and counselling session, so that private concerns may have been more difficult to raise. The denominator for the uptake calculation becomes questionable for both of these reports.

J-R, M-H and H provide the best descriptions of the chance of each unaffected individual inheriting the family's mutation, although using different terminology. If the first-degree relative of an affected proband (J-R) or of a cancer patient (H) can be assumed to have a 50% risk of inheriting the mutation (M-H), then all report similar results. In this group, 40–44% (H, J-R) attended for counselling, and 36% (J-R, M-H) proceeded to testing, but while there are less complete data for those at 25% risk, the proportion seen/tested is considerably lower.

Differences between females and males

With the far greater health implications for women of being a *BRCA1/2* mutation carrier, it is unsurprising that women tend to undergo testing more often than men. Without differentiating the results by study method or by sampling criteria, the ratio of women to men tested appears to be approximately 3 : 1, and this also applies when taking into account risk status and attendance records. It is difficult to be more precise than this because of the varying study methodologies.

Comparing prospective and retrospective studies

The difference between the level of interest in testing and actual uptake is much less for *BRCA* mutations than for Huntington's disease. This is well illustrated by the population studied by the BB group, who, in the 1995 report by Struewing, reported that 95% would definitely or probably want to be tested. The actual rate of test utilization was 55%, which is, as described by the author, probably due to the differences in the 'treatability' and preventive measures available for the two conditions.

Family studies

The BB group discusses family cohesion as a predictor of test utilization, while the S group looking at sibships, investigates the effect of family position and how this affects the psychosocial impact. The other authors mentioned concur that parents are more likely to be tested than non-parents (M-H), and affecteds more than unaffecteds (R).

The differences in uptake of predictive testing between kindreds, and especially in nuclear families, may be due in part to their experiences of the disease of cancer, and not just to the number of diagnoses. The measurement of the impact the disease has had on each individual and family group will be difficult, but must include psychological and psychosocial measures together with their own personal risk. The development of such systems will allow the comparison of uptake in close and disparate families and kindreds, in those who have been closely involved in the affected's life, treatment and death, as well as in those family members who become aware of the disease during counselling.

Non-participants

In study families, non-participants have been identified by researchers, but the same cannot be said for non-research families. Without records linked between regional centres, it is difficult to ensure that every individual is aware of their risk or the opportunity to attend counselling. In a separate survey by Julian-Reynier et al. (1996), 14% of breast cancer patients refused to contact their relatives, and McAllister et al. (1998) showed that male family members were less likely to be informed about breast cancer risk than their female relations.

The studies reviewed here that concentrated on specific families provide some useful data regarding test-decliners or non-attenders, specifically Watson et al. (1995), who account for everybody. Smith et al. (1999) report that non-participants are younger (<35 years), when the risk may not seem as important (see also discussion above regarding risk). Bowles Biesecker et al. (2000) report that they were unaware of any eligible family member having a test outside the study, but unless this can be confirmed, especially in non-research families, both numerator and denominator (depending on the test results) in the calculation could be inaccurate.

Summary

A number of strengths and weaknesses in the research methodologies have been mentioned, all of which can be justified by the overall different aims of the authors. The eight reports to date can be grouped and sub-divided in any number of different ways to attempt to reach concordance in their results, but differences will always exclude at least one study. The following generalizations, based on the information in Table 19.3, use fractions rather than percentages to reflect approximate trends after the previously discussed tight criteria used for each statement have been applied.

$U_{f/c} = n/N$ at $t = 'X'$

In research families, $U_{f/c}$ is about two-fifths, in the time period allowed for the study.

In non-research families, $U_{f/c}$ is lower, at about one-third, with at least an 8-months period since the mutation was found.

$\Delta U_f = \Delta n/N \times \Delta t$

In non-research families, this will stabilize after about 1 year, but variations in family communication may result in sections of the family attending later. In research families, further review of non-testers' future actions may reveal a change.

$U_i = n/C$, where $A = C/N$

Once at clinic, four-fifths of individuals will undergo testing, but attendance in non-research families is only one-third, compared with two-thirds in families where active recruitment has taken place.

More people with a diagnosis of cancer will undergo testing than unaffecteds.

Conclusions

Defining the denominator and numerator is the most difficult part of measuring the uptake of testing. Without active recruitment, it is impossible to be sure that the denominator excludes uninformed family members, but in research families, reporting the rate amongst study participants only repeats this error. The numerator may or may not include those persons who have been affected by cancer, and who have attended clinic for counselling about their risk and the possibility of testing.

The trends indicated above reflect the current experience, with the range of surveillance options and insurance implications that are open to today's patient. These may change and improve, and influence the level of uptake of pre-symptomatic testing.

REFERENCES

Aktan-Collan K, Mecklin JP, Jarvinen H, et al. (2000). Predictive genetic testing for hereditary non-polyposis colorectal cancer: uptake and long-term satisfaction. *Int J Cancer* (*Pred Oncol*) **89**: 44–50.

Benkendorf JL, Reutenauer JE, Hughes CA, et al. (1997). Patients' attitudes about autonomy and confidentiality in genetic testing for breast–ovarian cancer susceptibility. *Am J Med Genet* **73**: 296–303.

Bowles Biesecker B, Ishibe N, Hadley DW, et al. (2000). Psychosocial factors predicting BRCA1/BRCA2 testing decisions in members of hereditary breast and ovarian families. *Am J Med Genet* **93**: 257–63.

Broadstock M, Michie S, Gray J, Mackay J and Marteau TM (2000). The psychological consequences of offering mutation searching in the family for those at risk of hereditary breast and ovarian cancer – a pilot study. *Psychooncology* **9**: 537–48.

Cappelli M, Surl H, Humphreys L, et al. (1999). Psychological and social determinants of women's decisions to undergo genetic counselling and testing for breast cancer. *Clin Genet* **55**: 419–30.

Craufurd D, Dodge A, Kerzin-Storrar L and Harris L (1989). Uptake of pre-symptomatic predictive testing for Huntington's disease. *Lancet* **2**: 603–5.

Evans DGR, Maher ER, Macleod R, Davies DR and Craufurd D (1997). Uptake of genetic testing for cancer predisposition. *J Med Genet* **34**: 746–8.

Hagoel L, Dishon S, Almog R, Silman Z, Bisland-Becktell S and Rennert G (2000). Proband family uptake of familial genetic counselling. *Psychooncology* **9**: 522–7.

Julian-Reynier C, Eisinger F, Vennin P, et al. (1996). Attitudes towards cancer predictive testing and transmission of information to the family. *J Med Genet* **33**: 731–6.

Julian-Reynier C, Sobol H, Sévilla C, Noguès C, Bourret P, and the French Cancer Genetic Network (2000a). Uptake of hereditary breast ovarian cancer genetic testing in a French national sample of BRCA1 families. *Psychooncology* **9**: 504–10.

Julian-Reynier C, Eisinger F, et al. (2000b). Disclosure to the family of breast/ovarian cancer genetic test results: patients' willingness and associated factors. *Am J Med Genet* **94**: 13–18.

Lalloo F, Cochrane S, Bulman B, et al. (1998). An evaluation of common breast cancer gene populations in a population of Ashkenazi Jews. *J Med Genet* **35**: 10–12.

Lerman C, Daly M, Masny A and Balsham A (1994). Attitudes about genetic testing for breast–ovarian cancer susceptibility. *J Clin Oncol* **12**: 843–50.

Lerman C, Seay J, Balshem A and Audrain J (1995). Interest in genetic testing among first-degree relatives of breast cancer patients. *Am J Med Genet* **57**: 385–92.

Lerman C, Narod S, Schulman K, et al. (1996). BRCA1 testing in families with hereditary breast–ovarian cancer. A prospective study of patient decision making and outcomes. *JAMA* **275**: 1885–92.

Lerman C, Hughes C, Trock BJ, et al. (1999). Genetic testing in families with hereditary nonpolyposis colon cancer. *JAMA* **281**(17): 1618–22.

McAllister MF, Evans DG, Ormiston W and Daly P (1998). Men in breast cancer families: a preliminary qualitative study of awareness and experience. *J Med Genet* **35**(9): 739–44.

Meijers-Heijboer EJ, Verhoog LC, Brekelmans CTM, et al. (2000). Presymptomatic DNA testing and prophylactic surgery in families with a BRCA1 or BRCA2 mutation. *Lancet* **355**: 2015–20.

Meiser B, Butow P, Barratt A, et al. (2000). Attitudes to genetic testing for breast cancer susceptibility in women at increased risk of developing hereditary breast cancer. *J Med Genet* **37**: 472–6.

Powers M (1993). Publication-related risks to privacy: ethical implications of pedigree studies. *IRB* **15**: 7–11.

Quaid KA and Morris M (1993). The reluctance to undergo predictive testing: the case of Huntington disease. *Am J Med Genet* **45**: 41–5.

Reichelt JG, Dahl AA, Heimdal K and Møller P (1999). Uptake of genetic testing and pre-test levels of mental distress in Norwegian families with known BRCA1 mutations. *Dis Markers* **15**: 139–43.

Schneider KA, Farkas Patenaude A and Garber JE (1995). Testing for cancer genes: decisions, decisions. *Nat Med* **1**: 302–3.

Schoenfeld M, Myers RH, Berkham B and Clark E (1984). Potential impact of a predictive test on the gene frequency of Huntington disease. *Am J Med Gen* **18**: 423–9.

Smith KR, West JA, Croyle RT and Botkin JR (1999). Familial context of genetic testing for cancer susceptibility: moderating effect of siblings' test results on psychological distress one to two weeks after BRCA1 mutation testing. *Cancer Epidemiol Biomarkers Prev* **8**: 385–92.

Struewing JP, Lerman C, Kase RG, Glambarrest TB and Tucker MA (1995). Anticipated uptake and impact of genetic testing in hereditary breast and ovarian cancer families. *Cancer Epidemiol Biomarkers Prev* **4**: 169–73.

Tambor ES, Rimer BK and Strigo TS (1997). Genetic testing for breast cancer susceptibility: awareness and interest among women in the general population. *Am J Med Genet* **68**: 43–9.

Tibben A, Niermeijer MF, Roos RAC, et al. (1992). Understanding the low uptake of presymptomatic DNA testing for Huntington's disease. *Lancet* **340**: 1416.

Ulrich CM, Kristal AR, White E, Hunt JR, Durfy SJ and Potter JD (1998). Genetic testing for cancer risk: a population survey on attitudes and intention. *Community Genet* **1**: 213–22.

Watson M, Murday V, Lloyd S, Ponder B, Averill D and Eeles R (1995). Genetic testing in breast/ovarian cancer (BRCA1) families. *Lancet* **346**: 583.

Winter PR, Wiesner GL, Finnegan J, et al. (1996). Notification of a family history of breast cancer: issues of privacy and confidentiality. *Am J Med Genet* **66**: 1–6.

20

Breast cancer genetics: ethical, social and insurance issues

Patrick J. Morrison[1] and C. Michael Steel[2]

[1]Belfast City Hospital NHS Trust, Belfast, UK
[2]University of St Andrews, Fife, UK

Background

A family history of breast cancer is now universally recognized as a potential risk factor, and demand for appropriate clinical services is fuelled by publicity in both the popular media and the professional literature. Within the past few years, breast cancer family clinics have sprung up in almost every major medical centre and all are hard-pressed to cope with the numbers of referrals (Thompson et al., 1995; Vasen et al., 1998; Hodgson et al., 1999). There has been little time to reflect on what constitutes an appropriate clinical service in this setting, while the pace of new developments on the molecular and epidemiological fronts has left clinicians struggling to interpret their relevance for patients. A critical reappraisal of the care currently offered to women who may be at increased genetic risk of breast cancer is therefore timely.

Are women misinformed?

Mammography and ovarian screening

Surveys in several countries have found that women coming forward to breast cancer family clinics want, above all else, access to mammographic screening (Julian-Reynier et al., 1996; Lalloo et al., 1998). For those judged to be above a certain level of risk, regular mammography is indeed usually provided, typically from age 30 or 35 years and at annual or 2-yearly intervals (Hodgson et al., 1999; Møller et al., 1999a). It remains the 'gold standard' for early detection of breast tumours but is far from perfect (Law, 1997). Data on the sensitivity of screening mammography for young women are very incomplete. The radiographic density of breast tissue tends to be greater (Ellwood et al., 1993) and there is evidence that breast cancers grow more rapidly in younger patients (Tabar et al., 1987), so that effective intervention calls for the detection of very small lesions on a dense background. The challenge to the radiologist is daunting and while, in many centres, additional resources have been applied to the genetics arm of multidisciplinary services (Beckman, 1999; Hodgson et al., 1999; Kristofferson, 1999), commensurate increases in support for diagnostic radiology have been conspicuous by their absence. Data accumulating slowly, notably from the EU Biomed 2 demonstration programme, do indicate that the majority of breast cancers arising in young women enrolled in 'high risk' surveillance programmes can be detected while still very small and node-negative (Møller et al., 1999b; Macmillan, 2000). Expert mammography plays an important part. However, the findings also highlight the importance of clinical examination and access to all the diagnostic modalities included within the 'triple assessment' protocol for breast lesions (Møller et al., 1999c).

Belief in the 'magical' properties of mammography is clearly misplaced and campaigns for more and better breast cancer family clinics should perhaps concentrate on the overall breadth of service provision rather than on mammography in isolation. Most importantly, is the local clinic able to ensure that 'annual review' visits actually take place annually, rather than at intervals of 15 months, that so easily slip to 18 months and beyond (Møller et al., 1999a)?

Where a risk of ovarian cancer is identified, regular screening by transvaginal ultrasound and/or serum CA125 measurement may be offered (Emery et al., 2000). There are as yet, however, no data to show that this type of surveillance results in improved prospects of survival for those in a high-risk category. Familial ovarian cancers are almost invariably epithelial and usually of serous type (Bewtra et al., 1992). These tend to behave aggressively and, even with annual screening, may not be detected while still localized to the ovary. Because even normal follicles are visible on ultrasound and because there is an appreciable rate of false-positive CA125 results, which then need to be repeated, women may be impressed by the sensitivity of the tests and assume that screening offers a higher degree of protection than has actually been shown (Cull et al., 2001).

Gene testing

The role of specific genes in hereditary cancers is becoming ever more widely recognized and enquiries about the availability of 'the gene test' are now commonplace. Indeed, some women attend a breast cancer genetics clinic for the first time under the impression that a 'gene test' will be undertaken as a matter of course. This should be a cause for concern as it highlights the readiness of at least some members of the public to accept the application of medical technology without question. It is, of course, one of the functions of a cancer genetics clinic to provide clear information about the practical limitations of molecular diagnostics and about the issues to be considered before any individual family member proceeds down this road. The restricted availability of facilities for molecular analysis of *BRCA1* and *BRCA2* imposes its own discipline on the practice of gene testing. As molecular technology advances, however, mutation detection may become rapid, efficient and widely available. There is a real danger that individuals may then embark on predictive testing without adequate counselling.

The scale of familial cancer risk

Not surprisingly, individual self-estimates of breast cancer risk among members of multi-case families vary widely and are probably influenced by emotional responses to personal experience rather than a dispassionate assessment of mathematical realities (Evans et al., 1994; Lloyd et al., 1996; Cull et al., 1999). In any event, women attending breast cancer family clinics, in the main, neither wish nor expect very precise risk estimates for themselves, even if that were possible. Widely quoted lifetime penetrance figures of more than 80%, for *BRCA1* or *BRCA2* mutations (Ford et al., 1998), contrast with values of 40–60% obtained more recently from population-based studies (Struewing et al., 1997; Thorlacius et al., 1998). There are undoubtedly many more women than we had thought, living long and fruitful lives, without cancer but with germline mutations in *BRCA1* or *BRCA2*. It seems likely that penetrance may be modified by other genetic and/or environmental factors (Narod et al., 1995a; Burke et al., 1999). Until these are defined, the projection of risk, even for someone with a proven *BRCA1* or *BRCA2* mutation, must remain very uncertain. Where this becomes important is in influencing decisions about management, for example when there is a choice between continued surveillance and prophylactic surgery.

Management options

Even before *BRCA1* or *BRCA2* were identified, a few women with strong family histories of breast and/or ovarian cancer requested prophylactic surgery and, after thorough assessment, a procedure has sometimes been carried out. As molecular diagnosis becomes more widely available, surgical options are considered more frequently. Where the surgery is limited to oophorectomy, the issue may not provoke much controversy, although occasionally requests come from patients in their thirties or even younger. The risk of ovarian cancer before the age of 40 years is very low, even in carriers of *BRCA1* or *BRCA2* germline mutations (Ford et al., 1998) and the long-term consequences of very early oophorectomy (with prolonged use of HRT) are uncertain. Hence prophylactic oophorectomy is very hard to justify before that age. The procedure also carries some morbidity – and potentially some mortality – even in the best centres and is not to be promoted lightly. It does, however, appear to have a place in the management of familial breast/ovarian cancer, probably reducing the incidence of both tumours among *BRCA1/2* mutation carriers (Møller et al., 1999a; Rebbeck et al., 1999; Emery et al., 2000).

Bilateral total or subcutaneous mastectomy, with or without reconstruction, is a much more daunting procedure for both surgeon and patient (Baildam, 1999). The single large retrospective study published to date (Hartmann et al., 1999) indicates that the procedure reduces subsequent breast cancer risk by at least 90% and therefore it is not an unreasonable choice for those at very high risk. There is, however, no close correlation between objective estimate of risk and demand for prophylactic mastectomy. The extent of demand and the strength of feeling expressed by individual patients seem to be influenced by personal experience of cancer and by national or regional 'cultural norms' (Bebbington and Fallowfield, 1999; Eccles et al., 1999; Pasini and Pierotti, 1999). The popular media tend to highlight heroic surgery in stories related to familial cancer, and the perception that this is the first line of management may discourage some women from seeking referral to a cancer genetics clinic. In at least some instances, what is being managed by prophylactic surgery is anxiety rather than cancer risk per se. This is very evident, for example, in relation to requests for oophorectomy from women aged under 35 years. Nevertheless, anxiety can be seriously disabling and there is no escaping the message from women who have undergone prophylactic mastectomy that this is usually a highly successful operation, when measured by patient satisfaction.

Very high priority must be given to the collation of prospective data on the efficacy of surveillance and early detection for both breast and ovarian cancer so that management options can be presented in more concrete terms, balancing risks and benefits according to age, family history and molecular findings (Møller et al., 1999b).

Education

All of the foregoing issues relate to public perceptions of familial cancer risk. The past record of the medical profession in this regard does not inspire confidence. Many patients, on first attendance at a breast cancer genetics clinic, describe their family's longstanding concern about an abnormally high incidence of the disease and the repeated patronizing reassurance from doctors that there is no genetic component in breast cancer. We have a credibility gap to close.

At present, it is clear that highly educated professional women are over-represented and the most socially deprived groups under-represented among the clientele of cancer family clinics (Steel et al., 1999). If the early indications of health benefit from clinic attendance are confirmed, this social imbalance will become an embarrassment and specific plans to correct it should be developed now. A number of patient support groups, including at least one 'familial breast cancer help-line', provide an invaluable service in distributing educational material and answering frequently asked questions (Møller et al., 1999a). In many countries, these voluntary organizations are closely integrated with health services and this is demonstrably sound policy, particularly at the stage of rapidly evolving clinical practice. Strict separation of 'professional' and lay functions in other countries is perhaps connected with the traditional reluctance of doctors to admit uncertainty but, in the setting of the breast cancer genetics clinic, the pretence of omniscience cannot be sustained for long.

Where health services are organized on the basis of primary, secondary and tertiary care (as in the UK), the 'general practitioner' or 'family doctor' is expected to act as 'gatekeeper', regulating access to genetics clinics. It is a matter of some concern that GPs vary widely in their willingness to undertake this function, the level of training they have received, and the degree of interest they may express in clinical genetics (Emery et al., 1999; Watson et al., 1999a,b). Education must therefore extend beyond the general public if equity of access to clinical services is to be assured.

Exacerbating and alleviating anxiety

A frequent criticism of the publicity surrounding hereditary cancer risk is that it simply promotes anxiety while doing nothing practical to counter it. Setting aside the fact that publicity is generated largely by the popular media, over which cancer geneticists have no control, several studies of patients who have made use of cancer family clinical services provide a measure of reassurance. They have, in the main, confirmed that perceptions of risk before clinic attendance are often unrealistic, that there is some improvement in accuracy after attendance and that levels of anxiety tend to decline, at least in the short term, regardless of changes in risk perception. Hence there is some justification for the claim that cancer family clinics are responding to a pre-existing and hitherto unmet need and that they fulfil a useful function, even before they have been shown to influence cancer morbidity or mortality (Evans et al., 1994; Lloyd et al., 1996; Cull et al., 1999).

It is clear that, for many women referred to a cancer family clinic, simply having the legitimacy of their concerns acknowledged represents a significant advance. In this setting, those who can be told, after due investigation, that they are not at significantly increased risk, usually accept this reassurance. While access to mammography is often the most overt objective, the opportunity to discuss familial breast cancer rationally and in depth is greatly appreciated. Many clinics have gone to considerable lengths to develop clear and effective means of communicating quite difficult concepts of risk and management options, in the form of personal-ized letters, leaflets and videos (Cull et al., 1998; Skirton, 1999). Best practice is freely copied within the community of cancer family clinics. The genetics associate or genetics nurse specialist has a crucial role (Hodgson et al., 1999). Families will often form a close bond with one member of the clinic team and, in most instances, this is the nurse specialist. She/he needs protected time to be accessible in person and by telephone, to repeat information not fully 'taken on board', to answer questions and to receive news of any further developments in the family history. Patients' expectations of what a breast cancer family clinic can offer are, typically, modest. Many will state openly that their hopes are directed towards their children's generation rather than their own and that they gain real satisfac-tion from the opportunity to participate in long-term clinical research pro-grammes. This is reflected in a gratifying response rate for complex questionnaires and in remarkable patience with painfully slow progress towards universal avail-ability of molecular testing.

Eligibility criteria

Most breast cancer genetics clinics will accept referrals of women between the ages of 35 and 50 years if their lifetime risk of breast cancer is at least 20%. There is general agreement that this represents a pragmatic balance between the desire to satisfy demand and the need to 'ration' limited resource. The actual computation of risk (see Chapter 8) generally follows one of the widely accepted algorithms, based on the number, ages of onset and relationship of affected relatives with breast and/or ovarian cancer (Gail et al., 1989; Claus et al., 1991). Very precise figures can be generated by computer (Chapman, 1999) but few clinicians will wish to be guided by these alone. It is important to remember that current understanding of genetic risks is far from complete and that a modicum of built-in flexibility in referral policy will allow advances to be accommodated as they arise. For example, instances of ovarian cancer in the family are invariably taken into account but, at present, there is no formal procedure for considering pancreatic, prostate, bowel or other cancers, although it is clear that these too can be manifestations of germline mutations in *BRCA1* and/or *BRCA2* (Stratton, 1996).

One difficult issue is the weight that should be placed on anxiety, as distinct from assessed risk. If, as seems to be the case, attendance at a cancer family clinic and careful assessment of the family history by 'experts' can relieve both ('low-risk') patient and GP of a persistent problem, then this would appear to be a sensible use of clinic resources. It also contributes to a mutually supportive relationship between clinic and local GPs, to the benefit of both.

A further question is when to discontinue surveillance. With advancing age, the likelihood that a given unaffected family member is a carrier of a high-risk germline mutation diminishes (Ford et al., 1998). Furthermore, the biology of breast cancer implies that mammography and clinical examination need to be repeated at less frequent intervals in older women (Tabar et al., 1987). However, there is no sharp cut-off at the age of 50 years and, particularly if several relatives have been diagnosed in their early fifties, women are understandably reluctant to accept discharge from a cancer family clinic surveillance programme as soon as they become eligible for 3-yearly mammographic screening under a national or workplace-based scheme. Most clinicians will be guided by the pattern of cancers previously recorded in each family before making a judgement on when it is 'safe' to reduce intensity of screening, but objective guidance, from the analysis of a large body of clinical data, will be welcome.

The flexibility in enrolment policy referred to above means that, as adjustments are made in the light of experience, some women who were accepted in the early days of the clinics no longer satisfy eligibility criteria. Equally, as more information emerges about particular families, or as further cancers occur, some, who had been assured that special surveillance was not required, will have to be recalled and given different advice. In both situations, experience shows that most women react to the change in policy with understanding.

At present, different criteria tend to be applied for enrolment in a clinical surveillance programme and for molecular screening. In part, this reflects the need, in most centres, for blood DNA from a living affected relative before molecular analysis can be attempted. However, there is also a separate issue of limited laboratory resources, which means that rather stringent conditions (e.g. four close relatives affected) tend to be set before a complete screen for *BRCA1* and *BRCA2* mutations will be undertaken (Narod et al., 1995b; Gayther and Ponder, 1997; Ford et al., 1998; Stoppa-Lyonnet et al., 1999; Eccles et al., 2000). This position is expected to evolve rapidly as molecular screening techniques become faster and more efficient. In certain centres, where there are characteristic local 'founder' mutations, a quick and inexpensive preliminary screen for those particular mutations is carried out on almost all referred families.

Cost-effectiveness

Whether cancer family clinical services and associated laboratory facilities are provided through national, insurance-based or privately funded healthcare systems, the actual costs are large. There is, therefore, an obligation on all those involved to audit their activity. It would be invidious to attempt to place a cash value on a life saved or even on a 'quality-adjusted life year' gained. However, it is perfectly legitimate to point out that a substantial proportion of women affected by familial breast and ovarian cancer are in 'the prime of life', contributing to the work-force and the community as well as raising young families. The potential economic and social gain, if mortality and morbidity can be reduced, is thus enormous (Heimdal et al., 1999). Preliminary data from the EU Demonstration Programme indicate that the majority of breast cancers arising in young women under surveillance through a family history clinic can be detected at an early pathological stage and that prognosis is substantially improved thereby (Møller et al., 1999a). The task now is to refine the operation of these clinics and their associated laboratories so that services are directed precisely at those who will benefit most. The disposal of personnel, the mechanics and timing of clinical, mammographic and new alternative modes of screening and the development of laboratory protocols for mutation detection are all capable of streamlining so that resources are deployed most effectively. It may be some years before the 'ideal' system for running a breast cancer family service can be determined but, provided data are gathered, collated and analysed from a large number of existing clinics pursuing the same aims, real progress in that direction can be predicted with confidence.

As the contribution of molecular diagnostics grows, the proportion of breast cancer families in whom a causal germline mutation has been identified will increase. Assuming that many 'at-risk' members of these families will opt for predictive testing (Lerman et al., 1996; De Vos et al., 1999; Pasini and Pierotti, 1999; Reichelt et al., 1999), the mean level of risk for those enrolled in cancer family clinics will rise. By targeting resources more accurately, cost-effectiveness will be improved. There will remain, however, very substantial numbers of women at increased genetic risk of breast cancer, who do not belong to *BRCA1* or *BRCA2* mutation families. It is authoritatively estimated that the greater part of heritable breast cancer risk is attributable to common low-penetrance mutations in genes ('*BRCAx*') that have yet to be identified (Friend, 1996; Peto et al., 1999). Many women carrying these mutations will not have a family history striking enough to make them eligible for enrolment in a breast cancer family clinic screening programme. There is therefore a strong case for allocating resources to identifying '*BRCAx*'. If this should prove to be a single locus or even a small number of distinct loci, then it is possible that the mutations or polymorphisms conferring a three- or four-fold increase in lifetime risk of breast cancer may be identifiable by molecular screening of the population, rather than relying on family history – a reversal of the current policy in relation to *BRCA1* and *BRCA2*. That, in turn, will require a radical revision of clinical services for those at increased genetic risk, in anticipation of much increased demand for clinical/mammographic surveillance.

Confidentiality of family medical history

A recurring theme in clinical genetics is the difficulty of balancing an individual's right to privacy against the duty to share relevant information with the wider family. The enormous increase in the potential for genetic analysis in recent years has raised public awareness of the risks of 'genetic discrimination' in education, employment, insurance and access to health care. These are genuine concerns that society must address but the initial reaction, which is often to propose legislation that gives highest priority to confidentiality, may not secure the greatest good for the greatest number. Restricting access to medical records is well-intentioned but may achieve little in terms of protection of individual rights while negating efforts to gather epidemiological data of profound importance for improving the future health of all (Vandenbroucke, 1998; Wadman, 1998; Peto et al., 1999; White, 1999; Al-Shahi and Warlow, 2000; Strobl et al., 2000).

The very essence of clinical genetics is the taking of a verbal family history. At present, the prior consent of family members is not a statutory requirement and it is difficult to envisage a workable formula that would make it so. We therefore start with a family tree as described by the proband. It may well be both incomplete and inaccurate. This is certainly a common experience when dealing with familial breast/ovarian cancer. Good medical practice dictates that the information given should be checked and amplified so that risk assessment, advice and management are as soundly based as possible (Floderus et al., 1990; Theis et al., 1994; Kerber and Slattery, 1997; De Vos et al., 1999; Steel and Smyth, 1999). The great majority of families are cooperative and relatives readily give consent for confirmation of relevant diagnoses via hospital records or cancer registries. However, it does not require a great feat of imagination to recognize the potential for unnecessary distress when a reported mastectomy for breast cancer proves to have been a biopsy for benign disease. Some family members may be difficult, or impossible, to trace, though the place and date of previous surgery may be known. For a variety of reasons, a few relatives refuse permission to examine their hospital notes. Thus, not infrequently, we must rely, at least in part, on data that are unconfirmed. This problem may grow as legislators become more outspoken in their campaigns 'to safeguard individual privacy'. Existing and proposed laws often include a vague clause that permits release of information without formal consent 'for sound medical reasons' but it seems that what is envisaged is protection of the public against infectious diseases or other identifiable medical dangers. There is no indication, as yet, that provision of genetic information to other family members would constitute a 'sound medical reason' for obtaining limited access to the medical records of a third party (Reilly, 1996; Steel and Smyth, 1999). Yet, provided the information obtained is used for specific genetic purposes and is handled within the established conventions of medical confidentiality, it is difficult to see what benefit accrues to anyone from privacy legislation that 'protects' records in this way. The long-established practice of collecting and storing heelprick blood samples from all newborn infants in the UK (initially for phenylketonuria screening) would probably not be permitted if proposed today. It is interesting to note that organizations representing families affected by genetic disorders (i.e. those with the most profound stake in both the benefits and the disadvantages of medical secrecy) are among the strongest advocates of openness in recording genetic information (Hunt, 1992).

Very occasionally, a family history of breast (or other) cancers may be concocted or grossly embellished by a patient seeking attention or as a variant of Munchausen syndrome (Evans et al., 1998). The underlying psychological disturbance may not be obvious, though a refusal to permit approaches to relatives to confirm the reported diagnosis may arouse suspicion.

Given the stringent criteria for access to molecular analysis of *BRCA1* and *BRCA2*, there could be a temptation for patients to err on the side of over-reporting cases of cancer among their relatives, in order to obtain a 'gene test'. It will be interesting to find out what level of family history confirmation may be required by public or insurance-based health services who provide (and pay for) molecular testing. Similarly, it may be instructive to observe what effect, if any, this consideration may have on the framing and interpretation of medical privacy legislation.

Confidentiality of molecular genetic data

Once a germline mutation (for example in *BRCA1* or *BRCA2*) has been identified in one family member, then we enter more complex ethical and legal territory (Human Genetics Advisory Commission (UK), 1997; American Society of Human Genetics, 1998; Müller et al., 2000). A life assurance company is entitled to ask any questions it wishes about illnesses or causes of death among relatives (in much the same way as a clinical geneticist) and could repudiate cover if these were shown subsequently to have been answered untruthfully. The company's rights of access to predictive molecular genetics test results are, however, much less clearcut and vary widely from country to country (as discussed in Chapter 12). Similarly, while there may be a moral obligation to share the test result with other family members, reluctance to do so can be justified on the grounds that, compared with family medical history, molecular information is much more likely to lead to discrimination. It is therefore crucial to obtain genuinely informed consent for disclosure of the result to relevant members of the family before setting in train the process of analysing DNA from one key individual. It has been argued that, once the result is known, that information becomes the property of the whole family (Royal College of Physicians of London, 1991; Pembrey and Anionwu, 1996) but this concept has yet to be validated in law. As cascade testing proceeds through the family, it is quite possible that certain individuals will either decline to be tested or will refuse to allow anyone else access to their result (De Vos et al., 1999). Others in the cascade (their daughters, for example) are, of course, entitled to seek testing on their own account and the outcome may allow the 'private' result to be inferred, but this is an issue that arises in many areas of genetics and the ethical position – that A cannot obstruct access of B to a genetics test simply because it may reveal the status of A – is reasonably clear (Royal College of Physicians of London, 1991; Pembrey and Anionwu, 1996).

It is generally accepted that *BRCA1/2* testing should not be undertaken on minors since there is no proven advantage in knowing the result long before there is a measurable risk. The question of pre-natal testing arises only occasionally and, as a rule, prospective parents accept that it would be inappropriate.

Communicating and recording molecular test results can present more difficulties than are immediately apparent. Within a given family, the individual chosen to be the DNA donor for the initial mutation screen will usually have been affected herself and thus will anticipate a positive result. Sometimes, however, he or she is an unaffected obligate carrier and, while the implications may be clear to the geneticist, it is vital that the situation is spelled out with great care and that consent for the test and all its ramifications is truly informed. If the mutation is found in a 'research' sample that has been handled many times, perhaps over several years, it is mandatory that the test be repeated in a fresh specimen, ideally from the same individual, or, if that is impossible, from another affected member of the same family. Once the mutation is known, virtually all centres insist on formal counselling before any at-risk family member is offered a predictive test. When agreement to test has been reached, it is important that there should be minimal delay (no more than 2 weeks) before the result is obtained. Most clinics will make every effort to give the result in person rather than by post or telephone, and follow-up counselling should be available to both mutation-carriers and non-carriers.

Because of the special position of molecular test results, in relation to life assurance and employment, there is some uncertainty as to how and where they should be recorded. Hospital notes are, by their nature, not particularly secure. They are handled by clinical staff, by secretaries and by personnel in records departments. Without impugning the integrity of any of these, it must be admitted that, as the files are passed from department to department and even between hospitals, opportunities for unauthorized access to their contents must arise. One possible solution would be to hold the relevant data under lock and key, for example in the genetics department, recording in the notes only the fact that a result has been obtained and the place where it is stored. This, however, would inevitably complicate clinical management of the family and there would be many occasions – for example when sending samples to the laboratory for testing, or when discussing prior probabilities of genetic status with at-risk individuals – when the demands of accuracy would require extraction of the data from storage. Each such occasion would renew the risk of breaching security. Thus, complete protection of privacy is incompatible with good medical practice. A more fruitful approach might entail passing laws that impose severe penalties for attempting to gain unauthorized access to medical records or for making improper use of medical information obtained without consent. That could not only provide effective safeguards against discrimination but might also reverse the climate of fear placing obstacles in the way of data gathering for legitimate medical research.

Duty of care

The unit of currency in clinical genetics is, typically, the family rather than the individual and in the vast majority of instances there is mutually beneficial collaboration between the family members and the clinicians involved in their care. However, in the course of verification of a family history, pedigrees may be constructed that include relatives not personally known to those attending the clinic. Questions then arise about the extent of the clinicians' responsibilities (Müller et al., 2000). An easy answer might be that clinicians have a duty of care only to those family members who have approached them for professional advice. This might reasonably be extended to other family members in direct contact with the original proband(s) but not to more distant relatives whose existence might be known but for whom further details, such as addresses, are not readily available. What, then, is the position of very close relatives whose whereabouts are known but who are estranged from the proband(s)? Again, it may be argued that the clinician should not become involved in old family quarrels – 'let sleeping dogs lie'. Yet, suppose the genetic diagnosis in question is retinoblastoma. Where the germline mutation is known, at-risk infants can be tested at birth and, if carriers, can be examined at very frequent intervals so that incipient tumours can be eliminated by laser photocoagulation, so preserving both life and sight (Murphree, 1996). When such a mutation is discovered in any branch of a family, is it really consistent with medical ethics for a geneticist to restrict dissemination of that information to the immediate family – and then only to those who are speaking to each other? Do we therefore modify our concepts of what is ethical according to the scope for useful intervention? Perhaps we must but, if so, we should be aware that there are few fixed points in clinical genetics. Familial breast cancer is a typical case. It is not unreasonable to hope that the coming generation will reap great benefits, in terms of effective preventive measures, from current research. Failure to pass on now to distant branches of a family the fact that a *BRCA1* or *BRCA2* germline mutation has been discovered could have regrettable consequences in 20 or 30 years' time. Social trends suggest that family coherence is declining and world-wide mobility is certainly increasing so that opportunities for communication of relevant genetic information are unlikely to improve. Clearly, there are limits to what can be achieved and even to what can reasonably be expected of geneticists in reaching out to the extended family. At present, queries are received intermittently in most clinical genetics centres about families believed to originate from that region. In a few cases it is possible to make the desired connection but the process is very much 'hit or miss'. It might, however, be possible to establish in every country or state a central registry, which could be informed that genetic information was available about a family believed to be resident there. Identifying details of the original family and contact information about the clinical centre holding the relevant genetic data could be lodged, but not the actual data. Then, if a family in New Zealand, for example, believed that they might carry a predisposition to breast cancer and they knew that their forebears came from Scotland, they could consult the registry to see whether there was an entry relating to their distant cousins and, if so, make contact with the clinic concerned.

Gene patenting

Obviously, as the human genome project and concurrent advances in molecular technology broaden the impact of clinical genetics on the general population, the speciality is having to concern itself increasingly with matters of law, ethics and social organization. One of the most pressing current issues is the prospect of gene patenting and its implications for clinical practice. Despite existing law and directives on both sides of the Atlantic, the principle that gene sequences should be patentable is still being challenged (Directive 98/44/EC of the European Parliament and the Council (1998); Knoppers, 1999; Balter, 2000; Michel, 2000; Senior, 2000). Many geneticists worry that clinically important research and development will be stultified by companies who hold patents on particular sequences and who wish to recoup their investment in this field by controlling access to diagnostic tests and to new therapies based on knowledge of these sequences.

In relation to *BRCA1*, for which a patent application has been filed by Myriad Genetics Inc., the company has been prepared to enter into relatively liberal agreements with publicly funded health providers so that current clinical practice is unaffected. In the longer term, however, the fact that genes may be 'owned', even for a limited period, by any agency – commercial, governmental or charitable – is a cause of deep unease. It seems to contravene the principle that only a new invention should be patentable (Knoppers, 1999). A gene sequence is not an invention and its complete specification is usually the end result of a long process that has involved contributions from a number of (knowingly or unwittingly) collaborating groups. There is ample scope for the invention of diagnostic or other applications of the sequence and these processes may indeed be the subjects of patent applications. That would leave the field open for the development of newer, faster and less expensive alternative techniques. Something of that kind is going on at present in the field of *BRCA1* and *BRCA2* diagnostics. There could be major benefits for breast cancer families but, as matters stand, large-scale introduction of new *BRCA1* tests could be impeded by the patent-holder.

Commercial genetic testing

In a number of countries, commercial operators provide the bulk of medical laboratory services. They compete with each other, and sometimes with non-commercial laboratories, on the basis of quality and cost. Several such companies are now entering the genetics field (Farrell, 1997). In one sense, this is simply a logical extension of established practice, but there are some new concerns. Because predictive testing may have profound implications for the individual undergoing the test and for his/her family – implications that may not be fully apparent before the result is obtained – public access to genetic testing services should perhaps be regulated. In the case of commercial screening for *BRCA1* and *BRCA2* mutations, there is a requirement that samples should be submitted via a registered medical practitioner and that professional pre-test counselling should be provided (Barber, 1998). It is, however, unclear as yet what qualifications (if any) in clinical genetics the referring practitioner must have. Furthermore, among the sources of demand for commercial testing will be families judged not to be at sufficient risk to be eligible for mutation testing within a publicly funded or insurance-based service. In many cases, paying for a private test will be a reasonable option, but if the clinical geneticist feels that this is neither sensible nor in the interests of the individual seeking the test, does he/she have the right to refuse to forward a sample to the commercial laboratory or to provide pre- and post-test counselling?

Paternity testing

The current perspective in clinical practice when non-paternity is suspected following mutation testing is not to tell the husband directly of a non-paternity result (Lucassen and Parker, 2001). The committee on assessing genetic risks of the Institute of Medicine (1994) in the USA recommended that the woman herself should be informed as 'genetic testing should not be used in ways that disrupt families'. Most problems in practice are solved by raising the possibility at the outset as this minimizes the ethical dilemmas encountered when the tests suggest non-paternity. In Australia, this is often done with an information leaflet (Medical Research Council, 1992). Whatever way paternity is (or is not) broached following results, a sensitive approach to the discussion of the facts is needed.

Insurance issues

R.A. Fisher predicted the use of genetic information in assessing insurance risks as long ago as 1935 (Harper, 1992). Several genetic tests are now available routinely. For testing in familial breast and ovarian cancer, the main tests asked for are *BRCA1* and *BRCA2*, and less frequently *PTEN*, familial adenomatous polyposis and *TP53*. Occasionally FAP and HNPCC (hereditary non-polyposis colon cancer) tests may also involve some cases of ovarian and occasionally breast cancer (see Chapter 5). Huntington disease (HD), an autosomal dominant neurodegenerative disorder, has been a role model for this type of testing. Several ethical and legal problems have already been recognized (Huggins et al., 1990; Harper, 1993). In 1995, the American Society of Human Genetics published a statement to help understanding of insurance issues (The Ad Hoc Committee on Genetic Testing/Insurance Issues, 1995). Clearly, there is a difference between more highly penetrant autosomal dominant diseases such as HD, and such diseases as breast cancers. Life tables and penetrance have been worked out for HD and it is possible to predict the age of death within a narrow range. Cancers due to single genes, such as breast cancer, which constitute only 5–10% of a predominantly non-familial common cancer, present more difficulty, as few accurate lifetime risk tables are available or are difficult to compile with limited accurate penetrance data (MacDonald et al., 2000a,b). If genetic tests for *BRCA1* and *BRCA2* are used in insurance, they should only be used in conjunction with other information.

Several European countries have no legislation or guidelines on insurance and genetic testing. Countries that have some guidelines have a moratorium on the use of genetic tests. For example, in France the moratorium is up to 5 years, whilst in the Netherlands it has been extended indefinitely. Once a moratorium has been introduced, it is difficult to find sufficient scientific evidence to justify lifting a ban on the use of genetic testing in underwriting practice (Morrison, 1998a).

Definition of a genetic test

A genetic test has been defined as 'an examination of the chromosome, DNA or RNA to find out if there is an otherwise undetectable disease related genotype, which may indicate an increased chance of that individual developing a specific disease in the future' (Association of British Insurers, 1997).

The UK Advisory Committee on Genetic Testing (ACGT) (1997) definition defines it as 'a test to detect the presence or absence of, or change in, a particular gene or chromosome'.

Family history data have been used for years and are generally accepted by insurance companies, although there may be considerable inaccuracy in family history data. Using such history without good validated reasons is bad practice and should be challenged; further evidence needs to be collected to demonstrate whether such use is really fair or effective.

What percentage of policies are affected?

In the UK, 95–97% of life insurance policies are accepted at no increased premium. Only about 1% are declined, and 2–4% are rated up (LeGrys, 1997; MacDonald, 1997). There is no analysis of these figures for specific diseases. The main reason for refusal or 'loaded' premiums is the above-average sum assured, and not the type of 'high-risk' individual assessed. Risks for insurers will be small if the policy value is low (Human Genetics Advisory Commission, 1997), for example under £100 000.

The recent UK experience of insurance and genetic testing

In the UK the main concern is about the consequences of cancer genetic testing on the eligibility for life assurance (Morrison, 1998a,b). The recent history and development of the insurance and genetic testing situation in the UK is interesting and relevant, because it is the only country in Europe to have had a recent major change in insurance recommendations. Insurance companies have driven the changes. This contrasts with the Netherlands and other EU countries, which have legislation generated by the government. Before 1995, the insurance industry paid little attention to progression of genetic testing. A House of Commons Science and Technology Select Committee reported on human genetics in 1995 (Science and Technology Committee, 1995) and included insurance issues. The committee found a lack of published research on underwriting and adverse selection, with the insurance industry relying on the principle of the 'right to underwrite'.

Shortly after the publication of the report, the UK government gave the Association of British Insurers (ABI) 1 year to formulate proposals that would meet demands for access to insurance. At the same time, they announced the formation of a Human Genetics Advisory Commission (HGAC). The HGAC was established in December, 1996, as a non-statutory advisory body to report to the government on various developments in genetics. It concentrated on insurance as its first task. The insurance industry, in 1997, announced the appointment of a

Table 20.1. Recommendations on genetic testing and insurance of the Human Genetics Advisory Commission of the UK (1998)

1. A permanent ban on the use of genetic testing is not appropriate. Recommendation is for the introduction of a moratorium on genetic testing for at least 2 years.
2. There is not sufficient predictive ability of genetic tests at the moment to allow accurate risk assessment.
3. The life insurance industry could currently withstand limited adverse selection if non-disclosure of test results was current policy.
4. There is a perception of unacceptable discrimination – this may deter testing that may lead to beneficial treatment.
5. Arrangements for confidentiality of data are adequate under current practice.
6. No company should require taking of a test as a prerequisite of obtaining cover.
7. Increased research and collaboration between industry and science is required to improve knowledge of actuarial implications of genetic factors.
8. There should be a robust appeals procedure as part of any new system.
9. Recommendations are primarily relating to life insurance but the above principles should apply to other types of health insurance.

genetics adviser and drafted a code of practice. The first HGAC report was published in December, 1997 (Human Genetics Advisory Commission, 1997). The report recommended a 2-year moratorium on genetic testing. Its conclusions are shown in Table 20.1. The ABI, a body representing around 95% of insurers in the UK, also reported their recommendations at the same time as the HGAC (Association of British Insurers, 1997). The ABI code of practice for genetic testing came into effect in January, 1998. The code had several important features (Table 20.2) and applied to all insurance, including life, permanent health, critical illness, and long-term care and medical expenses. Most 'relevant' UK insurance is predominantly life insurance linked to personal pensions, and property insurance (mortgage cover). As the UK NHS provides free health care, health insurance is less frequently purchased than in the USA, although there has been a recent increase in sales of personal health insurance cover policies. The situation differs from the USA insurance market, which is dominated by private health insurance.

The Government responded to the HGAC in late 1998, and although it did not accept the proposed moratorium, it established a Genetics and Insurance Advisory Committee (GIAC) in April, 1999, in an attempt to validate genetic tests proposed by the ABI. The ABI had listed matrices of autosomal-dominant, autosomal-recessive and X-linked recessive diseases for potential validation. Initially a list of about 30 tests was drafted, and then shortened to eight autosomal-dominant diseases. Adult polycystic kidney disease was then dropped as a test as ultrasound scanning was found to be reliable and easier to institute than a genetic test. The list

Table 20.2. Association of British Insurers' principles for genetic testing (1998)

1. Insurance companies will not insist on genetic tests.
2. Genetic test results will only affect insurance if they show a clearly increased risk of illness or death. A low increase in risk will not necessarily affect the premium.
3. Insurance companies will always seek expert medical advice when assessing the impact of genetic test results on insurance.
4. Insurers may take account of a test result only when reliability and relevance have been established.
5. Applicants for insurance will not be asked to take a genetic test, but existing test results should be given to the insurance company when it asks a relevant question, unless it has stated that this information is not required.
6. Existing genetic test results need not be disclosed in applications for life insurance up to £100 000[a] that are directly linked to a new mortgage for the purchase of a house to be occupied by the applicant(s).
7. An applicant will not be required to disclose the result of a genetic test undertaken by another person (such as a blood relative), and one person's test information will not affect another person's application.
8. The reason for an increased premium or rejection of an insurance application will be provided to the applicant's doctor on request.
9. Insurers will not 'cherry pick' by offering a 'preferred life' lower than normal premiums on the basis of their genetic test results.
10. An independent adjudication tribunal is being set up to consider complaints that are unresolved.
11. Each year, chief executives will need to demonstrate how they have complied with the code.

[a]Extended to £300 000 for all classes of insurance in May 2001.

of seven conditions (Table 20.3) includes Huntington disease, multiple endocrine neoplasia, breast cancer (*BRCA1/2* genes), FAP, Alzheimer's disease, hereditary motor and sensory neuropathy, and myotonic dystrophy. The list was never openly published.

The role of the GIAC was in validating the tests proposed by the ABI. It deemed a test suitable for use in assessing insurance proposals if it met three conditions:

1 Technical relevance – is the test technically reliable and does it accurately detect the specific changes sought for the named condition?
2 Clinical relevance – does a positive result in the test have any implications for the health of the individual?
3 Actuarial relevance – do the health implications make any difference to the likelihood of a claim under the proposed insurance product?

The first condition for validation – Huntington disease – was approved in

Table 20.3. List of seven conditions and genetic tests recommended by the ABI as relevant for insurance purposes

Condition	Genes tested for
*Huntington disease	HD
*Early-onset familial Alzheimer's disease	*APP, PS1* and *PS2*
*Hereditary breast and ovarian cancer	*BRCA1* and *BRCA2*
Myotonic dystrophy	*MDPK*
Familial adenomatous polyposis	APC
Multiple endocrine neoplasia	RET
Hereditary motor and sensory neuropathy	PMP22

*Reduced to only these three by end December 2000.

October, 2000, as reliable and relevant. The insurance companies accepted this ruling and disclosed that they would not use tests that were not received for approval by the GIAC by the end of 2000. Two more conditions were submitted and are currently being processed: early-onset familial Alzheimer's disease and hereditary breast/ovarian cancer. Regrettably, the insurance companies took the view that although they had withdrawn other tests, including those for the cancers FAP and MEN-2, as they felt genetic testing by middle age was not going to add much to family history and clinical examination, they refused to allow the results of negative tests (i.e. not carrying a family mutation), which would have been advantageous in securing normal rates in those penalized by family history of these diseases. Although there was a large amount of public opposition to the first approval of HD by the GIAC, the role of GIAC has been useful in that it forced the ABI to consider the topic seriously, rather that its previous view that no problem existed. It also put the onus on insurers to produce facts and made a case for submitting evidence to the GIAC regarding reliability; for just these reasons, five of the eight tests have now been dropped. The GIAC has all types of insurance as its remit and not just life insurance, which is most problematic in the UK and has forced the consideration of health and critical illness and long-term care issue onto the agenda (issues that are particularly relevant in the USA).

Other issues, including ethical and social issues in relation to insurance, are not covered by the GIAC and are the remit of the Human Genetics Commission (HGC). The HGC was established in May, 1999, following a major government reorganization of committees, and it absorbed several predecessor committees, including the Human Genetics Advisory Commission (HGAC), which stopped functioning in December, 1999. In December, 2000, the HGC published a consultation on public opinion on several issues and showed that there was strong opposition to the use of genetic test results by insurance companies (Human Genetics Commission, 2000). This was confirmed in a MORI opinion survey published by the HGC in March, 2001 (Human Genetics Commission, 2001), and the HGC concluded that the level of public concern over the issue required a response. This information coincided with the new House of Commons Science and Technology Committee (2001) report, also in March, 2001. The committee took both oral and written evidence from several bodies, including the insurance companies within and outside the ABI. The report was severely critical of the insurance companies, and the conclusions (including recommending a 2-year moratorium) are listed in Table 20.4.

The HGC published a statement in May, 2001, recommending interim recommendations on the use of genetic information in insurance (Table 20.5). These included an immediate moratorium on the use of genetic tests by the insurance companies for a period of not less than 3 years. This would allow time for a full review of evidence and regulatory options. The use of family history information was allowed but the HGC specified that they would discuss this and address how insurers use family history information. They also placed a ceiling on the recommended moratorium of £500 000, to protect the insurance industry from significant financial loss. They recommended that legislation might be needed to enforce the moratorium because of the failings of the current system.

The ABI responded by issuing, on the same day, an extension to their existing moratorium to include all classes of insurance up to £300 000 (previously only mortgage-related policies up to £100 000).

The UK government response to both the House of Commons Select Committee report and the HGC interim recommendations was published on 23 October, 2001 (Government response to the report from the House of Commons' Science and Technology Committee, 2001). The key features are summarized in Table 20.6. The government and the ABI have announced a 5-year moratorium on the use of genetic test results by insurers. The moratorium will apply to life insurance policies up to £500 000 and critical illness, long-term care insurance and income protection up to £300 000 for each type of policy. In policy applications above these limits, the insurance industry may use genetic test results where these tests have been approved by the GIAC. Legislation has not been introduced; however, independent monitoring of the ABI code of conduct will take place possibly through an enhanced role for GIAC in monitoring both insurance compliance and customer complaints. It is also to review the composition of the GIAC committee with extension of its membership. The moratorium has not been extended to use of family history data, and the whole moratorium will be reviewed after 3 years. An important note from the patients' perspective is that the use of negative test results is encouraged by the insurer, subject to confirmation in most cases by a geneticist of the relevance of the result.

Table 20.4. Some of the House of Commons' Science and Technology Committee recommendations (May 2001)

1. Insurance companies should detail exactly which genetic tests they will consider (both positive and negative) for what conditions and under which circumstances as soon as possible.
2. Commerical insurance companies should have access to the same information as applicants, where it is relevant and reliable – but only if there are no adverse consequences for society as a whole.
3. It is not certain at present that the information obtained from positive genetic tests is relevant to the insurance industry.
4. Insurers have given test results a predictive significance that cannot at present be justified.
5. Insurers appear to be more interested in establishing their future right to use genetic test results in assessing premiums than in whether or not they are reliable or relevant.
6. Insurers must publish more data that unequivocally support the changes made to insurance premiums based on positive genetic test results.
7. Insurers should publish clear explanations as to exactly how such factors as early diagnosis and treatment are factored into their actuarial calculations.
8. The small number of cases involving genetic test results could allow insurers to ignore all genetic test results with relative impunity, allowing time to establish firmly their scientific and actuarial relevance.
9. The view that ignoring genetic test results is costly is contradicted by the actions of at least three insurers who chose to ignore tests for the short term.
10. We recommend that insurers take into account negative test results.
11. Insurers should explain how they use family history in assessing premiums and publish the supporting data.
12. Adequate independent research to discern the impact of the use of genetic test results by insurance companies should be carried out.
13. The distinction between research and diagnostic tests should be clearly understood by those seeking to use the results.
14. The statement that 'results from research will not be used' should be incorporated into the ABI code of practice.
15. The Government and the industry must collaborate to provide an alternative form of insurance for those who would be denied it because of their genetic make-up.
16. The ABI must act to convince the government and public that the code of practice is being complied with, and insurers must prove that they are capable of regulating themselves effectively and thoroughly.
17. We do not believe that legislation that denies insurers access to all genetic test results would be appropriate.
18. The best way forward would be a voluntary moratorium for at least 2 years to allow more research and the relevance of genetic testing to be established.

Table 20.5. HGC moratorium recommendations (May 2001)

1. No insurance company should require disclosure of adverse results of any genetic tests, or use such results, in determining the availability or terms of all classes of insurance.
2. Recommendation is for the introduction of a moratorium on genetic testing for not less than 3 years. This will allow time for a full review of regulatory options and afford the opportunity to collect data, which are not currently available. The moratorium should continue if the issues have not been resolved satisfactorily within this period.
3. The moratorium will not affect the current ability of insurance companies to take into account favourable results of any genetic test result, which the applicant has chosen to disclose.
4. HGC will address the issue as to how family history information is used by insurers.
5. An exception is made for policies greater than £500 000 as protection from significant financial loss.
6. Only genetic tests approved by the Genetics and Insurance Advisory Committee (GIAC) should be taken into account for these high-value policies. There remains a need for an expert body of this kind.
7. In view of the failings of self-regulation, independent enforcement of the moratorium will be needed. The HGC believes that legislation will be necessary to achieve this.

Table 20.6. Government- and ABI-agreed moratorium (October 2001)

1. There will be a 5-year moratorium on the use of genetic test results by insurers.
2. The moratorium will apply to life insurance policies up to £500 000 and critical illness, long-term care insurance and income protection up to £300 000 for each type of policy.
3. In policy applications above these limits, the insurance industry may use genetic test results where these tests have been approved by the GIAC.
4. Legislation has not been introduced. However, independent monitoring of the ABI code of conduct will take place through an enhanced role for the GIAC in monitoring both insurance compliance and customer complaints.
5. The moratorium has not been extended to the use of family history data.
6. The whole moratorium will be reviewed after 3 years.
7. The use of negative test results in obtaining normal premiums is encouraged by the insurer, subject to confirmation in most cases by a geneticist of the relevance of the result.

The situation in other European countries

There is a plethora of measures in other European countries. Some have legislation, some a moratorium on the use of genetic testing.

In Austria, the 1994 gene technology law states that employers and insurers are forbidden to obtain, request, accept or use results of genetic analyses.

In Belgium, a 1992 non-marine insurance law allows medical examinations, etc., to be based only on past medical history establishing the applicant's medical state, and not on genetic analysis techniques capable of determining *future* state of health.

In Denmark, the amendment to the Insurance Contracts Act, 1997, allows insurers only to ask for HIV tests and family history when the sum insured is high and over a certain level.

In France, the 1994 French Federation of Insurance Companies issued a statement saying that, for 5 years, the Federation would not use genetic information when determining applicants' insurability, even if *favourable* information is brought by applicants.

The German insurance system does not use genetic information to reach decisions about awarding coverage.

In the Netherlands, it is considered that strict regulation will be needed. In 1995, a 5-year moratorium was extended indefinitely and insurers have agreed not to use genetic tests or existing genetic information for policies below 300 000 guilders. Individual responsibility is seen as being extremely important. Limitations on the collection and use of genetic information are derived from the medical treatment and medical checks acts.

In Norway, a 1994 biotechnology law allows strict use of genetic tests. It states that it is 'forbidden to request, receive, retain or make use of genetic information from a genetic test result, and it is forbidden to ascertain if a genetic test has been performed'. This may not apply to diagnostic tests.

In 1997, Poland introduced a law that established a general inspectorate for personal data protection.

In Sweden, genetic discrimination can be subject to penalty by fine or prison sentence up to a maximum of 6 months. An agreement was reached with the insurance companies in 1999 not to require insurance applications to undergo genetic tests up until 2002.

Following the national referendum in Switzerland in June, 1998, to limit genetic experimentation, in which the vote went against the proposal, there are no plans to introduce genetic legislation for the time being. Insurers are not allowed to demand pre-symptomatic or pre-natal investigations as a condition of insurance.

There is no legislation in Finland, Greece, Hungary, Iceland, Italy, Portugal or Spain. In Ireland, the situation is similar to the UK, and although there is no specific legislation, most Irish insurance companies have organizational links to the ABI and follow the ABI code where possible.

Regulation of genetic testing and insurance in other countries

In the USA and other countries without national health services, the main concern is about health insurance, where a positive predictive test would have great relevance, although predictive genetic tests are rarely able to determine the time at which someone will become ill. In the USA, most health insurance is purchased on a group basis by employers, and the unemployed or low-income groups are often not insured. There is no obligation on an employer to insure a high-risk employee who would raise their costs. Thus, 31–36 million people in the USA have no health insurance (Brett and Fischer, 1993). The most significant legislation is the Health Insurance Portability and Accountability Act, 1996. This federal law provides some protection from genetic discrimination but only to employer-based and commercially issued group health insurance. President Clinton, in February 2000 (Josefson, 2000), signed an executive order forbidding the USA federal government from using genetic information in general employment decisions. Eventually, national legislation in the USA is likely in order to prevent discrimination. Indeed this has been proposed for some time (Hall et al., 2000). In the interim, 28 states have already introduced fairly restrictive legislation, including the recent Massachusetts law, which prohibits genetic discrimination by employers and health insurance agents (Anonymous, 2000). Interestingly, there does not appear to be any advantage taken of the gap in those states without laws. The situation in the USA is covered partly by the Discrimination Act, 1996. Current bills passing through the US government include one on genetic information and non-discrimination in health insurance (Rothenberg et al., 1997; Wadman, 1998).

Australia has an Insurance Contracts Act 1984 that allows insurers to take into account existing genetic information as well as family history. Insurers generally are against forcing individuals to take genetic tests. The Life, Investment, and Superannuation Association of Australia is currently revising further guidelines in 1997. The genetic privacy and non-discrimination bill, 1998, explicitly prohibits genetic discrimination by insurers. Canada has no legislation. New Zealand issued guidelines in April, 1997, on insurance and genetic tests.

Benefits of genetic testing

As in Huntington disease, if the genetic nature of the condition is sufficiently well defined, individuals may be unable to obtain insurance because they are at 50% risk, irrespective of DNA tests (Harper, 1993). This may prompt those at risk to request testing in the hope that their 50% prior risk will be reduced to the point of being able to obtain insurance. This has not been found to be a particularly important reason for opting for a test (Tyler et al., 1992); nonetheless we are aware of at least one woman who has tested positive for *BRCA1* whose weighted premiums have been reduced to normal after prophylactic mastectomy and oophorectomy.

The finding of negative test results (i.e. non gene carriers) has been used to lower already high premiums, as in Austria (Hauser and Jenisch, 1998). However, as in the UK, insurance companies cannot insist that applicants should have genetic tests. Many individuals at risk and on a higher premium will organize genetic tests at their own expense. Confirmation by genetic testing of a disease, such as Friedreich's ataxia or HD, does not increase the existing premium, but a negative test result has led to a reduced premium for some applicants.

Some insurers consider that genetic information is not essential for underwriting life insurance, and are not requesting information about genetic tests. Most applicants who were requested to provide further information were not rated at a higher premium or rejected. Some companies consider that they can absorb this small extra load: only 1 in 20 policies are actually claimed on death, which is not an excessive amount.

Evidence of discrimination

Our survey of European genetic centres involved in breast cancer testing showed that all the UK centres surveyed had had patients who refused testing because of fear of penalty or being unable to obtain insurance. Two (40%) of the UK centres had experience of patients who refused genetic testing because of fear of employment discrimination (Morrison et al., 1999a,b). Interestingly, although Norway has extremely strict laws, and there is no particular need to discuss insurance issues prior to testing, instances of refusal of testing due to both fear and employment were seen. This may reflect anxiety because of strict legislation, as people may consider there must be something behind the legislation. Most of the non-UK centres did not appear to have any major discrimination problems. This finding supports the HGAC statement that 'there is a perception of unacceptable discrimination in the UK' (Human Genetics Advisory Commission, 1998). The majority of the non-UK centres did not feel the need to discuss insurance issues before testing. The four centres (in the Netherlands) that have discussed this have an existing 5-year moratorium on genetic tests.

Six cases of actual discrimination were documented. All were from UK centres. Examples (some details slightly modified to maintain confidentiality) include a 40-year-old female with relatives with breast and ovarian cancer who could not get insurance, but was able to do so after preventive mastectomy and oophorectomy. A 33-year-old man with a family history of von Hippel–Lindau disease in a sibling, probably a new mutation, would not consider an exclusion test for fear of discrimination by the insurance company if positive. A 28-year-old woman with a family history of HNPCC was refused insurance on the grounds of family history. She is having a genetic test, in the hope of obtaining insurance if the result is negative. A 39-year-old female with a *BRCA1* family history, who divorced from her husband, was denied insurance and mortgage cover for a new house unless she had a negative *BRCA1* test. Three cases were also documented in which, on application for heath insurance, excessive details of other family history and genetic test results were requested (Morrison et al., 1999a,b; Morrison, 2001).

A recent postal survey found that up to 33% of respondents in patient support groups may have experienced problems when applying for life insurance (Low et al., 1998). Such findings can easily be over-interpreted due to a high non-response rate by more satisfied customers.

In the rest of Europe, where most countries have restrictive legislation, there is little evidence of discrimination (Morrison et al., 1999), although in Norway there is evidence of increased premiums for HNPCC, but not for *BRCA1/2* (Norum and Tranebjaerg, 2000).

There is little evidence of discrimination in obtaining health insurance in the USA for pre-symptomatic individuals (Hall and Rich, 2000); nonetheless, health insurers are unwilling to pay for testing of, for instance, *BRCA1*, with only 15% covering the costs (Anonymous, 2000), and this is likely to increase if the tests are targeted in the high-risk situation, such as a family with a known mutation (Schoonmaker et al., 2000). Unless more is done to encourage insurers, they may not to be prepared to pay for, for example, an FAP predictive test, thus denying those on lower incomes the opportunity for testing in the first place. Further work in the USA has also shown that the insurance industry's fears about adverse selection may be groundless. Women testing positive for BRCA1 mutations did not take out higher levels of life insurance (Zick et al., 2000).

In Australia, families with hereditary bowel cancer experienced genetic discrimination. In a survey of families on the hereditary bowel cancer register, Barlow-Stewart et al. (2001) found 8% discrimination – predominantly HNPCC related – and included a number of areas: refusal of life insurance, denial of an increase in life insurance for a pre-existing policy, refusal of income protection and trauma insurance, reduction of superannuation and loading on premiums for travel insurance. One interesting case was that of a civil servant who reported that her application for a senior position in the public service was subject to a negative FAP test result. She had to discontinue her application, as she would have been forced to have a test that would have revealed her mutation status. The issue had been picked up following her checking of a regular colonoscopy box on the health form.

As a result of release of this evidence, the Australian government has initiated several enquiries to determine the direction for future law or other policy development.

Conclusion

The rapidly evolving practice of clinical genetics is throwing up many questions to which we do not yet have clear answers. This is nowhere more apparent than in the genetics of common cancers, including breast cancer, which is the fastest growing area of genetic medicine. If this chapter has dwelt on problems rather than solutions, this is a reflection of the current 'state of the art' rather than of any underlying pessimism. We live in exciting and, above all, hopeful times. Given the pace of progress over the past decade, those involved in developing clinical and laboratory services for cancer families, in partnership with the families themselves, look forward with great confidence to a transformation scene within the next 20 years.

REFERENCES

Advisory Committee on Genetic Testing (1997). *Code of Practice and Guidance on Human Genetic Testing Services Supplied Direct to the Public.* London: Dept of Health.

Advisory Committee on Genetic Testing (1998). *Report on Genetic Testing for Late Onset Disorders.* London: Dept of Health.

Al-Shahi R and Warlow C (2000). Using patient-identifiable data for observational research and audit. *Br Med J* **321**: 1031–2.

American Society of Human Genetics (1998). ASHG statement: professional disclosure of familial genetic information. *Am J Hum Genet* **62**: 474–83.

Anonymous (2000). Private matters, public affairs. *Nat Genet* **26**: 1–2.

Association of British Insurers (1997). *Genetic Testing ABI Code of Practice.* London: ABI.

Baildam AD (1999). The role of bilateral prophylactic mastectomy (BPMX) in women at high risk of breast cancer. *Dis Markers* **15**: 197–8.

Balter M (2000). European science policy – France rebels against gene patenting law. *Science* **288**: 2115.

Barber JCK (1998). Code of practice and guidance on human genetic testing services supplied direct to the public. Advisory committee on genetic testing. *J Med Genet* **35**: 443–5.

Barlow-Stewart KK, French JA, O'Donnell SM and Spigelman AD (2001). *Genetic Discrimination Experienced by Australian Families Affected by Hereditary Bowel Cancer.* Proceedings of the 3rd Joint Meeting, Leeds Castle polyposis group and international collaborative group for hereditary non-polyposis colorectal cancer, Venice, Italy.

Bebbington HM and Fallowfield LJ (1999). Psychosocial implications of prophylactic bilateral mastectomy (abstr.). *Dis Markers* **15**: 154.

Beckman MW (1999). Clinical services for familial breast and ovarian cancer in Germany (abstr.). *Dis Markers* **15**: 48.

Bewtra C, Watson P, Conway T, et al. (1992). Hereditary ovarian cancer: a clinicopathological study. *Int J Gynecol Pathol* **11**: 180–7.

Brett P and Fischer EP (1993). Effects on life insurance of genetic testing. *The Actuary* **10**(3): 11–12.

Burke W, Press N and Pinsky L (1999). BRCA1 and BRCA2: a small part of the puzzle. *J Natl Cancer Inst* **91**: 904–5.

Cabinet Office (1999). *The Advisory and Regulatory Framework for Biotechnology*. Report from the Government's review. London: Office of Science and Technology.

Chapman CJ (1999). Risk estimation and pedigree analysis (abstr.). *Dis Markers* **15**: 119.

Claus E, Risch N and Thompson D (1991). Genetic analysis of breast cancer in the Cancer and Steroid Hormone Study. *Am J Hum Genet* **48**: 232–42.

Cull A, Miller H, Porterfield T, et al. (1998). The use of videotaped information in cancer genetic counselling: a randomised evaluation study. *Br J Cancer* **77**: 830–7.

Cull A, Anderson EDC, Campbell S, et al. (1999). The impact of genetic counselling about breast cancer risk on women's risk perceptions and levels of distress. *Br J Cancer* **79**: 501–8.

Cull A, Fry A, Rush R and Steel CM (2001). Cancer perceptions and distress among women attending a familial ovarian cancer clinic. *Br J Cancer* **84**(5): 594–9.

De Vos M, Poppe B, Delvaux G, et al. (1999). Genetic counselling and testing for hereditary breast and ovarian cancer: the Gent(le) approach. *Dis Markers* **15**: 191–5.

Directive 98/44/EC of the European Parliament and the Council (1998). The legal protection of biotechnological inventions. *J Officiel*: L213.

Eccles DM, Simmonds P, Goddard J, et al. (1999). Management of hereditary breast cancer. *Dis Markers* **15**: 187–9.

Eccles DM, Evans DGR, Mackay J and the UK Cancer Family Study Group (2000). Guidelines for a genetic risk based approach to advising women with a family history of breast cancer. *J Med Genet* **37**: 203–9.

Ellwood JM, Cox B and Richardson AK (1993). The effectiveness of breast cancer screening by mammography in younger women. *Online J Curr Clin Trials*, Document no. 32.

Emery J, Watson E, Rose P and Andermann A (1999). A systematic review of the literature exploring the role of primary care in genetic services. *Fam Pract* **16**: 426–45.

Emery J, Murphy M and Lucassen A (2000). Hereditary cancer – the evidence for current recommended management. *Lancet Oncol* (*Preview*): 9–16.

Evans DGR, Blair V, Greenhalgh R, Hopwood P and Howell A (1994). The impact of genetic counselling on risk perception in women with a family history of breast cancer. *Br J Cancer* **70**: 34–8.

Evans DGR, Kerr B, Foulkes W, at al. (1998). False breast cancer family history in the cancer family clinic – a report of 8 families. *Eur J Surg Oncol* **24**: 275–9.

Farrell S (1997). Screen yourself by mail order. *The Times* (*London*), Wednesday 24 September.

Floderus B, Barlow L and Mack TM (1990). Recall bias in subjective reports of familial cancer. *Epidemiology* **1**: 318–21.

Ford D, Easton DF, Stratton M and the Breast Cancer Linkage Consortium (1998). Genetic heterogeneity and linkage analysis of the BRCA1 and BRCA2 genes in breast cancer families. *Am J Hum Genet* **62**: 676–89.

Friend S (1996). Breast cancer susceptibility testing: realities in the post-genomic era. *Nat Genet* **13**: 16–17.

Gail M, Brinton L, Bryar P, et al. (1989). Projecting individualised probabilities of developing breast cancer for white females who are being examined annually. *J Natl Cancer Inst* **81**: 1879.

Gayther SA and Ponder BAJ (1997). Mutations of the BRCA1 and BRCA2 genes and the possibilities for predictive testing. *Mol Med Today* **3**: 168–74.

Government response to the report from the House of Commons' Science and Technology Committee (*Genetics and Insurance*) (2001). London: Dept of Health.

Government response to the Human Genetics Advisory Commission's report on the implications of genetic testing for insurance (1998). Department of Trade and Industry Office of Technology, and the Department of Health, London, UK.

Hall MA and Rich SS (2000). Laws restricting health insurers' use of genetic information: impact on genetic discrimination. *Am J Hum Genet* **66**: 293–307.

Harper PS (1992). Genetic testing and insurance. *J R Coll Phys Lond* **26**: 184–7.

Harper PS (1993). Insurance and genetic testing. *Lancet* **341**: 224–7.

Hartmann L, Jenkins R, Schaid D, et al. (1999). Efficacy of bilateral prophylactic mastectomy in women with a family history of breast cancer. *N Engl J Med* **340**: 77–84.

Hauser G and Jenisch A (1998). Laws regarding insurance companies. *J Med Genet* **35**: 526–8.

Heimdal K, Maehle L and Møller P (1999). Costs and benefits of diagnosing familial breast cancer. *Dis Markers* **15**: 167–73.

Hodgson S, Milner B, Brown I, et al. (1999). Cancer genetics services in Europe. *Dis Markers* **15**: 3–13.

Huggins M, Bloch M, Kanani S, et al. (1990). Ethical and legal dilemmas arising during predictive testing for adult-onset disease: the experience of Huntington disease. *Am J Hum Genet* **47**: 4–12.

Human Genetics Advisory Commission (UK) (1997). The implications of genetic testing for insurance. London: Dept of Health.

Human Genetics Commission (2000). *Whose Hands on your Genes?* A discussion document on the storage, protection and use of personal genetic information. London: Department of Health.

Human Genetics Commission (2001). *Public Attitudes to Human Genetic Information.* Peoples panel quantitative study conducted for the Human Genetics Commission. London: Department of Health.

Hunt A (1992). The patient's viewpoint. *Dis Markers* **10**: 205–10.

Institute of Medicine (1994). In *Assessing Genetic Risks*, ed. Committee on assessing genetic risks. Washington DC: National Academy Press.

Josefson J (2000). Clinton outlaws genetic discrimination in federal jobs. *Br Med J* **320**: 168.

Julian-Reynier C, Eisinger F, Chabal F, et al. (1996). Cancer genetics clinics: target populations and consultees' expectations. *Eur J Cancer* **32A**: 398–403.

Kerber RA and Slattery ML (1997). Comparison of self-reported and database-linked family history of cancer data in a case-control study. *Am J Epidemiol* **146**: 244–8.

Knoppers BM (1999). Status, sale and patenting of human genetic material: an international survey. *Nat Genet* **22**: 23–6.

Kristofferson U (1999). Clinical cancer genetic service in Sweden. *Dis Markers* **15**: 49.

Lalloo F, Boggis CRM, Evans DGR, et al. (1998). Screening by mammography, women with a family history of breast cancer. *Eur J Cancer* **34**: 937–40.

Law JA (1997). Cancers detected and induced in mammographic screening: new screening schedules and younger women with family history of breast cancer. *Br J Radiol* **70**: 62–9.

LeGrys J (1997). Actuarial considerations on genetic testing. *Phil Trans R Soc Lond* **B352**: 1057–61.

Lerman C, Narod SA, Schulman K, et al. (1996). BRCA1 testing in families with hereditary breast–ovarian cancer. A prospective study of patient decision making and outcomes. *JAMA* **275**: 1885–92.

Lloyd S, Watson M, Waites B, et al. (1996). Familial breast cancer: a controlled study of risk perception, psychological morbidity and health beliefs in women attending for genetic counselling. *Br J Cancer* **74**: 482–7.

Low L, King S and Wilkie T (1998). Genetic discrimination in life insurance: empirical evidence from a cross-sectional survey of genetic support groups in the United Kingdom. *Br Med J* **317**: 1632–5.

Lucassen A and Parker M (2001). Revealing false paternity: some ethical considerations. *Lancet* **357**: 1033–5.

MacDonald AS (1997). How will improved forecasts of individual lifetimes affect underwriting? *Phil Trans R Soc Lond* **B352**: 1067–75.

MacDonald AS, Waters HR, Wekwete CT (2000a). The genetics of breast and ovarian cancer. I. A model of family history. Research report No 00/01 of the Swiss Re/Heriot-Watt genetics initiative. Edinburgh: Heriot-Watt University.

MacDonald AS, Waters HR, Wekwete CT (2000b). The genetics of breast and ovarian cancer. II. A model of critical illness insurance. Research report No 00/02 of the Swiss Re/Heriot-Watt genetics initiative. Edinburgh: Heriot-Watt University.

Macmillan RD (2000). Screening women with a family history of breast cancer – results from the British Familial Breast Cancer Group. *Eur J Surg Oncol* **26**: 149–52.

Medical Research Council (1992). *Ethical Aspects of Human Genetic Testing: An Information Paper*. Sydney, Australia: Medical Research Council.

Michel H (2000). Allowing gene patents could be an expensive mistake for the US. *Nature* **407**: 285.

Møller P, Evans DGR, Haites NE, et al. (1999a). Guidelines for follow-up of women at high risk for inherited breast cancer: consensus statement from the Biomed 2 demonstration programme on inherited breast cancer. *Dis Markers* **15**: 207–11.

Møller P, Reis MM, Evans G, et al. (1999b). Efficacy of early diagnosis and treatment in women with a family history of breast cancer. *Dis Markers* **15**: 179–86.

Møller P, Evans D, Anderson E, et al. (1999c). Use of cytology to diagnose inherited breast cancer. *Dis Markers* **15**: 206.

Morrison PJ (1998a). Genetic testing and insurance in the UK. *Clin Genet* **54**: 375–9.

Morrison PJ (1998b). Implications for genetic testing for insurance in the UK. *Lancet* **352**: 1647–8.

Morrison PJ (2001). Insurance, genetic testing and familial cancer. *U Med J* **70**: 79–88.

Morrison PJ, Steel CM, Vasen HFA, et al. (1999a). Insurance implications for individuals with a high risk of breast and ovarian cancer in Europe. *Dis Markers* **15**: 159–65.

Morrison PJ, Steel CM, Nevin NC, et al. (1999b). Insurance considerations for individuals with a high risk of breast cancer in Europe: some recommendations. CME *J Gynaecol* **5**: 272–7.

Müller H, Eeles RA, Wildsmith T, McGleenan T and Friedman S (2000). Genetic testing for cancer predisposition; an ongoing debate. *Lancet Oncol* **1**: 118–24.

Murphree AL (1996). Retinoblastoma. In *Emery and Rimoin's Principles and Practice of Medical Genetics*, ed. D.L. Rimoin, M. Connor and R.E. Peyritz, 3rd edn, pp. 2585–2609. New York: Churchill Livingstone.

Narod SA, Goldgar D, Cannon-Albright L, et al. (1995a). Risk modifiers in carriers of BRCA1 mutations. *Int J Cancer* **64**: 394–8.

Narod SA, Ford D, Devilee P, et al. (1995b). An evaluation of genetic heterogeneity in 145 breast–ovarian cancer families. *Am J Hum Genet* **56**: 254–64.

Norum J and Tranebjaerg L (2000). Health, life and disability insurance and hereditary risk for breast and colorectal cancer. *Acta Oncol* **39**: 189–93.

Pasini B and Pierotti MA (1999). Familial breast and ovarian cancer: genetic counseling and clinical management in Italy. *Dis Markers* **15**: 41–3.

Pembrey M and Anionwu E (1996). Ethical aspects of genetic screening and diagnosis. In *Emery and Rimoin's Principles and Practice of Medical Genetics*, ed. D.L. Rimoin, M. Connor and R.E. Peyritz, 3rd edn, pp. 641–53. New York: Churchill Livingstone.

Peto J, Collins N, Barfoot R, et al. (1999). Prevalence of BRCA1 and BRCA2 mutations in patients with early onset breast cancer. *J Natl Cancer Inst* **91**: 943–9.

Rebbeck TR, Levin AM, Eisen A, et al. (1999). Breast cancer risk after bilateral prophylactic oophorectomy in BRCA1 mutation-carriers. *J Natl Cancer Inst* **51**: 1475–9.

Reichelt JG, Dahl AA, Heimdal K and Møller P (1999). Uptake of genetic testing and pre-test levels of mental distress in Norwegian families with known BRCA1 mutations. *Dis Markers* **15**: 139–43.

Reilly P (1996). Legal issues in genetic medicine. In *Emery and Rimoin's Principles and Practice of Medical Genetics*, ed. D.L. Rimoin, M. Connor and R.E. Peyritz, 3rd edn, pp. 655–66. New York: Churchill Livingstone.

Rothenberg KH, et al. (1997). Breast cancer, the genetic 'quick fix' and the Jewish community. *Health Matrix* **7**: 97–124.

Royal College of Physicians of London (1991). *Ethical Issues in Clinical Genetics.* London: Royal College of Physicians.

Schoonmaker MM, Bernhardt BA and Holtzman NA (2000). Factors influencing health insurers' decisions to cover new genetic technologies. *Int J Technol Assess Health Care* **16**: 178–89.

Science and Technology Committee (1995). *Human Genetics. The Science and its Consequences.* Third report of the Science and Technology Committee, House of Commons, HC41-I. London: HMSO.

Senior K (2000). Patent and be damned: the new slogan for human genetics? *Mol Med Today* **6**: 225–6.

Skirton H (1999). Genetic nurses and counsellors – preparation for practice with families at risk of familial cancer. *Dis Markers* **15**: 145–7.

Steel CM and Smyth E (1999). Molecular pathology of breast cancer and its impact on clinical practice. *Schweiz Med Wochenschr* **129**: 1749–57.

Steel CM, Smyth E, Vasen H, et al. (1999). Ethical, social and economic issues in familial breast cancer: a compilation of views from the EC Biomed II Demonstration Project. *Dis Markers* **15**: 125–31.

Stephens JC, Reich DE, Goldstein DB, et al. (1998). Dating the origin of the CCR5-32 AIDS-resistance allele by the coalescence of haplotypes. *Am J Hum Genet* **62**: 1507–15.

Stoppa-Lyonnet D, Caligo M, Eccles D, et al. (1999). Genetic testing for breast cancer predisposition in 1999: which molecular strategy and which family criteria? *Dis Markers* **15**: 67–8.

Stratton MR (1996). Recent advances in understanding of genetic susceptibility to breast cancer. *Hum Mol Genet* **5**: 1515–19.

Strobl J, Cave E and Walley T (2000). Data protection legislation: interpretation and barriers to research. *Br Med J* **321**: 890–2.

Struewing JP, Hartge P, Wacholder S, et al. (1997). The risk of cancer associated with specific mutations of BRCA1 and BRCA2 among Ashkenazi Jews. *N Engl J Med* **336**: 1401–8.

Tabar L, Fagerberg G, Day NE and Holmberg L (1987). What is the optimum interval between mammographic screening examinations? *Br J Cancer* **55**: 547–51.

The Ad Hoc Committee on Genetic Testing/Insurance Issues (1995). Background statement. Genetic testing and insurance. *Am J Hum Genet* **56**: 327–31.

Theis B, Boyd N, Lockwood G and Tritchler D (1994). Accuracy of family cancer history in breast cancer patients. *Eur J Canc Prev* **3**: 321–7.

Thompson JA, Weisner GL, Sellers TA, et al. (1995). Genetic services for familial cancer patients: a survey of National Cancer Institute centers. *J Natl Cancer Inst* **87**: 1446–55.

Thorlacius S, Struewing JP, Hartge P, et al. (1998). Population-based study of risk of breast cancer in carriers of BRCA2 mutation. *Lancet* **352**: 1337–9.

Tyler A, Morris M, Lazarou L, Meredith L, Myring J and Harper PS (1992). Presymptomatic testing for Huntington's disease in Wales 1987–90. *Br J Psychiatry* **161**: 481–8.

Vandenbroucke JP (1998). Maintaining privacy and the health of the public. *Br Med J* **316**: 1331–2.

Vasen HE, Haites NE, Evans DG, et al. (1998). Current policies for surveillance and management in women at risk of breast and ovarian cancer: a survey among 16 European family cancer clinics. *Eur J Cancer* **34**: 1922–6.

Wadman M (1998). Privacy bill under fire from researchers. *Nature* **392**: 6.

Watson EK, Shickle D, Quereshi N, et al. (1999a). The 'new genetics' and primary care: GP's views on their role and their educational needs. *Fam Pract* **16**: 420–5.

Watson E, Andermann A, Clements A, et al. (1999b). Development and evaluation of educational materials for primary care on familial breast and ovarian cancer (abstr.). *Dis Markers* **15**: 156.

White MT (1999). Underlying ambiguities in genetic privacy legislation. *Genet Testing* **3**: 341–5.

Zick CD, Smith KR, Mayer RN and Botkin JR (2000). Genetic testing, adverse selection and the demand for life insurance. *Am J Med Genet* **93**: 29–39.

Gene therapy for breast and ovarian cancer

Richard Kennedy and Patrick G. Johnston

Belfast City Hospital Trust, Belfast, UK

Introduction

Cancer results from a succession of genetic mutations that result in activation of oncogenes or inactivation of tumour suppressor genes. These changes can occur both early in the process of malignant transformation, and later, as the tumour becomes invasive. The success in the development of the technology for the transfer of genetic material into mammalian cells has raised the possibility of treating cancer at a molecular level. Despite initial enthusiasm, gene therapy has still not become a standard treatment modality for cancer. In this chapter we will review the approaches that have been attempted and consider why gene therapy is still an experimental approach.

Principles of gene therapy

Several strategies have been developed that involve the insertion of genetic material into cancer cells or immune cells involved in tumour cell kill. The success of these approaches depends on the ability to deliver the genetic material to the target cells. The transfer of genetic material to a cell is termed 'transduction' and the delivery systems used to transfer genes to target cells are called 'vectors'. Transduction of adequate amounts of genetic material into tumour cells represents one of the most challenging areas of gene therapy, and vector technology is one of the most important areas of current research.

For a vector to be practical for everyday clinical use, it must be:

1 Easy to manufacture
2 Specific to tumour cells or host cells that may benefit from modification
3 Efficient at transducing genetic material
4 Able to cause expression of the transduced gene for a sufficient period of time to be effective
5 Non-immunogenic, so it is not destroyed by the host's immune system

Table 21.1. Gene therapy vectors

Vector	Advantages	Disadvantages
Retroviruses Single-stranded RNA viruses	• Integrate into target cell DNA, causing prolonged gene expression • Small host immune response • Specific for dividing cells • Easy to manufacture	• Require rapidly dividing cells (breast and ovarian tumours may be indolent) • May cause mutations in normal cells
Adenoviruses Double-stranded DNA virus	• Highly efficient at gene transduction into target cell • Can transduce a cell at any stage of cell cycle • Very easy to manufacture at high titres	• Cause a host immune response • Can be toxic to the host • Lack target cell specificity (newer conditionally replicative adenoviruses are more specific) • Transient expression of transduced gene
Liposomes Positively charged lipid membrane complex surrounding DNA	• No immune response • Easy to manufacture • Can carry large amounts of genetic material	• Relatively inefficient at gene transduction • No target cell specificity • Transient expression of transduced genes
Molecular conjugate A protein/DNA complex	• Highly specific delivery of genetic material to target cell • Can carry large amounts of genetic material	• Difficult to manufacture • Transient expression of transduced genes
Naked DNA Direct injection or bombardment of target cells with DNA	• Simple • No immune response • Targeted	• Can only be used where tumour cells can be easily accessed • Unable to transduce a large number of cells

Unfortunately, the perfect vector still does not exist, leading to severe limitations on current gene therapy strategies. As there is no vector that is clearly superior, the choice depends on the amount of genetic material to be transferred, the length of time the foreign gene needs to be expressed and the route of vector delivery (Table 21.1).

Once a vector has been developed and adapted to carry a therapeutic gene, the next stage is its delivery to the target cell or organ. In the treatment of breast or ovarian cancer, three main strategies are used: (1) local delivery, (2) systemic delivery, and (3) *in vitro* delivery.

Local delivery

For ovarian cancer, intraperitoneal injection of the vector is often the preferred approach. This allows the vector to be in direct contact with tumour deposits at a relatively high concentration and results in less immunogenicity than systemic approaches. Local delivery increases the efficacy of gene transfer and reduces the exposure of normal cells to the treatment. However, the vector will not enter tumour cells outside the peritoneal cavity and therefore this approach is less effective for widespread metastatic disease. The vector is also unlikely to penetrate bulky peritoneal disease.

In breast cancer, direct injection of vector into a tumour may be possible as this can also result in a high local concentration. However, metastatic disease, including local lymph node involvement, may not be adequately treated by this approach.

Systemic delivery

Systemic delivery has the advantage of treating both primary and metastatic disease. Potential difficulties may arise with a host immune response, resulting in the vector becoming ineffective or adding to its toxicity. There is also a danger of introducing foreign genetic material into normal cells. Newer developments of conditionally replicative viral vectors and the use of antibodies to target vectors to cell receptors or other surface antigens may, in the future, make systemic gene therapy more specific to cancer cells.

In vitro delivery

In this method the aim is to beneficially alter normal host cells (typically cytotoxic T-cells) by gene therapy ex-vivo in the laboratory. The modified cells are then reintroduced systemically to the patient. This procedure allows great flexibility in the manipulation of target cells and is very specific. However, cells for this have important biological requirements to be maintained during processing, making it very labour intensive and expensive. It also cannot be used to directly target cancer cells.

Gene therapy treatment strategies

Over the past 10 years there have been extensive studies into several gene therapy strategies. Three major approaches have been proposed in the treatment of breast and ovarian cancer.

The first approach is to try to *correct the genetic mutations* that have resulted in the cancer cell phenotype, either by replacing defective tumour suppressor genes or by deactivating oncogenes.

There are many defective tumour suppressor genes in breast and ovarian cancer and many of these do not occur with sufficient frequency or predictability as to be useful targets in gene therapy. However, certain gene mutations, e.g. *TP53* or *BRCA1*, occur regularly enough to have a therapeutic potential.

Multiple oncogenes have also been identified in the development of breast and ovarian cancer. These are activated at varying frequencies in different tumours but certain oncogenes, such as HER2/neu, may be expressed regularly enough to be useful targets for gene therapy.

A problem with this approach is that neoplastic cells are genetically unstable, resulting in a multitude of genetic targets in any tumour population. Also, once a target has been identified it may become irrelevant as the next generation of cancer cells develop further abnormalities. Gene therapy designed to correct genetic abnormalities must be directed at mutations that are shared by all the cancer cells within a population in order to be effective. Genetic mutations in the apoptotic pathway or chemotherapy-resistance genes may be sufficiently common in tumour cell populations to be the targets of choice in the future.

The second approach is to selectively target cancer cells with a cytotoxic gene. *Molecular chemotherapy* involves the transduction of a gene into tumour cells, making them either produce a toxin or become susceptible to a systemically administered pro-toxin. This has the advantage of being only cytotoxic to the target cells, unlike conventional chemotherapy that can also affect normal cells.

Unfortunately, limitations in vector technology have limited the effectiveness of the strategies discussed so far as selective cancer cell transfection and sustained gene expression is difficult. A possible method for targeting cancer cells more accurately may be the use of *conditionally replicative adenoviruses.* Adenoviruses readily infect both dividing and non-dividing cells and do not integrate into the host genome. Modification of the viral genes can alter viral metabolism and function, depending on the characteristics of the host cell, resulting in better cell targeting. The modified virus can also carry foreign genetic material that will only be expressed in the target cell.

The third commonly used approach is to use gene transfer techniques to improve the effectiveness of immunotherapy or chemotherapy. As this strategy does not require the genetic modification of all cancer cells and is less reliant on sustained gene expression, it may be more easily attained with modern vector techniques. *Immunopotentiation* is an approach designed to make the host immune system recognize tumour-associated antigens, leading to a selective antitumour response. This mechanism is promising as the immune system has the potential to recognize and specifically kill metastatic cancer cells, resulting in fewer side-effects than conventional chemotherapy. Immunopotentiation can involve *passive* or *active* immunotherapy. Passive immunotherapy is where the existing immune response to a tumour is modified to make it more efficient. An example would be the use of tumour-infiltrating T-lymphocytes, which are harvested from a patient, cultured *in vitro* and genetically altered before being reintroduced. T-cells are appealing as a target for gene therapy as they are highly specific in recognizing antigenic peptides and have the capacity to destroy tumour cells. They also differentiate into memory cells that continue to circulate and may stop the recurrence of a tumour.

Active immunotherapy refers to the initiation of an immune response to a previously unrecognized or poorly immunogenic tumour antigen. This involves techniques to increase the expression of a tumour antigen or to cause local release of cytokines that enhance the immune system's ability to recognize antigens.

The difficulty with immunological techniques is that cancer cells possess a variety of defects in the processing and presentation of antigens. Certain human tumour cells have been shown to have defective histocompatibility and transport molecules, resulting in a failure of the immune response (Sanda et al., 1995). Cancer cells also are known to release factors that suppress the immune system (Grimm et al., 1988).

Another potential strategy is to improve the effectiveness of conventional chemotherapy. In this approach a *chemoprotectant gene* is introduced into normal bone marrow stem cells in order to protect them from the effects of cytotoxic chemotherapy. This may prevent haematological toxicity, allowing a greater dose intensity of treatment. There are, however, some potential problems with this approach. Higher doses of chemotherapy do not necessarily translate to higher tumour response rates, non-haematological toxic effects may be dose limiting, and there is the danger of transducing cancer cells with the resistance gene.

Studies of gene therapy for breast and ovarian cancer

Over the past 10 years there has been a large amount of research into gene therapy for ovarian and breast cancer. It is important to appreciate that many of these studies have only been involved in cell culture or animal models and have yet to be studied in human subjects. Others have proven initially successful in pre-clinical models but have failed to show a benefit in the treatment of humans. Unfortunately, as many of the clinical studies have been disappointing, the results are often only published in abstract form.

Correction of genetic mutation in cancer cells

The p53 tumour suppressor gene encodes a protein in response to DNA damage that leads to cell cycle arrest at the G1/M phase and may result in apoptosis or DNA repair. Mutation of this gene is found in about half of ovarian and breast cancers (Kohler et al., 1993; Vogelstein et al., 2000) and is associated with a decrease in sensitivity to chemotherapy along with aggressive tumour behaviour. Reintroduction of the wild type p53 gene is therefore a potential mechanism for treatment of chemoresistant tumours. Using this approach, Kigawa et al. (2000) demonstrated cisplatin sensitivity when a p53-containing adenovirus was introduced into a transplanted human ovarian tumour with p53 mutation (Kigawa and Terakawa, 2000).

Nielsen et al. (1998a) demonstrated a reduced number of tumour metastases in a murine model of metastatic breast cancer after the intravenous administration of recombinant-adenovirus-expressing p53. This approach, however, resulted in significant liver damage that was thought to be due to the adenoviral vector. New conditionally replicative adenoviral vectors with E1 and E4 gene deletions are much less hepatotoxic and may be useful for p53 transduction in the future.

Increased sensitivities to paclitaxel, cisplatin, doxorubicin, 5-fluorouracil, methotrexate and etoposide chemotherapy have been demonstrated in breast and ovarian cell-lines treated with an adenovirus-carrying wild-type p53, and this has been proposed as a mechanism to overcome resistance to these drugs (Nielsen et al., 1998b; Gurnani et al., 1999).

The human breast and ovarian cancer susceptibility gene *BRCA1* is a tumour suppressor gene that is mutated or lost in hereditary breast and ovarian cancer. In sporadic breast and ovarian cancer, the normal gene is usually present but its expression is decreased. Introduction of a *BRCA1*-containing vector into breast or ovarian cancer cell-lines has a growth-inhibiting effect that is not found in other tumour cell-lines. This suggests a specific action against breast and ovarian cancer for *BRCA1*-expressing vectors that may be therapeutically relevant. Initial work with a retroviral vector containing *BRCA1* showed prolongation of life in mice with an intraperitoneal human breast cancer (Holt, 1997).

A phase I trial of an intraperitoneal injection of a retrovirus containing a *BRCA1* gene into patients with advanced ovarian cancer demonstrated stable disease in 8 out of 12 patients, of which 3 showed tumour reduction (Tait et al., 1997, 1998). Unfortunately, a follow-up phase II trial did not demonstrate any response or disease stabilization after six patients were treated, and the study was discontinued (Tait et al., 1999).

The HER2/neu oncogene encodes a membrane-associated receptor protein and is over-expressed in 30% of breast cancer. Its over-expression is associated with an increase in tumour metastatic potential and resistance to chemotherapy (Kolata, 1987). Reduction of HER2/neu expression may result in decreased metastatic spread and increased chemosensitivity in breast cancer. An adenoviral vector containing a gene that encodes an antibody to HER2/neu has been developed and has been given, by intraperitoneal injection, to patients with ovarian cancer. The antibody was successfully detected in cells over-expressing HER2/neu and resulted in down-regulation of the receptor (Deshane and Siegal, 1997).

The adenovirus 5 E1A gene is the first viral gene to be expressed in the cell after infection. It codes for a protein that down-regulates the expression of HER2/neu and therefore may be used in gene therapy. In a phase I trial, 12 patients with ovarian cancer were treated intraperitoneally with a liposomal complex containing the E1A gene. Two patients developed down-regulation of HER2/neu within their tumour cells (Ueno et al., 1998).

Conditionally replicative adenoviruses

The adenovirus E1b gene is responsible for coding for a protein that deactivates p53 in the host cell allowing viral replication. An adenovirus (ONYX-015) has been engineered that is deficient in this gene and therefore is unable to replicate in normal cells. In cancer cell-lines containing mutant p53, this virus is able to divide and cause cell lysis.

Disappointingly, intraperitoneal administration of ONYX-015 has resulted in no responses in ovarian cancer patients, although work with other human tumours suggests that there may be a synergistic action with cytotoxic chemotherapy (Gomez-Navarro and Curiel, 2000). This virus may have a role in the future as a vector for delivery of therapeutic genetic material specifically to cancer cells.

Molecular chemotherapy

A pre-clinical molecular chemotherapy approach has been the introduction of the herpes virus thymidine kinase (TK) enzyme into tumour cells. Systemically administered ganciclovir is phosphorylated by TK and becomes incorporated into the cellular DNA and RNA, causing cell death. Normal cells are unaffected by ganciclovir as they do not express TK. Interestingly, when this mechanism was tested in cell-lines, tumour cells that had not been transduced with the TK initially also responded to ganciclovir. This 'bystander effect' may be due to transfer of phosphorylated ganciclovir between cells via gap junctions (Freeman et al., 1993).

Link and Mooreman (1995) have proposed the intraperitoneal use of a retroviral vector to transfect ovarian cancer cells with the TK enzyme. This may cause the ovarian tumour cells to respond to ganciclovir as well as leading to a bystander effect. Initial work with ovarian cell-lines demonstrates effective transfection of tumour cells with the retrovirus.

Another approach was the injection of an adenoviral vector containing TK into rat mammary ducts followed by systemic ganciclovir treatment. The rats were then exposed to carcinogens with no development of breast cancer. This work suggested a potential mechanism for prevention of breast cancer by the elimination of dividing ductal cells without the need for mastectomy (Sukumar and McKenzie, 1996).

A vector containing the TK gene with a radiation-sensitive transcriptional control element has been engineered and used to transfect a human breast cancer cell-line. The altered cells became sensitive to ganciclovir after being irradiated. This approach may increase the effectiveness of local radiotherapy to breast cancer (Marples et al., 2000).

In a phase I study, irradiated TK-transduced ovarian cancer cells were injected into the peritoneum of patients with ovarian cancer. The aim was to produce a bystander effect, leading to ganciclovir sensitivity in the patient's tumour: 4 out of 18 patients had a response to ganciclovir (3 complete, 1 partial) (Ramesh et al., 1998).

Another proposed molecular chemotherapy approach is the intraperitoneal injection of an adenoviral vector containing the TK gene. Provisional work with ascites taken from women with ovarian cancer suggested good TK transduction. This was also expected to cause tumour sensitivity to ganciclovir as well as to cause a bystander effect. A phase I study of this approach together with topotecan chemotherapy for recurrent ovarian carcinoma demonstrated some effect (Hasenberg et al., 1995; Rosenfeld et al., 1995).

An alternative type of molecular chemotherapy has been developed that takes advantage of the over-expression of HER-2/neu in tumour cells. In this approach the vector carries a cytosine deaminase gene that is regulated by the tumour-specific *erb*-B2 promoter. When the genetic material is introduced into a tumour cell that is over-expressing HER-2/neu, it is activated, producing the enzyme cytosine deaminase that converts the inactive pro-drug fluorocytosine to the chemotherapy drug 5-fluorouracil. Direct injection of a plasmid containing the HER/neu-regulated cytosine deaminase gene has been performed with human breast tumours. This resulted in a 90% expression of the enzyme in the tumour tissue (Pandha et al., 1999).

Immunotherapy

Irradiated murine ovarian tumour cells have been transduced with the interleukin-2 (IL-2) gene *in vitro*. These cells, when injected into ovarian-tumour-bearing mice, cause an immune response to the tumour. Future work will involve the IL-2 transduction of human tumour taken at surgery and vaccination with these postoperatively in order to cause an immune response to remaining ovarian cancer cells (Berchuck and Lyerly, 1995).

Marr et al. (1997) have developed an adenovirus containing the tumour necrosis factor alpha gene and injected this directly into a murine breast tumour, resulting in tumour regression. These animals also developed tumour specific immunity that would be expected to prevent metastatic disease.

In another immunological strategy a gene encoding a chimeric protein, consisting of an antibody to ovarian cancer plus a T-cell-receptor signalling chain, has been engineered. T-cells, which have been transduced with a retrovirus containing this gene, specifically cause lysis of ovarian tumour cell-lines. A phase I study (Hwu et al., 1995) using this technology has been commenced for treatment of advanced ovarian cancer. Patients are given intravenous infusions of T-cells transduced with the Mov-γ receptor gene, a chimeric receptor derived from the Mov18 antibody to ovarian cancer and T-cell-receptor signalling chains.

The use of a recombinant adenovirus expressing the human IL-2 gene has been investigated in the phase I trial setting. The virus was injected into metastatic breast cancer tumour sites with the aim of producing very high local tumour concentrations of IL-2 with low systemic levels. Some tumour regression was seen in 24% of patients and the treatment was well tolerated (Stewart et al., 1999).

Chemoprotection

The multi-drug resistance (MDR) protein is a drug efflux pump that leads to chemotherapy resistance in some tumours of epithelial origin. This protein causes resistance to anthracycline and taxoid cytotoxic drugs that are commonly used to treat breast or ovarian cancer. Pre-clinically, the MDR gene has been introduced into haemopoeitic stem cells *in vitro* to cause resistance to chemotherapy (Hania and Deisseroth, 1994).

In a phase I study, stem cells were collected from 10 patients with metastatic breast cancer and exposed to a retrovirus carrying the MDR-1 gene. The patients were then treated with high-dose cyclophosphamide and the stem cells reintroduced. Following re-engraftment the patients were treated with 12 cycles of paclitaxel chemotherapy. Six patients had a complete response after high-dose chemotherapy and a further three patients had a complete response after the paclitaxel treatment. The paclitaxel was well tolerated with no bone marrow failure (Rahman et al., 1998).

Gene therapy: the future

Several promising gene therapy approaches to treating breast and ovarian cancer are under investigation. To date, however, despite the growing number of positive pre-clinical studies, the activity in human subjects has been disappointing, reflected by the relatively few publications of successful phase II clinical studies. This may partly be explained by a failure in laboratory models to adequately predict human *in vivo* tumour behaviour.

Potential reasons for this are:

- Cell culture lines and animal tumour models often replicate rapidly, resulting in faster uptake of vectors such as retroviruses. Human tumours may spend a longer period of time out of the cell division cycle.
- Cell culture lines and animal tumour models are often more antigenic than human *in-vivo* tumours, which often evolve to lose their antigen expression.
- Certain vectors for gene therapy may be destroyed by an immune response in human subjects that could not be predicted *in vitro*.
- Animal immune systems may not respond to cytokines or viral vectors in the same manner as the human immune system.

The biggest challenge to effective gene therapy is the inadequacy of current vector technology. The efficacy of genetic transfer remains low for tumours *in vivo* and the expression of the transduced genes can be highly variable. A better understanding of viral genetics in the future may allow development of more tailored vectors with a greater ability to infect tumour cells specifically. Information must be taken from phase I clinical trials on how vector systems behave and the action of the introduced genetic material. These data can be used to design more relevant pre-clinical models that represent the behaviour of human tumours *in vivo* more accurately (Olopade, 1996).

To date, the vast majority of human trials of gene therapy in ovarian and breast cancer have been limited to patients with advanced incurable disease. It is unrealistic to expect a single gene therapy strategy to be able to radically treat advanced cancers, given the difficulty in delivering the genetic material to all cancer cells as well as the large genetic variance within the tumour population. It is more likely to be effective as a treatment for microscopic early disease, where tumour bulk is at a minimum and genetic abnormalities may be more predictable. Future trials may be better aimed at surgically resected breast or ovarian cancer, where adjuvant gene therapy may prevent disease recurrence.

The past decade has seen rapid advances in the understanding of the molecular basis of cancer. The challenge ahead is to apply this knowledge to cancer treatment in the form of gene therapy. With adequate resources to fund the necessary translational research, the development of useful gene therapy in breast and ovarian cancer seems likely in the next decade.

REFERENCES

Berchuck A and Lyerly H (1995). A phase I study of autologous human interleukin 2 (IL-2) gene modified tumour cells in patients with refractory metastatic ovarian cancer. *Human Gene Transfer Protocols*. Office of Recombinant DNA Activities, Bethesda, Maryland: National Institutes of Health.

Deshane J and Siegal GP (1997). Transduction efficacy and safety of an intraperitoneally delivered adenovirus encoding an anti-erbB-2 intracellular single-chain antibody for ovarian cancer gene therapy. *Gynecol Oncol* **64**(3): 378–85.

Freeman S, Abboud C, Whartenby KA, et al. (1993). The 'bystander effect': tumour regression when a fraction of the tumour mass is genetically modified. *Cancer Res* **53**: 5274–83.

Gomez-Navarro J and Curiel DT (2000). Conditionally replicative adenoviral vectors for cancer gene therapy. *Lancet Oncol* **1**: 148–58.

Grimm EA, Crump WL, Durett A, Hester JP, Lagoo-Deenadalayan S and Owen-Schaub LB (1988). TGF-beta inhibits the in vitro induction of lymphokine-activated killing activity. *Cancer Immunol Immunother* **27**(1): 53–8.

Gurnani M, Lipari P, Dell J, et al. (1999). Adenovirus-mediated p53 gene therapy has greater efficacy when combined with chemotherapy against human head and neck, ovarian, prostate and breast cancer. *Cancer Chemother Pharmacol* **44**(2): 143–51.

Hania E and Deisseroth A (1994). Serial transplantation shows that early haemopoietic precursor cells are transduced by MDR-1 retroviral vector in mouse gene therapy model. *Cancer Gene Ther* **1**: 21–5.

Hasenberg A, Tong XW, Rojaz-Martinez, et al. (1999). Phase I study of adenovirus mediated HSV-TK gene therapy followed by concomitant chemotherapy with topotecan after optimal debulking surgery for recurrent ovarian cancer. *Proc Am Soc Clin Oncol* **18**: 366a (abstract).

Holt JT (1997). Breast cancer genes: therapeutic strategies. *Ann N Y Acad Sci* **833**: 34–41.

Hwu P, Yang JC, Cowherd R, et al. (1995). In vivo antitumour activity of T cells redirected with chimeric antibody/T-cell receptor genes. *Cancer Res* **55**: 3369–73.

Kigawa J and Terakawa A (2000). Adenovirus-mediated transfer of a p53 gene in ovarian cancer. *Adv Exp Med Biol* **465**: 207–14.

Kohler MF, Marks JR, Wiseman RW, et al. (1993). Spectrum of mutation and frequency of allelic deletion of the p53 gene in ovarian cancer. *J Nat Cancer Inst* **85**(18): 1513–19.

Kolata G (1987). Oncogenes give breast cancer prognosis. *Science* **235**: 160.

Link C and Mooreman D (1995). Clinical protocols: a phase I trial of in vivo gene therapy with the herpes simplex thymidine kinase/ganciclovir system for the treatment of refractory or recurrent ovarian cancer. *Cancer Gene Ther* **2**: 230–1.

Marples B, Scott SD, Hendry JH, et al. (2000). Development of synthetic promoters for radiation-mediated gene therapy. *Gene Ther* **7**(6): 511–17.

Marr RA, Addison CL, Snider D, et al. (1997). Tumour immunotherapy using an adenoviral vector expressing a membrane-bound mutant TNF alpha. *Gene Ther* **4**(11): 1181–8.

Nielsen LL, Gurnani M, Syed J, et al. (1998a). Recombinant E1-deleted adenovirus-mediated gene therapy for cancer: efficacy studies with p53 tumour suppressor gene and liver histology in tumour xenograft models. *Hum Gene Ther* **9**(5): 681–94.

Nielsen LL, Lipari P, Dell J, et al. (1998b). Adenovirus mediated p53 gene therapy and paclitaxel have synergistic efficacy in models of human head and neck, ovarian, prostate and breast cancer. *Clin Cancer Res* **4**(4): 835–46.

Olopade OI (1996). Genetics in clinical cancer care – the future is now. *N Engl J Med* **335**(19): 1455–6.

Pandha HS, Martin LA, Rigg A, et al. (1999). Genetic prodrug activation therapy for breast cancer. A phase I clinical trial of erbB-2-directed suicide gene expression. *J Clin Oncol* **17**(7): 2108–9.

Rahman Z, Kavanagh J, Champlin R, et al. (1998). Chemotherapy immediately following autologous stem-cell transplantation in patients with advanced breast cancer. *Clin Cancer Res* **4**(11): 2717–21.

Ramesh R, Marrogi AJ and Freeman SM (1998). Tumor killing using HSV-tk suicide gene. In *Gene Therapy and Molecular Biology, Vol. I*, ed. T. Boulikas, pp. 253–63. USA: Gene Therapy Press.

Rosenfeld ME, Feng M, Michael SI, Siegal GP, Alvarez RD and Curiel DT (1995). Adenoviral-mediated delivery of the herpes simplex virus thymidine kinase gene selectively sensitizes human ovarian carcinoma cells to ganciclovir. *Clin Cancer Res* **1**(12): 1571–80.

Sanda MG, Resitifo NP and Walsh JC (1995). Molecular characterization of defective antigen processing in human prostate cancer. *J Natl Cancer Inst* **87**(4): 241–3.

Stewart AK, Lassam NJ, Quirt IC, et al. (1999). Adenovector-mediated gene delivery of interleukin-2 in metastatic breast cancer and melanoma: results of a phase I clinical trial. *Gene Ther* **6**(3): 350–63.

Sukumar S and McKenzie K (1996). Breast cancer prevention strategies for the twenty-first century. *Mol Med Today* **2**(11): 453–9.

Tait DL, OberMeiller PS, Redlin-Frazier S, et al. (1997). A phase I trial of retroviral BRCA1 sv gene therapy in ovarian cancer. *Clin Cancer Res* **3**(11): 1959–68.

Tait DL, Obermiller PS, Jensen RA, et al. (1998). Ovarian cancer gene therapy. *Haematol Oncol Clin N Am* **13**: 539.

Tait DL, Obermiller PS, Hatmaker AR, et al. (1999). Ovarian cancer BRCA1 gene therapy: phase I and II trial differences in immune response and vector stability. *Clin Cancer Res* **5**(7): 1708–14.

Ueno N, Hung MC, Weiden P, et al. (1998). Phase I E1A gene therapy in patients with advanced breast and ovarian cancers. *Proc Am Soc Clin Oncol* **17**: 432.

Vogelstein B, Lane D, Levine AJ, et al. (2000). Surfing the p53 network. *Nature* **408**: 307–10.

Future directions

Patrick J. Morrison[1], Shirley V. Hodgson[2] and Neva E. Haites[3]

[1]Belfast City Hospital Trust, Belfast, UK
[2]Guy's Hospital, London, UK
[3]University of Aberdeen, UK

It is abundantly clear from the contents of this book that our understanding of the inherited aspects of cancer has increased enormously in the past decade. Epidemiological studies (Easton et al., 1995) demonstrate that familial clusters of common cancers could be due to: (1) germline mutations in rare, highly penetrant cancer susceptibility genes, (2) more common, less penetrant mutations, or (3) common environmental factors. It is likely that all of these mechanisms are important. Subsequent to the identification of *BRCA1* and *BRCA2* (Miki et al., 1994; Wooster et al., 1995), large collaborative studies of families with hereditary breast and ovarian cancer suggest that currently detectable germline mutations in these genes account for approximately 85% of families with six cases of breast cancer but only 41% of those with four to five cases, most families with two ovarian cancer (in addition to breast cancer) cases but 88% (69% due to *BRCA1* mutations) with only one ovarian cancer case, while 77% of families with four female cases and one male case of breast cancer are due to *BRCA2* and 19% of such families to *BRCA1* mutations (Easton et al., 1995; Ford et al., 1998; Thorlacius et al., 1998). Thus a significant proportion of smaller families, particularly those with no cases of ovarian cancer, are likely to be due to polymorphic variants in other genes. The search for a major, highly penetrant '*BRCA3*' gene has remained elusive (Hopper, 2001; Nathanson and Weber, 2001; Welcsh and King, 2001); initial evidence for the importance of a locus at 8p19–22 showing somatic allele loss has not been substantiated by larger linkage studies. A candidate locus at 13q21, identified by comparative genomic hybridization and linkage has been found in a small number of Scandinavian families (Kainu et al., 2000). Recent research from Finland has demonstrated preliminary evidence for linkage disequilibrium and loss of heterozygosity at a locus at 22q13 in breast cancer cases with only a minor family history of the condition (Hartikainen et al., 2001; Kujala et al., 2001). The failure of many studies to identify clear-cut evidence for a third major locus for hereditary breast and ovarian cancer may be because the remaining families are smaller, contain more phenocopies, are genetically heterogeneous, or their disease is due to unidentified mutations in *BRCA1* or *BRCA2*. Such families may be accounted for by less penetrant predisposing genes. Association studies are frequently used in an attempt to identify important aetiological polymorphisms, but caution is needed in interpreting small data sets (Anonymous, 1999); thus there is some evidence for an association between the prohibitin T allele (with an inactive product lacking anti-proliferative activity) and breast cancer in women with a single first-degree relative with the disease (odds ratio 2.5; $p = 0.005$), greater if they were diagnosed before 50 years of age (odds ratio 4.8; $p = 0.003$). The prohibitin gene locus is on chromosome 17q21, and the gene product binds to the retinoblastoma protein, repressing transcription mediated by E2F. In addition, the RNA encoded by the 3' untranslated region of this gene arrests cell proliferation by blocking G1 to S transition in the cell cycle. Frequent loss of heterozygosity is found at 17q21 in breast cancers, and prohibitin could be a tumour suppressor gene in this region (Jupe et al., 2001). Thus this study has a good candidate gene but low power and needs to be reproduced in other populations and with larger numbers.

Another recent (Ziv et al., 2001) association has been found between the T29 → C polymorphism in the transforming growth factor β1 gene and late-onset breast cancer. A cohort of 3075 women was ascertained at age 65 years and genotyped for this polymorphism; 1124 had the T/T, 1439 the T/C and 458 the C/C genotype. Prospective follow-up for breast cancer diagnosis demonstrated a decreased hazard ratio (HR) for breast cancer (HR 0.36; 95% CI 0.17–0.75) for women with the C/C genotype. The risks for women with T/C and T/T genotypes did not differ significantly from each other (rates adjusted for age, age at menarche and menopause, oestrogen use and parity). This suggested that the TGF-β1 genotype may be associated with breast cancer risk in women aged over 65 years, and that the protective allele is the rarer allele.

A single nucleotide polymorphism in the 5' untranslated region of the *RAD51* gene has also been shown (Levy-Lahad et al., 2001) to modify cancer risk in germline *BRCA2* mutation carriers, but interestingly not in *BRCA1* mutation carriers, in a sample of 254 Ashkenazi women carrying one of the ancestral mutations (HR for breast cancer of 3.46 in *BRCA2* mutation carriers who were *RAD51-135C* heterozygotes).

Other candidate lower penetrance genes with a proposed effect on breast cancer susceptibility include *ATM* (Lu et al., 2001), H-*ras* VNTR polymorphisms, HER2 and *PTEN* (Angele and Hall, 2000). Polymorphisms in *BRCA1* and *BRCA2* may also have an effect (Healey et al., 2000a). Germline mutations in p53 can cause early-onset breast cancer in a small proportion of families. Mutations in genes involved in metabolic pathways, such as carcinogen (CYP17, CYP1B1, CYP19, NAT1-10, NAT1-11) (Healey et al., 2000b; Millikan, 2000; Young et al., 2000; Xie et al., 2000) and oestrogen metabolism (CYP1B1, 5α-reductase) (Guillemette et al., 2000; Scorilas et al., 2001) may also be responsible for moderately increased breast cancer risks (Watanabe, 2000; Zheng et al., 2000). Chromosome instability and impaired DNA repair has been observed to occur more commonly in women with breast cancer (Baria et al., 2001), and genes underlying this phenotype (including *ATM*) may be important in causing cancer susceptibility (Alapetite et al., 1999). Indeed, a recent analysis by Peto and Mack (2000) has indicated that most women with breast cancer have an inherited susceptibility to this cancer.

The methods of detecting high-penetrance gene mutations are becoming more efficient; about 10% of germline mutations in *BRCA1* and *BRCA2* may be deletions or duplications (Puget et al., 1999; Rohlfs et al., 2000; Unger et al., 2000), and these should be excluded in any systematic mutation search. A beautiful novel technique using colour bar codes on combed DNA to detect large rearrangements has recently been utilized for *BRCA1* mutation detection (Gad et al., 2001). The pathogenicity of polymorphisms may be assessed by functional studies. Functional mutation analysis includes the yeast 2 hybrid transactivation Lacs assay in which functionally inactive mutations (Camplejohn and Rutherford, 2001) fail to 'turn on' reporter genes.

New techniques such as comparative genomic hybridization and gene expression profiling (Duggan et al., 1999; Khan et al., 1999) are powerful tools for dissecting out specific genetic pathways and the genes involved in directing cells down the tumorigenic pathway (Loveday et al., 2000).

The role of methylation in the silencing of tumour suppressor genes in carcinogenesis is becoming appreciated (Schofield et al., 2001; Costello and Plass, 2001). Patterns of CpG methylation are often altered in neoplasia, which may comprise both gene-specific hypermethylation in addition to more global methylation abnormalities. Aberrant DNA methylation of promoter regions is a mechanism for epigenetic silencing of tumour suppressor genes. Increasing numbers of examples of this phenomenon are being described, including – in the context of this volume – the *BRCA1* gene promoter (Catteau et al., 1999; Esteller et al., 2001). These epigenetic mechanisms could be one of the 'two hits' required for tumour suppressor gene inactivation.

It is clear that epigenetic silencing of tumour suppressors may occur early in tumorigenesis: for example, p16INK4A CpG island promoter hypermethylation occurs in pre-malignant stages of cancer, giving rise to a selective advantage to clones of cells containing this epigenetic change (Myohanen et al., 1998). This suggests the possibility of treating cancer patients with drugs that could reactivate tumour suppressor genes (Costello and Plass, 2001). Conversely, hypomethylation can lead to inappropriate activation of genes that are important for neoplastic growth, such as *CMYC* and H-*ras* (Del Senno et al., 1989). Hypomethylation may also lead to transcriptional activation of mobile genetic elements: transposons (Florl et al., 1999). These mobile genetic elements are abundant in the genome, and although they are rarely functional, Alu-mediated retrotransposon 'mutations' have been observed in *BRCA1* and *BRCA2*.

Activation of transposons could be related to genome hypomethylation (Miki et al., 1996). Retrotransposons may themselves alter the transcription of nearby genes, which could reduce tumour suppressor function. In addition, hypomethylation may be related to chromosome instability (Ehrlich, 2000), which is detected at increased frequency in breast cancer cases.

The public health implications of the detection of breast cancer susceptibility genes are likely to increase. Currently, genetic testing for germline *BRCA1* and *BRCA2* mutations can be offered in only a very small proportion of breast/ovarian cancer families. As it becomes possible to identify lower penetrance polymorphisms that may occur commonly in the population, population screening for such mutations may be considered. However, it will be important to evaluate the prophylactic and lifestyle measures needed to reduce cancer risks in women carrying such mutations in order to establish the usefulness of such a measure, which may be unwarranted if the mutation only confers moderately increased risks of breast/ovarian cancer. Ethical issues of confidentiality and concerns about the use of genetic testing by insurance agencies and employers must be taken into account when considering testing for such mutations, in addition to tests for high-penetrance mutations. Mammography has already dramatically reduced deaths due to breast cancer in the UK. Identification of high-risk individuals to target for surveillance will increase the efficiency of screening.

Information about differing biological behaviour of cancers arising in individuals with different genetic backgrounds is emerging and may have important implications for management. Thus, histological features of breast cancer are characteristically different in *BRCA1* and *BRCA2* mutation carriers (Chappuis et al., 2000; Pericay et al., 2001) and gene expression profiles in breast cancer have also been found to differ in carriers of these two types of mutation (Hedenfalk et al., 2001; Lakhani et al., 2001). Such biological differences may have implications with regard to prognosis and susceptibility to chemotherapy and radiotherapy. Conversely, the presence of specific histological types may indicate which gene is more likely to have caused the underlying susceptibility.

Surveillance and preventive strategies for high-risk women continue to require evaluation, such as the use of MRI imaging for breast cancer detection and analysis of nipple fluid aspirates, and this can only be done by the collection of large amounts of data in a large cohort of at-risk women over a long time-period. New interventions and cancer treatments are also being developed: these include gene therapy (see p. 372) and therapy to reduce the neovascularization in early tumours that is involved in the development of the malignant phenotype (Folkman, 1999; Im et al., 2001). Studies of treatments to reduce neovascularization in cancer have provided exciting early results (Locopo et al., 1998) and merit further research.

As such novel surveillance and therapeutic measures are being developed, their evaluation requires studies on large cohorts of affected women, well-documented genetically. The best way forward in the future is by multicentre collaborations such as that of the European Biomed 2 Group (from which the International Collaborative Group – Familial Breast/Ovarian Cancer [ICG-FBOC] group has evolved). Several chapter authors in this volume are members of this group.

REFERENCES

Alapetite C, Thirion P, de la Rochefordiere A, Cosset J-M and Mostacchi E (1999). Analysis by alkaline comet assay of cancer patients with severe reactions to radiotherapy: defective rejoining of radioinduced DNA strand breaks in lymphocytes of breast cancer patients. *Int J Cancer* **83**: 83–90.

Angele S and Hall J (2000). The *ATM* gene and breast cancer: is it really a risk factor? *Mutat Res* **462**: 167–78.

Anonymous (1999). Freely associating (editorial). *Nat Genet* **22**: 1–2.

Baria K, Warren C, Roberts SA, West CM and Scott D (2001). Chromosomal radiosensitivity as a marker of predisposition to common cancers? *Br J Cancer* **84**: 892–6.

Camplejohn RS and Rutherford J (2001). p53 functional assays: detecting p53 mutations in both the germline and in sporadic tumours. *Cell Prolif* **34**: 1–14.

Catteau A, Harris WH, Xu C-F and Solomon E (1999). Methylation of the *BRCA1* promoter region in sporadic breast and ovarian cancer: correlation with disease characteristics. *Oncogene* **18**: 1957–65.

Chappuis PO, Nethercot V and Foulkes WD (2000). Clinico-pathological characteristics of BRCA1- and BRCA2-related breast cancer. *Semin Surg Oncol* **18**: 287–95.

Costello JF and Plass C (2001). Methylation matters. *J Med Genet* **38**: 285–303.

Del Senno L, Maestri I, Piva R, et al. (1989). Differential hypomethylation of the c-myc protooncogene in bladder cancers at different stages and grades. *J Urol* **142**: 146–9.

Duggan DJ, Bittner M, Chen Y, Meltzer P and Trent JM (1999). Expression profiling using cDNA microarrays. *Nat Genet* **21** (Suppl.): 10–14.

Easton DS, Ford D and Bishop DT (1995). Breast and ovarian cancer incidence in BRCA1-mutation carriers. *Am J Hum Genet* **56**: 265–71.

Ehrlich M (2000). DNA methylation: normal development, inherited diseases, and cancer. *J Clin Ligand Assay* **23**: 144–6.

Esteller M, Corn PG, Baylin SB and Herman JG (2001). A gene hypermethylation profile of human cancer. *Cancer Res* **61**: 3225–9.

Florl AR, Lower R, Schmitz-Drager BJ and Schulz WA (1999). DNA methylation and expression of LINE-1 and HERV-K provirus sequences in urolithial and renal cell carcinomas. *Br J Cancer* **80**: 1312–21.

Folkman J (1999). Angiogenesis research: from laboratory to clinic. *Forum* **9**(3 Suppl. 3): 59–62.

Ford D, Easton DF, Stratton M, et al. (1998). Genetic heterogeneity and penetrance analysis of the BRCA1 and BRCA2 genes in breast cancer families. *Am J Hum Genet* **62**: 676–89.

Gad S, Scheuner MT, Pages-Berhouet S, et al. (2001). Identification of a large rearrangement of the BRCA1 gene using colour bar code on combed DNA in an American breast/ovarian cancer family previously studied by direct sequencing. *J Med Genet* **38**: 388–92.

Guillemette C, Millikan RC, Newman B and Housman DE (2000). Genetic polymorphisms in uridine diphospho-glucuronosyltransferase 1A1 and association with breast cancer among African Americans. *Cancer Res* **60**: 950–6.

Hartikainen J, Kujala H, Kataja V, et al. (2001). Linkage disequilibrium in chromosome 22q13 in Eastern Finnish breast cancer cases. *Eur J Hum Genet* **9**(Suppl. 1): 82.

Healey CS, Dunning AM, Teare MD, et al. (2000a). A common variant in *BRCA2* is associated with both breast cancer risk and prenatal viability. *Nat Gen* **26**: 362–4.

Healey CS, Dunning AM, Durocher F, et al. (2000b). Polymorphisms in the human aromatase cytochrome P450 gene (*CYP19*) and breast cancer risk. *Carcinogenesis* **21**: 189–93.

Hedenfalk I, Duggan D, Chen Y, et al. (2001). Gene-expression profiles in hereditary breast cancer. *N Engl J Med* **344**: 539–48.

Hopper JL (2001). More breast cancer genes? *Breast Cancer Res Treat* **3**: 154–7.

Im S-A, Kim J-S, Gomez-Manzano C, et al. (2001). Inhibition of breast cancer growth in vivo by antiangiogenesis gene therapy with adenovirus-mediated antisense-VEGF. *Br J Cancer* **84**: 1252–7.

Jupe ER, Badgett AA, Neas BR, et al. (2001). Single nucleotide polymorphism in prohibitin 3′ untranslated region and breast-cancer susceptibility. *Lancet* **357**: 1588–9.

Kainu T, Juo SH, Desper R, et al. (2000). Somatic deletions in hereditary breast cancers implicate 13q21 as a putative novel breast cancer susceptibility locus. *Proc Natl Acad Sci USA* **97**: 9603–8.

Khan J, Saal LH, Bittner ML, Chen Y, Trent JM and Meltzer PS (1999). Expression profiling in cancer using cDNA microarrays. *Electrophoresis* **20**: 223–9.

Kujala H, Anttila M, Hartikainen J, et al. (2001). Allelic imbalance in chromosome 22q13 in Eastern Finnish breast cancer patients. *Eur J Hum Genet* **9**(Suppl. 1): 126.

Lakhani SR, O'Hare MJ and Ashworth A (2001). Profiling familial breast cancer. *Nat Med* **7**: 408.

Levy-Lahad E, Lahad A, Eisenberg S, et al. (2001). A single nucleotide polymorphism in the *RAD51* gene modifies cancer risk in *BRCA2* but not in *BRCA1* carriers. *Proc Natl Acad Sci USA* **98**: 3232–6.

Locopo N, Fanelli M and Gasparini G (1998). Clinical significance of angiogenic factors in breast cancer. *Breast Cancer Res Treat* **52**: 159–73.

Loveday RL, Greenman J, Simcox DL, et al. (2000). Genetic changes in breast cancer detected by comparative genomic hybridisation. *Int J Cancer* **86**: 494–500.

Lu Y-J, Condie A, Bennett JD, Fry MJ, Yuille MR and Shipley J (2001). Disruption of the *ATM* gene in breast cancer. *Cancer Genet Cytogenet* **126**: 97–101.

Miki Y, Swensen J, Shattuck-Eidens D, et al. (1994). A strong candidate for the breast and ovarian cancer susceptibility gene BRCA1. *Science* **266**: 66–71.

Miki Y, Katagiri T, Kasumi F, Yoshimoto T and Nakamura Y (1996). Mutation analysis in the BRCA2 gene in primary breast cancer. *Nat Genet* **13**: 245–7.

Millikan R-C (2000). NAT1*10 and NAT1*11 polymorphisms and breast cancer risk. *Cancer Epidemiol Biomarkers Prev* **9**: 217–19.

Myohanen SK, Baylin SB and Herman JG (1998). Hypermethylation can selectively silence individual p16ink4A alleles in neoplasia. *Cancer Res* **58**: 591–3.

Nathanson KL and Weber BL (2001). 'Other' breast cancer susceptibility genes: searching for more holy grail. *Hum Mol Genet* **10**: 715–20.

Pericay C, Brunet J, Diez O, et al. (2001). Clinical and pathological findings of BRCA1/2 associated breast cancer. *Breast* **10**: 46–8.

Peto J and Mack T (2000). High constant incidence in twins and other relatives of women with breast cancer. *Nat Genet* **26**: 411–14.

Puget N, Stoppa-Lyonnet D, Sinilnikova OM, et al. (1999). Screening for germ-line rearrangements and regulatory mutations in BRCA1 led to the identification of four new deletions. *Cancer Res* **59**: 455–61.

Rohlfs EM, Chung CH, Yang Q, et al. (2000). In-frame deletions of *BRCA1* may define critical functional domains. *Hum Genet* **107**: 385–90.

Schofield PN, Joyce JA, Lam WK, et al. (2001). Genomic imprinting and cancer; new paradigms in the genetics of neoplasia. *Toxicol Lett* **120**: 151–60.

Scorilas A, Bharaj B, Giai M and Diamandis EP (2001). Codon 89 polymorphism in the human 5αreductase gene in primary breast cancer. *Br J Cancer* **84**: 760–7.

Thorlacius S, Struewing JP, Hartage P, et al. (1998). Population-based study of risk of breast cancer in carriers of BRCA2 mutation. *Lancet* **352**: 1337–9.

Unger MA, Nathanson KL, Calzone K, et al. (2000). Screening for genomic rearrangements in families with breast and ovarian cancer identifies *BRCA1* mutations previously missed by conformation-sensitive gel electrophoresis or sequencing. *Am J Hum Genet* **67**: 841–50.

Watanabe J, Shimadu T, Gillam EMJ, et al. (2000). Association of *CYP1B1* genetic polymorphism with incidence to breast and lung cancer. *Pharmacogenetics* **10**: 25–33.

Welcsh PL and King MC (2001). BRCA1 and BRCA2 and the genetics of breast and ovarian cancer. *Hum Mol Genet* **10**: 705–13.

Wooster R, Bignell G, Lancaster J, et al. (1995). Identification of the breast cancer susceptibility gene BRCA2. *Nature* **378**: 789–92.

Xie D-W, Shu X-O, Deng Z-L, et al. (2000). Population-based, case-control study of HER2 genetic polymorphism and breast cancer risk. *J Natl Cancer Inst* **92**: 412–17.

Young IE, Kurian KM, MacKenzie MAF, et al. (2000). A polymorphic tetranucleotide repeat in the *CYP19* gene and male breast cancer. *Br J Cancer* **82**: 1247–8.

Zheng W, Xie D-W, Jin F, et al. (2000). Genetic polymorphism of cytochrome P450-1B1 and risk of breast cancer. *Cancer Epidemiol Biomarkers Prev* **9**: 147–50.

Ziv E, Cauley J, Morin PA, Saiz R and Browner WS (2001). Association between the T29 → C polymorphism in the transforming growth factor β1 gene and breast cancer among elderly white women: the study of osteoporotic fractures. *JAMA* **285**: 2859–63.

Index